CONTRIBUTORS

Patricia M. Feeney, RN, BSN, MSW
St. Louis, Missouri

Lynda S. Hilliard, MBA, RN, CNAA
Pleasanton, California

Elizabeth Hogue, JD
Silver Spring, Maryland

T. M. Marrelli, MSN, MA, RNC
Kent Island, Maryland

Sandra B. Martin Whittier, BSN, RN
Everett, Massachusetts

Margaret Sharp Woodard, RN, BSN
Richmond, Virginia

The
NURSE MANAGER'S
SURVIVAL GUIDE

Practical Answers to Everyday Problems

THE
NURSE MANAGER'S
SURVIVAL GUIDE

Practical Answers to Everyday Problems

T. M. Marrelli, MSN, MA, RNC

Health Care Consultant
Kent Island, Maryland

With Assistance from

Lynda S. Hilliard, MBA, RN, CNAA

Second Edition

 Mosby

St. Louis Baltimore Boston Carlsbad Chicago Naples New York Philadelphia Portland
London Madrid Mexico City Singapore Sydney Tokyo Toronto Wiesbaden

Mosby

Dedicated to Publishing Excellence

A Times Mirror Company

Executive Editor: N. Darlene Como
Associate Developmental Editor: Dana L. Knighten
Project Manager: Carol Sullivan Weis
Production Editor: David Stein
Designer: Jen Marmarinos
Manufacturing Supervisor: Karen Lewis

Printed in the United States of America
Composition by Top Graphics
Printing/binding by R. R. Donnelley

Mosby–Year Book, Inc.
11830 Westline Industrial Drive
St. Louis, Missouri 63146

International Standard Book Number 0-8151-5672-3

97 98 99 00 01 / 9 8 7 6 5 4 3 2 1

ABOUT THE AUTHOR

T. M. Marrelli, MSN, MA, RNC, received a bachelor's degree in nursing from Duke University School of Nursing in Durham, North Carolina, and a master's degree from Central Michigan University. Ms. Marrelli also is the author of *Handbook of Home Health Standards and Documentation Guidelines for Reimbursement* and *Nursing Documentation Handbook,* as well as co-author of *Home Care and Clinical Paths: Effective Care Planning Across the Continuum, Home Health Aide: Guidelines for Care,* and *Home Health Aide: Guidelines for Care Instructor Manual.* Ms. Marrelli is the president of Marrelli and Associates, Inc., and editor and publisher of *Home Care Nurse News.*

Ms. Marrelli has extensive experience in hospital, home health, and hospice administration and has worked for the Health Care Financing Administration, where she received the Bureau Director's Citation. Ms. Marrelli is listed in the World Who's Who of Women, 1993/1994. Ms. Marrelli provides consultation services on various aspects of health care, especially the areas of documentation, operations, and management. Correspondence, including feedback about this text, may be directed to the author at Health Care Consulting, Suite 159, 3 Church Circle, Annapolis, MD, 21401.

PREFACE

When I first became a new manager, no one told me many of the things that, in retrospect, I needed to know. From the running of successful staff meetings to dealing with hospital administration, I learned to manage by trial and, many times, by error. To ease your journey and to refresh and reinforce management skills you may have already developed is the goal of this book. Staff nurses sometimes receive more extensive orientation and planned educational programs than the managers who supervise them! As managers, we and our staffs deserve better. I hope this book fills this gap.

The Nurse Manager's Survival Guide is a practical guide to day-to-day operations for nurses who manage people, care plans, or groups of patients. This book is designed to assist nurses recently placed in management positions. It also serves as a refresher for more experienced nurse managers. As hospitals and other patient care settings experience decreasing lengths of stay and increasing patient acuity, the professional nurse must manage more responsibilities in a shorter time frame.

It is unfortunate that some of us have encountered ineffective managers and unproductive or unpleasant management environments. My hope is that this book will help you become a competent, communicative manager and help you take the steps needed to improve your work circumstances, if necessary.

Some important information, usually not included in nursing books, has been incorporated, such as how to market yourself, how to honestly evaluate your own capabilities and needs, and how to manage stress for both you and your staff.

Many of the specific guidelines and descriptions included in the book address nursing management in various practice settings. The general management principles and techniques described can be applied to any nursing care delivery setting, including the increasingly important areas of home care, ambulatory care, hospice, and long-term care. For example, principles of effective time management and communications are relevant regardless of the particular practice setting. Likewise, hiring and other human resource skills are needed and appropriate to all health settings. Because nursing management of day-to-day operations in home care and in hospitals differs significantly, I have written Chapter 11, "The Nurse Manager in Home Care and Hospice," which describes how to effectively manage day-to-day nursing activities in home care settings. In addition, at the end of most chapters is a box entitled "Considerations for Home Care Managers."

Some other special features have been included to make this book easy to use. Helpful "Manager's Tips," listed as behavioral strategies, are listed in every chapter. Glossaries to help you more easily understand unfamiliar terms are included for both Chapter 7, "Resource Management and Budgeting Basics," and Chapter 8, "Legal Issues and Risk Management." A summary concludes each chapter. Resources for further professional development, including lists of relevant conferences and certification programs, as well as a list of suggested readings, are provided at the end of each chapter.

Because contemporary health care facilities are continuing to evolve at a rapid pace, the extensively revised second edition includes suggestions for coping with the changes and stresses brought about by restructuring, reorganizing, and reengineering. It also addresses the major health care issues and concerns that have arisen as a result of the widespread adoption of managed care and case management. In response to recent trends, this book also places increased emphasis on the unique needs and concerns of home care managers and expands its coverage of delegation. Rather than treat continuous quality improvement (CQI) in a separate chapter, as does the previous edition, the second edition carries the quality theme throughout the book to reflect its importance as an integral part of all management functions and day-to-day operations.

The process of becoming a competent and effective manager is a growth journey, unique to each nurse and to each specific work environment. This book was created to facilitate this process.

T. M. Marrelli

CONTENTS

5   Day-to-Day Operations, 105
Lynda S. Hilliard
T. M. Marrelli

THE
NURSE MANAGER'S
SURVIVAL GUIDE

Practical Answers to Everyday Problems

CHAPTER 1

THE NURSE MANAGER ROLE TODAY

T.M. MARRELLI

When the first edition of this book was published in 1993, health care was starting its massive evolutionary process. Since then, the core of nursing management has remained the same; however, many more internal and external events are affecting the role of the nurse manager. Managed care has become a reality for most areas of the country and with it have emerged large regional and national health care networks dominating the marketplace. The role of staff nurses as supervisors of paraprofessional staff is being scrutinized at the judicial level as nursing unions and hospital management grapple with further unionization efforts. Hospital closures and mergers with other institutions or networks, along with the downsizing or reengineering of patient care staff to better meet patient care needs in a constrained financial environment, are refocusing the way in which managers are trained, viewed, evaluated, and compensated for their endeavors to maintain stability in the face of change. This book seeks to provide the information needed to assist nurse managers in this tumultuous time in the health care industry.

Congratulations! Because of your clinical expertise, education, and other valued traits, you were promoted to a management position. Yet the process of becoming an effective manager does not happen overnight. It is a growth process unique to each nurse and specific environment. Whether you are a new manager or new to a facility with a new team, you need to know you are not alone and you may need some insights to help you through this period of transition. The team members you will be managing are unique and are the most positive part of this position. Manager and staff all work together to meet the organizational goals, as defined in your employer's mission statement and nursing philosophy. Any new role is exciting, but it can also be anxiety producing.

MIDDLE MANAGEMENT DILEMMA

The new nurse manager must remain flexible in order to survive in the health care industry, and the most valuable tool in her/his arsenal is the combination of clinical and business expertise. As reported by Weil and Jorgensen, ". . . The U.S. healthcare system, focusing on regional networks and HMOs, could have a negative impact on earlier manpower projections for health services management (HSM) . . . the 1993 estimate suggesting that about 3,000 new health services management jobs will be required annually during the 10 year period through 2005 . . . business-oriented, middle management positions are being eliminated throughout healthcare—promotions are being extended to those with strong clinical and management backgrounds to minimize overlap in responsibilities and to cut costs."[1] In other words, sharp clinical skills and a business acumen for financial, time, and other resource management make the trained nurse manager a prime choice for promotion to middle and senior management.

As hospitals and other patient areas experience decreasing lengths of stay coupled with increased patient acuity and turnover, the professional nurse in a leadership role must manage more responsibilities in a shortened time frame. The learning needs of managers are varied and complex, covering various fields of study. In addition, as health care delivery has changed, so too has the diversity of settings in which nurses manage. Nurses may practice in more than one of the following settings over the course of their careers: hospitals, community health programs, hospices, urgent care centers, outpatient surgical centers, subacute units, extended care facilities, and home health agencies. Other areas include day care programs, office practices, health maintenance organizations (HMOs), and preferred provider organizations (PPOs), as well as other clinical centers.

Traditional nursing middle management as we have known it during the past 30 years is slowly being dismantled. With increased demands from senior management to improve quality, decrease costs, and enhance customer service, it is sometimes difficult to aspire to a management role. Because staff nursing pay has increased over the years, the financial rewards of being a manager are not as enticing as they once might have been. We sometimes wonder if it is worth the hassle to work extra hours (without additional overtime pay); to be the recipient of the grievances of patients, staff, physicians and management; and to carry the burden of making sure a unit functions smoothly with competent caregivers. Some nurses decline management positions because they desire continued patient contact and do not want the added responsibility of 24-hour accountability. However, for the nurse who truly desires to make a positive change in the care of patients and has the endurance and motivation to continually challenge the status quo, as well as the ability to maintain excellent clinical skills, nursing management in the twenty-first century can be the perfect job.

ROLE TRANSITION

Too often, professional nurses in any health care setting receive little formal management training before being promoted to the management team. It is the nurse's education that ultimately facilitates the role transition to manager. Once a nurse is promoted, it is thought that some skills may have to be changed or even unlearned. The challenge is to provide new managers with the information and skills needed to develop fundamental and successful behaviors and thought processes that effectively contribute to work accomplishment.

Luckily, most new nurse managers bridge parts of this gap using the clinical and educational experiences they bring to the new position. These skills are what nurses do well everyday, including communicating, planning, organizing, prioritizing, and documenting. All are talents that lend themselves well to the new role of nurse manager. Further expansion into the nurse manager role is based on learned management behaviors including planning, organizing, directing, controlling, and evaluating.

The nurse manager's orientation should follow a formal plan. It is important to note that no program, however well thought-out, can address all the issues that will confront the new nurse manager in any setting. Some skills develop fully only after a period of time with the integration of knowledge and practice. These good habits become "automatic" only with use.

All change is stressful, even though it may be experienced as good or bad. Some of the most frequently cited causes of stress include vague role descriptions and adapting to what may be perceived as continual change. We know that all nurses experience stress. The new nurse manager has the additional stress of changing roles and integrating herself/himself into the organization as a manager. It is important at the onset for the new manager to always look for opportunities in every problem. (For an in-depth discussion of stress and its management, see Chapter 9, "Taking Care of Yourself and Your Staff.")

Example of a Position Description for a Nurse Manager

We have all seen position descriptions for a nurse manager that enumerate various responsibilities. The nurse manager is responsible for:

1. Staffing, organizing, and coordinating patient care 24 hours a day.
2. Developing, administering, and evaluating goals and objectives for the unit.
3. Providing for cost-effective use of human and material resources consistent with goals of cost containment and productivity, while providing outcome-oriented quality patient care.
4. Participating in the management process.
5. Problem-solving.
6. Directing the activities of subordinates.
7. Identifying systems problems.
8. Providing for the continuing education of staff.
9. Developing and evaluating staff.
10. Providing clinical assistance and consultation.
11. Developing, administering, and ensuring compliance with policies and procedures and any applicable governmental and accreditation regulations.
12. Assuming other responsibilities as assigned by the supervisor.

Reading this list and reflecting on what the nurse manager actually does on a daily basis can make the job seem overwhelming. The actual activities may include attending or chairing meetings, evaluating and counseling staff members, assigning or reassigning schedules, and myriad other functions. Appendix 1-1 presents a detailed description of the nurse manager's responsibilities as delineated by the American Nurses Association. As we move towards a greater focus on outcomes or predetermined activity levels of patients at time of discharge (i.e., a satisfied patient whose needs have been met successfully by discharge), we see why this new role is stressful. The nursing staff comfort and care for patients 24 hours a day. The nursing staff coordinate all activities related to the patient. These activities are multifaceted and complex and range from clinical tests to therapeutic interventions.

Because of increased specialization of health care providers and complexity of patient problems and associated technology, multiple and varied services are provided to patients. Patients and their families and friends look to the professional nurse for quality care.

Health Care Changes Affecting Nursing Management

Four major factors contribute to the changes that are affecting nursing management.

1. The current economics of the health care system including managed care, capitation, and utilization management
    *   In response to spiraling health care costs, third-party payers (government, commercial, and business self-insurers) have increased their scrutiny of expensive hospital and other health services. Capitation, case management, and utilization management have all been influential in decreasing lengths of hospital stays.
    *   Decreased lengths of stay typically cause patients to have acute nursing care needs met in a shorter time frame. The phrase sometimes heard to describe this phenomenon is "quicker and sicker," referring to the patient's status at discharge. Ten years ago the same patient population would have been hospitalized for longer periods. Today much hospital care is provided on an outpatient-only basis.
    *   Clinical documentation often is the basis on which third-party payers make payment or denial decisions. Nursing documentation often becomes the core or foundation for providing substantiating documentation for a payment or denial determination.
2. The emphasis on quality and outcomes in health care
    *   As health care quality improvement and management programs have evolved, patient care outcomes are recognized as valid indicators of quality of care.
    *   The Joint Commission for the Accreditation of Healthcare Organizations (JCAHO) has focused on interdisciplinary planning across a care continuum

to create an atmosphere for the entire health care network to work together to achieve desirable patient outcomes. JCAHO standards and an in-depth discussion of the outcome-oriented quality management and the improvement of organization performance processes are discussed throughout this text.

3. The emphasis on standardization of care, practices, protocol, and clinical pathways and the increasing recognition and empowerment of the nursing profession

- All patients are entitled to a certain level, or standard, of nursing care. As patients become proactive consumers in the purchase of health care, patient satisfaction with care becomes key to a health care network's reputation and ultimate survival. Nurses, because of their healing skills and proficiency and the considerable amount of time spent with patients and families, are pivotal in achieving patient satisfaction. It is also known that, generally, satisfied patients are less likely to pursue legal methods to resolve disputes. The nursing roles of patient advocate, listener, and teacher have become even more significant in recent years.

- All professions, including nursing, have recognized standards of care. As society has become more litigious, the professional nurse must be aware of State Nurse Practice Acts and other accepted standards of care. Other standards include health care institution policies and procedures, state and federal regulations, and the published standards of professional nursing organizations. It is important to keep current and informed of professional standards in nursing specialties or other groups and to be aware of the standards of professional nursing practice.

- Health care settings, such as hospitals, also have their own nursing standards of care. Some examples are:
  - Every patient shall have a nursing assessment that is comprehensive, addresses specific patient needs, is performed by a registered nurse at least every _____ hours, and is documented in the patient's record.
  - Discharge planning will begin on admission and includes collaboration with other members of the health team and involves the patient, family, and caregivers.

- Through complete and effective documentation, nursing demonstrates that the standard of care has been met.

- Even with the specter of mergers and downsizing there continues to be a great need for qualified nurses in the workplace. Recently the *American Journal of Nursing*[2] stated that the demand for nurses will increase by 38.9% by the end of the century. The U.S. Department of Labor projects that 613,000 new registered nurse (RN) positions will be created during this same time.

4. The emphasis on effectiveness and efficiency in health care

- As health care settings and hospitals continue to streamline, administrative tasks historically performed by nurses are being examined. Repetitive or duplicative activities, which can be found in some documentation systems, are inefficient. Better ways are being explored to meet patient needs while freeing nurses for other important activities. Patient care redesign, or reengineering, is one of many ways that patient care functions are being examined and reviewed for appropriate use of expensive staff resources.

- Considering these tumultuous changes in the current health care environment, we see why the nurse manager role is so important today. All these factors create an environment where the nurse has more responsibilities and less time in which to do them. Because of the many tasks that must be undertaken or delegated, flexibility is a necessity for effective nurse managers.

WHAT DOES THE NURSE MANAGER DO?

Core duties that nurse managers assume, regardless of setting, include assignments, delegation, meetings, performance evaluations, budgets, writing and interpersonal skills, and 24-hour accountability for the area. Nurse managers must blend business and clinical skills and perspectives. Because the bulk of the manager's education focused on clinical nursing, it is the business side that usually needs additional educational emphasis. The nurse manager, to be effective, creates an environment that empowers staff to grow professionally. The staff are encouraged to identify problems, recommend and implement solutions, and evaluate outcomes. The staff "own" their issues and work as a group for resolution. Most importantly, the staff achieve patient goals while adhering to policies and the mission statement of the health care setting. The nurse manager is the link between staff and upper management. This role, by definition alone, imparts significant influence and power.

The actual day-to-day operational duties of the nurse manager can be as varied as the practice area of responsibility. In a hospital or a home health agency, for example, the activities are focused on the patient, the consumer of the needed services. The nurse manager, by position and personality, sets the tone for the effective completion of these activities. In patient care settings, the goal of these activities is a satisfied customer.

UTILIZING POWER EFFECTIVELY

Being new to management, the nurse manager needs to understand power and how to use it effectively. Leah Curtin in her editorial, *Power: The Trap of Trappings,* gives a very short but succinct definition of power: ". . . the ability to *do* something."[3] The corporate culture of an organization may be very subtle, but either through observation of formal structures (e.g., the organizational chart) or informal structures (e.g., seeing who really controls the place) the new manager should try to identify where the power is located and learn how to access that power to get a job done.

Just as important as gaining and developing power is the ability to do what is right with power—not only to use it for personal gain. As Ms. Curtin explained in the above article, the concept of power includes action, knowledge, position, judgment, and perception. Power is not static; it is not a place. Power is intoxicating and its results can be devastating to staff and an organization if used in a nonproductive manner. It needs to be activated for the good of the group.

A new manager has the power that is associated with the hierarchy of position. However, that power can be eroded if not used effectively or if allowed to be usurped by another. Power becomes another tool for the manager to manage a department effectively. Even though it may appear superficial, it is important for nurse managers to look the part in order to receive the power that is due them. Dress as a manager, act as a manager—body language and communication styles exude power. That is not to say that aggressive behavior denotes power. Knowing when to use which behavioral style (e.g., aggressiveness, assertiveness, passivity, submission) is an important element of gaining a power base.

Power should never be used to dominate or totally control subordinates. Respect the individuality, responsibility, and creativity of staff and use power to develop and mentor them to be more involved in team efforts. Delegate, mentor, and manage through performance goals and expectations. Leadership (as described in depth in Chapter 2, "Management: An Overview") is intertwined with effective use of power.

Just as important as communicating power to subordinates is the need to gain power with superiors. An old management saying goes, "the job of a manager is to make her/his boss look good." The purpose of a nursing middle management position is to manage a patient care department, meeting quality, regulatory/accreditation, and financial objectives. The senior manager is responsible for a number of departments, overseeing the strategic direction and leadership. A good manager is aware of the familial relationship and nurtures positive growth of that important relationship with a supervisor.

A senior manager can definitely give valuable feedback on various options to review for the management of a specific problem. However, the responsibility of the middle manager is to operate the area, abiding by legal and accrediting standards and regulations without continually complaining to the senior manager about the job's difficulty or needing to discuss *every* operational decision that must be made. By having strategic organizational goals and objectives that are filtered down to the appropriate departments, managers should have a general understanding of the status of the organization and receive the approval to operate within given parameters.

Senior management should be informed of the general direction of the unit and how it interacts and intersects with other departments. Problems that may affect another department or financially or legally affect the organization should also be brought to the attention of the senior manager. It is the responsibility of the middle manager always to inform her/his superior immediately of a potentially controversial or volatile situation, so that the senior manager isn't "broadsided" by an angry physician, family members, or other managers without having the appropriate information to respond or defuse the situation. Besides being frustrated, the senior manager faces embarrassment when caught unaware.

Be supportive of your supervisor; this, however, does not mean just saying yes to everything. Rather, provide insightful, positive feedback and try to view situations as your manager would—see the forest, instead of only the trees. If time and responsibilities permit, request special projects to work on. Accept new responsibilities that are delegated as a professional, providing your manager with both an analysis of what impact the new responsibilities will have on your ability to operate your unit and a possible solution that will allow you to accomplish the new tasks.

The nurse manager may possess and use the following types of power to achieve her/his goals:

Coercive power As implied, this is the power to inflict some type of punishment. This is universally seen as the weakest type of power.

Expert power The power commanded by special knowledge or competence. This may include degrees, certification, publication, or other skills.

Legitimate power The power given to exert authority because of a position or title.

Referent power The personal power of the individual. An example is a person with a motivating personality.

Reward power The power to bestow or withhold something valued by another person.

The nurse manager's clinical skills will be used in the management role—if only as a resource for staff members (expert power). Some people theorize that a nurse manager, to be effective, must have strong clinical skills. This strong knowledge base may command immediate respect from staff and physicians.

The new nurse manager has tools available to appear powerful (see Manager's Tip 1-1). Initially, the manager's title alone will lend some legitimate power. Manager's Tips 1-2 and 1-3 on p. 10 present long-range suggestions for maintaining personal power and making a successful transition to nurse manager.

CHANGE MANAGEMENT

Nurse managers are the "captain of the ship" in terms of assisting staff to view the positive element of change and leading staff towards positive growth. As the health care industry has grown and become a more competitive business, the public perception of the industry has changed from one of compassionate caring to a more profit-motivated enterprise. Consumers of health care want to be treated with

MANAGER'S TIP 1-1

SEVEN WAYS TO APPEAR MORE POWERFUL

- ✔ Powerful people usually appear to be calm and unflappable.
- ✔ Powerful people usually speak less and listen more.
- ✔ Powerful people exude confidence in themselves and in their problem-solving abilities.
- ✔ Powerful people are usually optimistic.
- ✔ Powerful people set appropriate limits for themselves, their resources, and their staff.
- ✔ Powerful people may not always feel that way, but they have learned to act powerful and know the behaviors and feelings will follow.
- ✔ Powerful people dress for the role, modeling a potential mentor or successful manager in the organization.

respect and "get their money's worth." They want positive, quantifiable results; however, it is not always easy to mesh positive outcomes, customer satisfaction, and cost reduction. The complexity of such a task can take its toll on managers, as well as frontline staff members.

As mentioned earlier in this chapter, hospitals are no longer the only place where health care is delivered to a large number of people. No longer can patient care or other health care staff go to school, graduate, be hired at a local hospital, and expect to remain there for the rest of their careers. In fact, some people believe that "job security" is an oxymoron in today's environment. The days of the large employer caring for all the needs of staff have gone with the wild stock market days of the 1980s. Health care organizations are big business and as such will be affected by the fluctuation of supply and demand and cannot remain impervious to what is going on in the local and national economies.

The old saying, "the only constant is change," has never been more apparent than in health care as the paradigm continues its shift from fee-for-service to managed and capitated care. In order to survive this tumultuous time, nurse managers must have a clear sense of where they want to go with their careers, as well as where their organization is going. Strategic direction and leadership have never been more important. Managers must recognize all their personal skills and be able to translate their worth to staff, superiors, and potential employers. Clinical expertise used to be the ticket to a management position. Now, in addition to maintaining clinical excellence, the nurse manager must exhibit financial acumen, human resource management, and customer service skills, as well as creative thinking. No one trait is more important than another and the nurse manager must understand and translate into objective behaviors a balance between all the needed skills. Most importantly, the manager must understand and know at what time and in what situation certain skills are needed.

THREE WAYS TO ACQUIRE POWER

✔ Ensure that an ongoing educational program is available and includes an orientation program for new staff RNs. Your attendance accomplishes two goals: you learn what new nurses are taught and learn more about the health system or institution.

✔ Participate in educational endeavors, such as pursuing a degree, certification, or learning in another area of interest. Information about certification is addressed in Chapter 12.

✔ Network with other nurse managers on an ongoing basis. This peer support is invaluable for problem-solving support and builds morale.

29 BEHAVIORS TO HELP YOU DURING THE TRANSITION

As a new nurse manager it is also important to recognize your own limitations while learning your new role. This can be accomplished initially with the following behaviors.

✔ Recognize and accept that, initially, it is okay to learn, listen, and observe.

✔ Resist the urge to immediately intervene and change how things have been done in the past, unless patient or staff safety is in jeopardy. Change may be needed, but it may be more successful and acceptable to staff members if their input is sought after you have become the nurse manager in practice and perception. This will also allow for a thorough assessment of the problem and identification of possible solutions and implications.

✔ Remember that the nursing or scientific process is an effective tool for problem-solving and evaluation.

✔ Use the initial weeks as time to gather data and learn about the organization, daily routines, and your new staff.

✔ Remember that it is okay to NOT have an answer for all problems or issues that staff members may want to lay at your door. Direct the staff, since they are close to the problems and therefore are often the best source for effective solutions, to develop possible solutions for problems. This approach empowers the staff by valuing their input and may lead to team problem resolution.

✔ Know that it is okay to ask your staff's input in the decision-making process whenever they are affected or know the problem. Let them "own" problems and solutions.

✔ Develop your own management style. You possess unique skills and traits that can be effectively used as a manager.

✔ Know that your unique individual presence will ultimately become your style. Observe managers you respect and add the behaviors you want to emulate to your repertoire. All managers have inherent personality traits. Make the best ones work for you.

✔ Seek ways to understand and motivate your staff. Dale Carnegie is credited with saying there is only one way to get anybody to do anything—by making the other person want to do it. There is no other way. With this statement in mind, a good manager learns what specifically motivates individual team members.

Continued.

✔ Ask for feedback from peer managers or others you trust.

✔ Create an environment of cooperation through your example.

✔ Act and look like a manager. It has been said that perception looks like reality. If you make this leap of faith initially and successfully, so too will others. Observe the behaviors, dress, manners, and people skills of managers and past and present mentors you respect.

✔ Cultivate a positive relationship with your boss. Keep in mind that this important relationship may affect your overall success with the organization in the future.

✔ Communicate clearly, both in writing and in speaking. Communications should be succinct and true. Always validate information before stating facts or committing them to paper.

✔ Practice visualizing yourself as an effective manager. See yourself dealing effectively in a given situation. Practice this by trying it out behaviorally; then evaluate your actions, the process, and the outcome achieved.

✔ Recognize and accept that you cannot have all the right answers and knowledge all the time.

✔ Believe that you are the best person for this job.

✔ Give up on trying to initially address all identified problems.

✔ Remember that, in time, role ambiguity will give way to role definition.

✔ Develop, maintain, and ultimately increase and use your sense of humor. All nurse managers must have a well-developed sense of humor as a stress management tool for self and staff and, where appropriate, for patients, families, and visitors. The inherent healing value of humor is finally being recognized.

✔ Prioritize and think through problems before acting. Some problems will resolve themselves, others may not be yours. Those remaining need to be acted on.

✔ Remember that earning respect and credibility from your staff may take time.

✔ Understand that your staff look to you as role model, teacher, and resource.

✔ Realize that sometimes you need to (diplomatically) rock the boat. Being a successful manager requires taking some risks.

✔ Remember that, although you may not think your boss is always right, she/he is still the boss and as such has an inherent power.

✔ Accept that some your decisions may not be popular. This does not mean that your decisions are wrong or that you are not a likeable person.

✔ Recognize that during the role transition, one of the most difficult realizations is that you are no longer a staff nurse but a manager. Former peers, now staff members, may no longer confide in you and you may feel isolated. New peer networks and relationships need to be established.

✔ Remember that there is always more to learn.

✔ Realize that your staff is the key to getting all work accomplished.

It is important for the nurse manager to look beyond herself/himself to those on the patient care team for support and the inner resources to meet the challenge of operating on a daily basis in a positive, caring atmosphere. As Roberta Nicholson strategized in her article on developing managerial resources, ". . . tapping these strengths and developing them can help nurse executives facilitate a widespread increase in psychic energy, which can be channeled towards carrying out the goals and objectives of the organization."[4] Ms. Nicholson described the nine essential guidelines for successful nurse manager behavior as such:

1. Use mature defense mechanisms whenever possible:
    *   sublimation
    *   altruism
    *   suppression
    *   anticipation
    *   sense of humor
2. Be able to give and receive love.
3. Exhibit a concern for the life and growth of those you love.
4. View responsibility as a voluntary act in response to your own needs.
5. Define respect as the ability to view the uniqueness of self and others.
6. Understand that knowledge of self and others is the cornerstone of respect.
7. Become committed—develop your mission statement in life.
8. Act with influence, or a sense of control through imagination, knowledge, skills, and choice.
9. View change as a stimulating challenge that enhances growth.[4]

Assuming the New Role

It is important from the onset that you firmly establish yourself as the new nurse manager. Hold a staff meeting as soon as possible after the announcement of your assumption of the position. Plan a meeting for each shift. For consistency, use the same agenda for all meetings. When in these meetings, keep in mind the "Seven Ways to Appear More Powerful" shown in Manager's Tip 1-1 on p. 9.

Your First Staff Meeting as New Nurse Manager

The meeting's goals are to formalize your new role with the staff members, introduce yourself, and begin meeting your staff. At this initial meeting:
*   Welcome everyone and introduce yourself
*   Have everyone introduce themselves
*   Speak briefly about your qualifications

An example would be, "As some of you know, I have my BSN and have worked at St. Elsewhere General for 7 years in cardiac rehab. I look forward to the challenge of being the nurse manager of your new cardiac step-down unit and to working with you. Please let me know any recommendations you may have, since I am open to better ways of doing things. Initially, I'll be in orientation and will be scheduling time on all shifts to get to know everyone and the patient routines." (See Manager's Tip 1-4 for suggestions about how to conduct the meeting.)

For a more in-depth discussion about conducting or leading meetings, please refer to Chapter 5, "Day-To-Day Operations."

MANAGER'S TIP 1-4

TIPS FOR CONDUCTING
INITIAL STAFF MEETINGS

✔ Be aware that staff meetings and their management can be difficult even for experienced nurse managers.
✔ Reassure your staff that you will not be making any changes initially and that you will be observing and speaking to patients and staff members to learn the daily operational routines. This reassurance is needed at this time to decrease staff anxiety about a new manager and more changes.
✔ Share that you will be having similar meetings with the rest of the staff (if that's your plan) and will make rounds on all shifts with team leaders as part of your orientation.
✔ Do say that change is difficult for everyone and you are interested in their input.
✔ Reassure them you will not be changing representatives (again, if true) to the nursing practice council, the product selection committee, or other committees.
✔ Do not be offended if all staff members don't attend. Some staff members may act out or be complacent or appear uninterested. Change is difficult for all!
✔ Keep brief minutes, including attendance, topics discussed, and outcomes accomplished to share with staff members who were not able to attend the meeting.
✔ Always open with a welcome and state how long the meeting will last. Start on time and, when the end of the meeting is near, start wrapping up. An example of a closing statement might be, "We have a few minutes left, we need to come to a decision."
✔ As nurse manager and often chairperson of the meeting, remember to plan for factors such as the logistics of time, place, and dates. Keep in mind also that the best attended and most successful meetings often include food. Some managers have luncheon meetings to capitalize on this fact.

YOUR ORIENTATION

By title you are now a part of the management team and will be oriented to the organization (see Manager's Tip 1-5 on p. 14). Some power has been transferred to you by your new position and by your knowledge before the promotion. As professionals, all nurses perform some management functions. Staff nurses manage teams of patients, equipment, and clinical environments. They delegate as team leaders and assign duties. The leadership role inherent in RN education moves the nurse to the head of the team. The successful nurse manager integrates these past roles with the knowledge base of sound principles in day-to-day operations. These behaviors coupled with learned skills make the nurse manager unique.

The new nurse manager has a special and well-known theory available throughout this transition. The nursing process can be readily applied to management in individual patient care scenarios and in the larger view of the health care or hospital system, which may span multiple departments, services, and geographic areas.

AN ORIENTATION CHECKLIST

The following basic information and resources should be readily available to you as a new nurse manager. If not, you may need to tailor an orientation program for yourself with the help of your supervisor.

✔ Typical hours of the nurse managers in the setting.
✔ Tour of the facility or other organization.
✔ The shifts available to staff (e.g., 8, 10, or 12 hours).
✔ Organizational chart.
✔ Position descriptions for nurse manager, staff, and other care providers.
✔ The facility's policy and procedure manuals (administrative and clinical).
✔ Human resource policy manuals.
✔ Information regarding other policies (e.g., if, when, and where smoking is permitted).
✔ Location and hours of staff library, and types of material available.
✔ Mentor, peer, or other manager orientation programs.
✔ Information regarding continuing education and reimbursement policy.
✔ Other, based on your specific learning needs.

MEETINGS WITH PEER MANAGERS OF OTHER AREAS

As a manager you need to understand the workings and specific functions of areas with which your unit or department frequently interacts. It is also helpful to get to know your peers, the managers of these areas. Setting up a meeting with these managers enables you to gather needed information and begin to network with your peers.

To be effective, a nurse manager needs information about the important services and departments listed in Appendix 1-2 at the end of this chapter. The suggestions presented in Manager's Tip 1-6 can help you maximize the value of your peer manager meetings. The peer managers you meet at these meetings may become part of your support group at work. They may become friends or important allies who can help you achieve your unit's and the organization's goals. They may have interpersonal, budgetary, or other skills you will want to learn.

TAKING TIME TO TAKE STOCK

During your learning and growth period it is appropriate and helpful to review your actions and accomplishments periodically. Questions may include:

• What did I accomplish or learn today?
• What did I learn from my staff, peer managers, and boss?
• On a scale of 1 to 10, how successful was I in achieving the goals I set for today?

MANAGER'S TIP 1-6

EIGHT TIPS TO LEARN MORE FROM SCHEDULED ORIENTATION MEETINGS

✔ See these meetings as informational and networking sessions.
✔ Decide what information you want to learn.
✔ Think about the specific questions you want answered.
✔ From these meetings, consider possible actions to improve operations on the unit.
✔ Ask specific questions.
✔ Write clear, detailed notes for future reference; these notes can also serve as a source of information in the orientation of new nursing staff members.
✔ These meetings should be informational and only for meeting peers; withhold any criticisms at these introductory meetings.
✔ Remember, first impressions are important. Put your best foot forward.

- What did I do especially well that makes me feel proud?
- What can I do better the next time?
- What do I need help with and who can I ask for help?
- Did I visualize my success before I acted it out?

Most importantly, recognize that every issue and its resolution adds to your knowledge base of experience and leads to more successes in the future.

Nurse Manager Competencies

As a new nurse manager, you must measure your own competency as well as that of subordinate staff. Although the nurse manager is responsible for a wide range of activities, in frontline or first-line management patient care competencies are just as important as managerial competencies during this time of restructure and change. (For further explanation of competency-based achievement, see Chapter 3, "Human Resource Management.")

According to a 1994 study of nurse managers by the American Organization of Nurse Executives (AONE), from rural to urban settings, ". . . human and leadership competencies are the most important for effectiveness in the nurse manager role." Effective communication and decision making were identified as the most significant skills necessary for nurse managers. Other strategies that ranked high included:

1. Effective staffing strategies
2. Counseling strategies
3. Performance evaluations
4. Team-building strategies

5. Delegation
6. Change process
7. Conflict resolution
8. Problem-solving[5]

Financial performance continues to be a major concern for new managers as they are confronted with increased pressure to adhere to tighter budgets. The ability to balance financial with quality and regulatory compliance goals becomes more of a challenge as health care moves into the future.

THE MODEL OF THE FUTURE: PATIENT-CENTERED CARE

Patient-centered care is a term that has been used for a number of years in psychiatric treatment settings. However, during the past few years it has become a term synonymous with patient care planning in all types of health care settings. For the new nurse manager it is very important to understand the meaning of the term and how it is or has been applied in your unique work environment.

Patient care redesign is the process a group of patient care team members undertake when analyzing the needs of patients and beginning the task of redesigning the implementation and flow of care a patient receives while in a particular setting. The implementation may include which team member does what, when, and where for the assigned patient. Patient-centered care is usually a goal of patient care redesign or reengineering and includes the integration of interdisciplinary care. Unfortunately, redesign, or reengineering, has gained a negative connotation because it is being used in many health care settings as the primary tool to downsize or right-size the number of care providers, particularly registered nurses, at the inpatient bedside.

Primary care, the nursing model of care from the mid-to-late 1970s until today, stressed the importance of the registered nurse in providing total care to an assigned group of patients, from giving bed baths, medications, and treatments to emptying bedpans; this allowed the registered nurse to assess the needs of a patient and to problem-solve, as appropriate. The financial impact of the prospective payment system (PPS), managed care, decreased hospital census, and increased pay rates for registered nurses converged until a crisis point arose and the system needed a solution.

With public demands for more patient involvement, increased competition among care providers, tighter reimbursement regulations, and the need for quantifiable patient care outcomes, patient-centered care was a model of care ripe for implementation. There are many ways to begin developing a patient-centered care model in a facility, but the most important element is placing the needs of the patient first. Quality of care and outcomes have to be the driver of this process and not just quick financial solutions for the health entity.

The professional nurse is the ideal manager for patient care teams because her/his education and orientation are geared towards caring for the whole patient, physically, psychosocially, and spiritually. The nurse manager must be constantly aware of the traditional "turf" issues surrounding other health care professionals who have worked alone in the past and now may resent being managed by a nurse. Reaching out and involving these staff members in the planning process as much as possible and having them interact with and get to know personally the other team members may often act as a catalyst in bringing the team together.

The improvement of organizational performance (IOP) and the continuous quality improvement (CQI) processes are ideal ways to present the patient care delivery issue for review. By having a multidisciplinary committee, composed of both clinical and administrative staff, systematically review current literature on practice patterns and standards of care, as well as analyze the customer service, quality outcomes, and financial resources required to attain a certain goal or outcome of care, more rational decisions can be made. The process allows the staff members who know the most about the needs and desires of their patients to verbalize their concerns, present their ideas, and assist in deciding what will be the "best" model for this institution.

Marianne Dunn et al described *The Expert Panel Nursing Staffing and Resource Management Model* developed at the Veterans Administration in 1991 to review the current nursing staffing model and revamp it for patient care in the 1990s. As the authors explain, ". . . the expert panel method is based on the beliefs that the best decisions about staffing are made by knowledgeable nurses themselves . . . who are able to consider the many elements that go into providing patient care (and) can make fair and equitable decisions about nurse staffing requirements using their 'professional judgment'."[6] In this model, the panel systematically reviewed the structure, process, and outcomes of all areas providing either direct or indirect patient care; it began with the appointment of an implementation coordinator and went through the identification of final staffing recommendations. The outcome of the project included a shifting of nursing resources from one area to another as the data gathered indicated; in some cases, skill mix change or staff reduction in certain areas occurred. The changes were met with less resistance by staff because of the existence of data that supported either the staff reduction or addition.

For the new nurse manager, it is important to understand the process of project development and staff involvement (as much as possible) in the decision-making process. A thorough comprehension of change theory, as noted earlier in this chapter, is helpful in assisting staff to understand and work with the team on this improvement of patient care systems. Collaboration with other health care managers undergoing redesign is also helpful as a means to vent frustrations, commend successes, and learn by experience. It is imperative that the new nurse manager refrain from complaining about the process or any of the individuals, either peer managers, senior management, or staff involved in the process, to subordinates. It is counterproductive to inform staff of dissent within the planning group and ultimately lends itself to feelings of undue concern and fear of future outcomes.

It is imperative to have the team act as one, assisting each other when necessary and crossing traditional professional boundaries to care for the patient. This is not to say one professional can act in the scope of practice for another such as a respiratory therapist (RT) medicating a patient for an RN, but rather the RT might assist the nurse in positioning the patient in bed (even though the patient is not receiving RT treatments at that time).

Using the management techniques described in this book will assist the new nurse manager in motivating and uniting her/his team to strive for improved patient care outcomes and any other goals and objectives of the patient care unit.

IMPORTANT REALIZATIONS

The following realizations may be helpful during your transition to your new nursing management role. Often it takes new nurse managers many months to reach these important and perhaps surprising realizations.

- Resources (financial, personnel, and material) are limited and they will probably become more limited in the future as health care facilities continue to face fiscal constraints.
- There are rarely (if ever) enough hours in the work day.
- One new nurse manager cannot fix all the problems that have plagued a particular unit for years, perhaps even decades.
- People, including your staff, manager, and staff from other departments, will want more from you than you can reasonably give. Learning how and when to say no diplomatically is essential to your health and well-being as well as to your success.
- Your health care institution may not adapt well to change.
- There is a "good-old-boy/girl" network in many work environments. You may be faced with one at your institution. If you cannot or do not want to join it, you will need to learn to work around it. Chances are you will not be able to be effective by ignoring it.
- What the institution or your supervisor says may be different from the behaviors and rules implemented; when this occurs remember that actions speak louder than words.
- You are not responsible for all of the problems at your workplace. Only own and work on those that are truly yours.
- Most nurses and nurse managers are women. If you are a woman, assumptions may be made that you will take care of and fix everything for everyone. It is up to nurse managers to be effective role models and to not reinforce the belief that women are selfless caretakers.

Considerations for Home Care Managers

THE MANAGER'S EVOLVING ROLE: DETERMINING COMPETENCY AND MENTORING

The role of the home care nurse manager continues to evolve as does her/his counterpart in the other health care settings. The most important elements that may affect that role are:

- Continued growth of home care as an industry and managed care contracting.
- Transition of hospital-based nurses to home health care.
- Imminent change from cost-based to prospective pay system.
- Intense scrutiny of the industry by government and especially consumers.
- Increased community violence and safety issues surrounding home care personnel.
- Increased computerization of home care and improved linkage with health care settings.
- Need for quantifiable, reliable, and valid home care outcomes.
- Risk management concerns unique to home care.

Strategically, the home care manager is in an enviable position of being in "the right place, at the right time." Home care nurse managers must be creative and think globally when strategically planning the future of their units within a larger organization. It is time that the individuals who understand the needs of the community take the lead in collecting the data and developing programs that will address the community health needs of the twenty-first century.

COMPETENCY ISSUES

The home care manager is in an enviable position as the industry continues to grow in terms of number of referrals, even if the number of visits per patient drops as managed care takes a stronger hold of visit utilization. It will become important for the home care manager to set up systems and processes to orient, train, and educate staff on new or revamped home care protocols. The determination of staff competency in home care is more important because staff members are usually in the home alone and do not have the backup of other staff in the same vicinity if a problem arises. As agencies grow, the tendency to hire quickly to meet referral needs must be weighed by the value of having qualified, competent, and oriented staff to provide safe, quality patient care.

MENTORING

Home care managers typically are clinicians who have been promoted from the staff ranks. The education and nurturing of good managers must begin before the individual is promoted. It is very important for nurse managers, and especially for women managers, to commit to providing leadership and mentoring services to those promising staff members who have the ability, ambition, and courage to pursue management. Even as the workday never seems to end, it is vital that we train the new generation of managers to successfully take charge of their own area.

Seek out opportunities to mentor—either at your own work place or through local professional, business, and clinical service organizations. A mentor can be of either sex and need not be in your direct chain of command. What is important is the dedication of time, energy, and commitment towards assisting a "budding" manager in developing the maturity, problem-solving skills, and networking abilities to successfully tackle projects and potentially challenging positions.

SUMMARY

Although management may have inherent pitfalls, effective nurse managers can make positive, lasting impressions on numerous patients, families, and staff. The new nurse manager may feel isolated and inadequate. Conversely, the successful resolution of problems and the delicate handling of personnel issues leave a feeling of accomplishment like no other. Nurses blend complex healing technology with nurturing care. This combination is why patients and their families marvel at the profession and those skills brought to the bedside.

However, problems are inevitable, and some days the hassles may seem overwhelming. Yet problems present opportunities for personal growth and satisfaction in problem resolution. Use your orientation time to get to know others in your facility and to learn from their experience. They will be glad that someone values their knowledge and expertise.

Transition from staff nurse to the leadership position of nurse manager can be a difficult process. The initial enthusiasm, pride, and fantasies to fix the system must ultimately be tempered with a realistic role identification and realistic goal setting.

References

1. Weil TP, Jorgensen E: Health manpower trends in a market-driven environment, *Journal of Healthcare Resource Management,* December 1995, pg. 17.
2. NewsCaps: 613,000 new RN jobs projected, *Am J Nurs* 90(1):74, 1990.
3. Curtin LL: Power: the trap of trappings, *Nursing Management,* June 1989, pg.7.
4. Nicholson R: Manager's primer for developing inner resources, *Nursing Management: Management Briefs* August, 1989, pg. 17-19.
5. Chase L: Nurse manager competencies, *JONA* 24(4S):63, 1994.
6. Dunn MG, et al: Expert panel method for nurse staffing and resource management, *JONA* 25(10):62, 1995.

For Further Reading

Boll ML: Middle management in nursing. Notes from the Field, *Nursing Management* 21(2): 1990.

Belasco JA, Strayer RC: *The flight of the buffalo: to excellence, learning to let employees lead,* New York, 1993, Waverly Books.

Clinical managers help agency staff cope with growth, stress, *Hospital Home Health* August 9(8):108, 1992.

Clinicians: manage your move to manager. Executive Advancement, *Hospitals* March 5, 1991; 60.

Curtin LL: Power: the trap of trappings, *Nursing Management* 20(6):7, 1989.

delBueno D, Vincent P: Organizational culture: how important is it? *Journal of Nursing Administration* 16(10):15, 1986.

Dunn MG, et al: Expert panel method for nurse staffing and resource management, *JONA* 25(10):35 1995.

Gage M: The patient-driven interdisciplinary care plan, *JONA* 24(4):44 1994.

Griest DL, Belles DR: Health care executives: a personality profile, *Hospitals* 64(3):74, 1990.

Hamilton JM, Kiefer ME: Personal power: your key to success, *Nursing 90* October 1990; 146-148.

Hood JN, Smith HL: Quality of work life in home care: the contribution of leaders' personal concern for staff, *Journal of Nursing Administration* 24(1):40, 1994.

Janz M: Perception of knowledge—what administrators and assistants know, *Journal of Gerontological Nursing* August 1992; 7-12.

Kaplan SM: The nurse as a change agent. Professional Perspectives, *Pediatric Nursing* 16(6):603, 1990.

Kison C: Leadership: how, who and what? *Nursing Management* 20(11):72, 1989.

Knollmueller RN: Reshaping supervisory practice in home care, *Nursing Clinics of North America* 23(2):353, 1988.

Lasater ME: Strategies for organizational change in home health care, *Home HealthCare Nurse* 11(2):38, 1993.

Levesque RF: Business planning in home health care agencies: a guide for nurse executives, *Columbia University Teachers College* 1991 ED. D.

Noone C, Szekay L: Working with consultants to achieve home health agency goals, *Journal of Nursing Administration* 21(10): 61, 1991.

Patz J, et al: Middle nurse manager effectiveness, *Journal of Nursing Administration* 21(1):15, 1991.

Rutledge DN, Donaldson NE: Building organizational capacity to engage in research utilization, *JONA* 25(10): 1995.

Scalzi CC, Wilson DL: Future preparation of home health nurse executives, *Home Health Care Services Quarterly* 12(1), 1991.

Sherry D: Coping with staffing shortages: strategies for survival, *Home Healthcare Nurse* 12(1):38, 1994.

Smith TC: Management skills for directors of nursing, *Journal of Nursing Administration* 23(9):38, 1993.

Werkheiser L, et al: The nurse manager resource peer: part II. *Nursing Management* 21(12):30, 1990.

APPENDIX 1-1

SCOPE AND STANDARDS FOR THE NURSE MANAGER

Nurse managers are responsible to a nurse executive and manage one or more defined areas of organized nursing services. In smaller settings, they may have responsibilities for management of the entire facility and its service. Nurse managers allocate available resources to promote efficient, effective, and compassionate nursing care; provide input into executive-level decisions; and keep staff informed of executive-level activities.

Nurse managers coordinate activities between defined areas, and provide clinical and administrative leadership and expertise. They facilitate an atmosphere of interactive management and the development of collegial relationships among nursing personnel and others. They serve as a link between nursing personnel and other health care disciplines throughout the organizations. Nurse managers have major responsibility for the implementation of the vision, mission, plans, and standards of the organization and nursing services within their defined areas of responsibility.

To fulfill the responsibilities described above, the nurse manager, in collaboration with nursing personnel and members of other disciplines, engages in the following activities:

1. Participates in nursing and organizational policy formulation and decision-making.
2. Facilitates participation of staff in nursing and organizational policy formulation and decision-making.
3. Accepts organizational accountability for services provided to recipients.
4. Evaluates the quality and appropriateness of care.
5. Provides guidance for and supervision of personnel accountable to the nurse manager.
6. Coordinates nursing services with the services of other health care disciplines.
7. Participates in the recruitment, selection, and retention of personnel.

8. Assumes responsibility for staffing and scheduling personnel. Assignments reflect appropriate utilization of personnel.

9. Assures appropriate orientation, education, credentialing, and continuing professional development for personnel.

10. Evaluates performance of personnel.

11. Participates in planning and monitoring the budget for her/his defined areas.

12. Participates and involves the nursing staff in evaluative research activities.

13. Fosters a climate conducive to educational experiences for nursing and other students.

14. Fosters peer review.

Nurse managers are accountable for the environment in which clinical nursing is practiced. The ability of nurse managers to enhance the practice environment is critical to the recruitment and retention of nurses with diverse backgrounds and appropriate education and experience. They contribute to the strategic planning process, day-to-day operations, and attainment of goals of the organization. Nurse managers collaborate with the nurse executive and others in organizational planning, innovation, and evaluation.

From *Scope and standards for nurse administrators,* Washington, DC, 1995, American Nurses Association.

CHECKLIST OF KEY INFORMATION ABOUT IMPORTANT SERVICES AND DEPARTMENTS

CHAPLAINCY SERVICES

____ Types of services (e.g., bereavement, remembrance, worship services, baptisms, other)
____ Hours the chaplain or other representative chaplaincy staff is available
____ How a referral is initiated
____ Ethics
____ Other

DATA PROCESSING AND INFORMATION SERVICES

____ Orientation to nursing and other information systems (hardware and software)
____ Video display terminal (VDT) password and confidentiality safeguards
____ Management reports and their retrieval
____ Other

DIETARY OR FOOD SERVICES

____ Schedule of meal and snack delivery times
____ Flexibility of menu based on specific patient needs (e.g., kosher, macrobiotic)
____ Location and hours of restaurants, cafeterias, and snack bars
____ Staff cafeteria hours
____ Other

CASE MANAGEMENT/DISCHARGE PLANNING

____ Resources available to patients, families, and staff
____ Policy of patients being evaluated on admission
____ The referral process
____ The schedule for discharge planning rounds held in the clinical area
____ Other

FINANCE

____ How often the unit financial and other utilization reports are generated
____ Your responsibilities regarding specific reports
____ The budget processes and time frames

____ The process for requesting new capital equipment
____ Your role in the budget process
____ The historic supply use baseline for the clinical area
____ The current occupancy rate
____ The facility's breakdown of types of payers
____ Percentage of charity care the facility provides annually and the amount that gets written off
____ The average length of stay
____ Other

HUMAN RESOURCES/PERSONNEL

____ The process of nurse selection
____ The nurse manager's interview occurs at what point after the nurse recruiter has validated licensure and references
____ Nurse recruiter responsibilities
____ Policies and procedures for counseling
____ Status of union involvement
____ Overtime and on-call salary guidelines
____ Availability of a professional nursing pool, either in-house or through nursing agencies on a temporary basis
____ Actions to take if you believe a nurse is impaired
____ The standard policy for hiring, evaluation, and termination
____ Grievance policy and process
____ Location on the unit of the institution's personnel handbook
____ Other

LABORATORY SERVICES

____ Hours of service, pick-up schedule, stat bloods, prn delivery schedule
____ Find out who is responsible for venipunctures, starting intravenous (IV) solutions, and maintaining IVs and other lines
____ Other

MEDICAL RECORDS

____ Policy on patients accessing their clinical charts
____ Protection of confidentiality if clinical records are data entered or keyed directly into a computerized system
____ Services and results accessible via the video display terminal (VDT)
____ Type of medical record system that is in place
____ Types of charting that are the standard or acceptable
____ Existence of an institution-wide charting process
____ Role of nurses pertaining to documenting in the same clinical note areas as physicians and other professional team members
____ The program's or hospital's use of problem-oriented medical record (POMR), SOAP, or focus charting
____ Requirements for computerized documentation in lieu of clinical entries or narrative notes
____ Other

QUALITY IMPROVEMENT/RISK MANAGEMENT

_____ The roles of these departments in the facility
_____ The process and use of incident reports
_____ When to call the risk manager
_____ Status of studies currently underway (e.g., on patient falls, medication errors, or the use of restraints)
_____ How the nursing manager and staff members receive feedback on the findings
_____ Your areas of responsibilities regarding quality improvement
_____ How nursing integrates with the overall quality improvement process of the hospital
_____ Other

REHABILITATION SERVICES

_____ Services available (e.g., physical, occupational, and respiratory therapies and speech-language pathology [SLP] services)
_____ How referrals are initiated
_____ Policy on all CVA patients receiving a swallowing evaluation on admission
_____ Ascertain which department does swallowing evaluations at the institution—occupational therapy (OT) or SLP
_____ Ascertain if the schedules for patient pick-up are posted for the nursing staff
_____ Learn who at the facility does chest PT (e.g., PT, RT, or RN)
_____ Length of time the patient is usually gone from the unit
_____ Accessibility of the charting entries by these professional associates
_____ The schedule for interdisciplinary team meetings
_____ Other

RADIOLOGIC SERVICES

_____ Hours of services
_____ Availability of MRI
_____ Location of services
_____ The process for scheduling and transport of patients
_____ Availability and policy for portable X-ray examinations
_____ Ascertain who holds patients in position for X-ray examinations after hours
_____ Ascertain which X-ray examinations are not done after certain hours
_____ Other

HOME HEALTH CARE

_____ The admission policies
_____ Which types (severity, diagnosis, specialty areas) of patients are appropriate for referral to the program
_____ The geographic boundaries
_____ The referral process
_____ Status of nurse-to-nurse communication for continuity of the plan of care before discharge
_____ Whether the patient meets her/his primary home care nurse, when possible, before discharge
_____ How soon after discharge the patient is assessed in the home setting

_____ Lists of supplies the in-patient nurse should send home with the patient for initial wound or other care
_____ Existence of 24-hour on-call service
_____ How patients are admitted on the weekends
_____ Other services available to support patients and their families at home, such as personal emergency response systems or private duty care
_____ Other areas of expertise offered, such as home IV administration or total parenteral nutrition (TPN)
_____ How the need for services at home is determined and who makes the determination
_____ How durable medical equipment or other needs are addressed
_____ Status of the agency (e.g., licensed, Medicare certified, and JCAHO or National League for Nursing [NLN] accreditation)
_____ Other

HOSPICE

_____ How a referral is initiated and the admission policies
_____ Where the patient goes if in-patient care is necessary
_____ When the hospice nurse meets the patient and family before hospital discharge for continuity of care
_____ The geographic boundaries
_____ Acceptance of both pediatric and adult patients
_____ The bereavement support process
_____ Support groups for the family
_____ Other

STAFF EDUCATION

_____ The organizational structure for staff development
_____ The scheduled conferences or resources planned for the next two quarters (or other specified time frame)
_____ Availability of clinical preceptors, instructors, or specialists to the staff
_____ Research that is currently occurring in the clinical setting
_____ Ascertain if the orientation program is competency-based and how competency is measured
_____ The needs assessment tools currently in use
_____ The mechanism for reevaluation and how often they are reevaluated
_____ Learn what program is currently employed to assist new graduates in their transitions to proficient, professional nurses
_____ The specific resources (e.g., human, fiscal, audiovisual) available to the nurse manager and her/his staff
_____ Ascertain if the manager of staff development is a peer resource for new nurse managers
_____ Ask if there is a peer support program for the staff development team
_____ Status of JCAHO or ANA Nursing Staff Development Standards in the program
_____ The resources available for specialty training (e.g., maternal/child, hospice, home care, operating room, or critical care staff)
_____ Other

Other areas could include housekeeping, facility management, and numerous specialty areas, depending on the size, resources, and structure of the facility.

CHAPTER 2

MANAGEMENT: AN OVERVIEW

SANDRA B. MARTIN WHITTIER

MANAGEMENT: WHAT IS IT?

New nurse managers are experienced at nursing but new to management. Management is constantly working to define itself in a positive manner. For a new nurse manager, it means collaborating with clinicians from other disciplines and health care colleagues to accomplish outcome-oriented activities. A new nurse manager must:

- Define her/his management/leadership style.
- Assess the culture of the group and management environment.
- Master the organization's philosophy, as well as policies and procedures.
- Define knowledge deficits to pinpoint continuing education topics.

New managers initially may require guidance from their own manager, and must be assertive enough to identify and operationalize behaviorally the expectations of the new position. It is for this reason that managers must have a clear understanding of the mission of the organization—in order to clearly communicate to subordinate staff and senior management. Initially, the new manager can focus on the following principles, outlined by McGregor[1]:

- Knowledge of organizational policies and management philosophy.
- Knowledge of organizational standards, regulations, and procedures.
- Knowledge of change theories.
- An atmosphere of approval.
- Subordinates' need for security.
- Consistent behavior, including discipline.

The purpose of the organization will enlighten the manager as to the management philosophy and reporting mechanisms of the agency or hospital. Departmental goals, documentation procedures, use of the nursing process, and any theoretic basis used for practice guidelines are communicated via the direct supervisor of the new manager.

Managers must have a clear understanding of the mission of the agency or organization and be able to communicate to staff in ways that promote understanding and adoption of that mission. Abilities and skills necessary for such communication are listed in Box 2-1.

What Is Leadership?

Nurse managers are chosen for their leadership ability and demonstrated clinical competence. Earlier in their careers, they performed well when "in charge," were complimented by staff or supervisors, and began to see themselves differently. At some point they discovered their innate leadership skills, a foundation on which to build and add new skills. Some believe that "leadership is viewed as larger and more important than management."[2]

Leadership is the key to management. According to Bethel,[3] a leader:
1. Has a mission that matters.
2. Is a big thinker.
3. Has high ethics.
4. Masters change.
5. Is sensitive.
6. Is a risk taker.
7. Is a decision-maker.
8. Uses power wisely.
9. Communicates effectively.
10. Is courageous.
11. Is a team builder.
12. Is committed.

Leading is guiding and directing the skills of others towards positive outcomes. Leaders must continually examine and develop their own skills to remain confident in their abilities.

Just as confidence and enthusiasm are contagious, insecurity can be sensed and targeted by some staff. Leaders must be perceptive and use their powers of observation when evaluating the group's cohesiveness. Divisive staff members challenge the manager to keep strengthening and reevaluating leadership skills. Leadership is essential to orderly direction in supporting the staff in quality patient care.

Types of Leaders

Excellent nursing leadership requires being action-, result-, or outcome-oriented.[4] Leading by example, being available to staff when needed, constantly sharpening skills, and having an earnest understanding of staff concerns are important to creating loyalty and respect between staff members and manager. Leaders are problem-solvers who do not see a problem as an obstacle to *overcome* but as a puzzle requiring thought to *solve*.

box 2-1

ABILITIES AND SKILLS NEEDED BY NEW NURSE MANAGERS

ABILITIES

- Influence workers to believe in themselves
- Develop individual staff strengths
- Create a desire for excellence and loyalty
- Work with staff behaviorally to improve weaknesses
- Provide challenges in the context of a busy day
- Evaluate performance constructively
- Mentor both staff members who display leadership characteristics and those who require coaching
- Communicate with their managers and staff to outline responsibilities and decision-making
- Lead by example
- Demonstrate knowledge of human behavior and its motivation
- Motivate staff members to work together
- Administer departmental budgets
- Communicate clearly and nonjudgmentally
- Be consistent
- Be flexible
- Take risks
- Demonstrate concern for staff
- Be open and honest with staff

SKILLS

- Demonstrate clinical excellence
- Make effective decisions
- Evaluate the clinical knowledge and skills of individual staff members to match staff to patients
- Implement reasonable staffing schedules on a timely basis
- Have vision to plan for next week or month while getting through today
- Create a stimulating environment that encourages staff autonomy
- Develop short- and long-term goals with your staff's input
- Acknowledge that staff members need to ventilate emotions and allow this in the proper setting
- Display commitment
- Build effective work groups
- Make performance evaluations a positive experience
- Empower your staff
- Provide positive reinforcement—often and loudly
- Choose not to be intimidated by a "potential" or "de facto" manager
- Encourage professional growth of staff by exposure to clinical seminars or conferences
- Successfully incorporate change theory principles

Two leadership concepts, as defined by Burns,[5] can assist the new manager to establish a style of leading. A transformational leader has a vision that, when shared with the staff, creates motivation for working to accomplish the goal. A transformational leader is dynamic, can see the end result, and can incorporate staff input, thereby illustrating staff creativity. Once staff members see that their suggestions have value, more suggestions will follow, and they will begin to originate their own solutions to other problems.

The transformational leader gives responsibility to employees at all levels to make the most of their talents. The transformational leader encourages learning, exploration, and creativity.[6] This type of leader could be important for another reason—organizations cannot afford to support nonproductive employees. The transformational leader is able to take the employee beyond the level of performance achieved by the more traditional, transactional leader.[6]

In contrast, the transactional leader is more involved with managing daily operations. The transactional leader negotiates with followers to meet immediate demands on a short-term basis. In transactional leadership, the exchange benefits both the leader and the follower but meets the immediate needs of the employee and management.

The transformational leader believes that cooperation, empowerment, vision, trust, and intuition are more valued than control, competition, and power wielding.[7]

THE MANAGEMENT ENVIRONMENT

All nurse managers face economic and professional influences that affect their work environment. These may be internal in the organization or external in the larger health care environments. Some of the most important contemporary influences are listed below.

Economic issues
- Increases in number of patients without health insurance coverage
- More acutely ill patients seeking care
- More pressure for staff members to work as more family members lose jobs in the current economic climate
- Third-party–payer restrictions on covered care
- Third-party payer's increased expectation of patient participation in care
- Spiraling cost of health care

Professional issues
- Ethical dilemmas
- Values clarification
- Redesign of organizations with change in patient care delivery model
- Rotation and weekend work, overtime requests, on call, other staffing needs
- "Quicker and sicker" syndrome causing the staff to respond by "doing the best they can"

- Managed care
- Customer service focus
- Outcomes management
- The need for more collaborative and interdisciplinary working relationships
- Professional development/continuing education
- Staff questioning of management decisions
- Staff, patient, and provider diversity issues

THE GROWTH OF A NEW MANAGER

Some new managers are fortunate enough to have worked for nurse managers who taught administrative as well as clinical skills. Those without this previous training will have to successfully develop these new skills.

Nurse managers report to managers themselves. Depending on the agency or organization, nurse managers are also influenced by layers of management and agendas, whose downward influence can determine a new manager's effectiveness and longevity. Good managers support, as well as develop, new managers and potential new managers.

Nursing management skills are vital to nursing's continued growth. Adverse economic and professional influences compound the difficulties seen by staff members as deterrents to managerial aspirations. The future of nursing management depends on the growth and positive leadership of staff. Nurse managers foster the development of future nurse managers by:
- Being managerially self-aware.
- Nurturing the staff's clinical and leadership potential.
- Leading by example.
- Demystifying managerial concepts with the staff to increase mutual understanding.
- Mentoring other nurses.
- Becoming a professional role model by both acting and dressing appropriate to the corporate culture of the organization.

As resources decrease and work stressors increase, nurse managers must use their individual strengths to promote loyalty in an atmosphere of trust. Creating a stable environment that promotes professional growth, excellence in patient care, and individual problem-solving and goal-setting is the role of the nurse manager.

The importance of effective nursing management must not be underestimated. New managers need guidelines and mentoring, especially through the classic management dilemmas, such as poor work performance or disruptive staff or behaviors. Without appropriate nursing direction, new managers will become discouraged and either return to patient care or leave nursing entirely. Nursing cannot afford to lose these potential managers who could have been effective leaders but who never fulfilled the manager role.

STYLES OF MANAGEMENT

Choosing one management style does not allow the nurse manager the flexibility required to meet her/his own needs or those of the staff. New managers will want to select a style that is satisfying and productive while continuously being developed (see Manager's Tip 2-1).

All new managers may incorporate the positive and negative aspects of their own previous managers. Many managers can be categorized based on the management style characteristics displayed. It is important to note that staff members also function at varying levels, depending on the management style and expectations of their former nurse managers.

The tasks of the area, unit, or organization must be reviewed when considering management styles. For example, the immediacy of response to life-threatening events may require some autocracy in management. Imperative to management

MANAGER'S TIP 2-1

MANAGEMENT STYLES

Research and development to design strategies for managerial use have defined four management styles:

✔ *Autocratic managers*
- Do not delegate.
- Make all decisions.
- Have little or no use for staff input.
- Use authority to accomplish goals.
- Foster reliance on the manager.

✔ *Laissez-faire managers*
- Provide little direction.
- Perform without structure or organization.
- Do not provide guidance.
- Do not foster group cohesion.
- Abdicate decision-making.

✔ *Democratic managers*
- Initiate staff participation.
- Delegate with the purpose of staff development.
- Encourage staff towards goal-setting.
- Allow individuals a degree of control.
- Provide frequent positive feedback.

✔ *Participative managers*
- Make final decisions, but include staff input.
- Negotiate as well as direct.
- Enlist staff suggestions.
- Provide staff members with opportunities to develop their careers.
- Transcend the manager—staff gap.

style development is the assessment of individual nurses' strengths and weaknesses. The same new critical care manager may have a disproportionate amount of new staff who require more supervision. Therefore a critique of staff performance can be a guide on which to base managerial style selection. In addition, the level of autonomy or professionalism in a particular staff member affects the choice of leadership style.

The concept of situational leadership can be used when considering which management style a group requires. All staff members and managers have various facets that influence their adaptability to change, new direction, or new management. Each staff member has strengths that rise to the surface, often based on clinical experience and problem-solving attributes, and these qualities can be matched by the manager to foster growth in other staff members who need improvement in these areas.

To adapt leadership to the situation, the workers' needs, the leader's abilities, and the methods chosen to direct or supervise should be based on whether the required tasks are clear-cut or ambiguous, whether staff members desire structure or independence, and whether the leader is a skilled group worker or an autocrat.[6] Autocracy has its place at times, but no manager of the 1990s can use autocracy as a prominent style. Assertiveness of individuals, disappearance of the handmaiden concept of nursing, and changing medical/nursing relationships prohibit managers from directing without staff participation.

Management philosophies focus on the manager's ability to attain cost-effective and productive quality results. Therefore a laissez-faire style, with its lack of focus and direction, is not a useful style for the new nurse manager to develop. This is true in any nursing setting, where the new nurse manager must by her/his presence and personality lead the staff to work towards development of their potential, as well as positive patient outcomes.

The new nurse manager must have a working knowledge of all leadership styles for use in multiple situations. Communication with confidence is crucial when incorporating a style into the nurse manager's daily repertoire. Consistent behaviors by the manager will help staff members adopt a style to use themselves.

Autocratic and laissez-faire managers are extremes in management styles, the former manager making all decisions without staff input, and the latter being unable to make swift and decisive management decisions. More balanced management styles are democratic and participative. These styles allow the manager to develop staff members to a degree that they are often asked, and feel comfortable giving, their opinions for problem-solving. Remember, the staff are closest to the identified challenges and therefore may have the most workable or practical solutions. Short- or long-term goals generated by the staff are more likely to be successfully achieved when the manager leads democratically. Staff members led by a democratic leader who takes and uses their advice project a feeling of being part of an effective group process. A leader's use of a democratic style in management will not stifle or stagnate the staff. A true leader may find a few specific uses for the autocratic rule, but she/he will generally depend on democratic and participatory leadership styles that can be blended with transformational styles. The last two styles promote in staff members the ability and confidence to identify problems and solve them, while evaluating effects of both solutions and processes.

Participatory leadership varies from the democratic style of management in several ways. This leader presents the identified problem with potential solutions. Staff input is then invited, but the manager may ultimately decide on the specific implementation. Participatory leadership has its drawbacks. By creating an illusion of participation through feedback solicitation, but then not using the staff suggestions, the nurse manager may unknowingly sabotage future efforts to promote participation. Positive aspects of participatory management involve the commitment of sharing authority and responsibility throughout an agency or organization. This is most effectively ensured when the entire organization values participatory management as their philosophy. In fact, many believe that the sign of an effective manager is the organization's ability to function efficiently in her/his absence.

Participatory leadership creates a dependency on the leader to identify problems, unlike the democratic style, which encourages staff to initiate and develop ideas as well as solutions. An illustration of the various styles in response to a familiar scene might be:

The autocratic leader "I have completed the schedule for the holidays, using the policy of staff members working every other holiday. There will be no switching of time among staff members."

The laissez-faire leader "The holiday schedule is completed by the scheduling office; I can't think of a better way to do it."

The democratic leader "Mary has an idea to present at the staff meeting about coverage for the upcoming holidays."

The participatory leader "We will have a staff meeting and complete the holiday schedule as a group."

It may be appropriate, depending on the situation, to use any or all of these styles. This choice of leadership styles can be pivotal in being an effective nurse manager. It is important to be aware that staff members will respond negatively to styles and responses that are not consistent. Conversely, even when managers give predictable responses, the staff is at least aware of managerial expectations in given circumstances. *The test of managerial success in nursing is successfully developing a comfortable and consistent management style that facilitates growth and satisfaction for both the manager and the staff.*

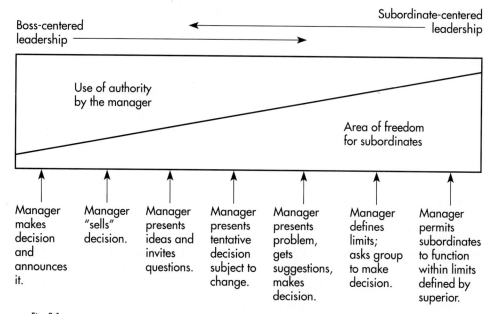

Fig. 2-1 Continuum of leadership behavior and participation. (From Tannebaum R, Schmidt WH: How to choose a leadership pattern, *Harvard Bus Rev* 51:164, 1973.)

The new manager, while studying management styles, may want to try out her/his initial responses to employees' performance and apply them to a behavior scale to characterize the style that surfaces. Several tools are available that categorize a manager's responses to the appropriate management style, such as Hersey and Blanchard[8] and Fiedler.[9] One classic example is Tannenbaum and Schmidt's continuum of behavior (Figure 2-1).[10]

Figure 2-1 enables the new manager to problem-solve when dealing with various prospective solutions to practical situations. Making use of her/his knowledge of individual staff members and their needs, as well as her/his own, the new manager can anticipate new problems while solving others and analyze her/his own behavior at the same time. The new manager must have enough personal confidence to allow new and seasoned nurses to flourish without feeling that her/his power or knowledge is usurped or threatened. Nurse managers cannot control the environment by their presence alone and must be able to take a vacation with confidence that daily activities will continue smoothly. A key sign of an effective nurse manager is that the staff functions well whether or not the manager is present.

COMMUNICATION (REGARDLESS OF MANAGEMENT STYLE)

Communication, negotiation, the ability to understand the political process and economics, sensitivity to organizational process, knowledge of how to form alliances, critical thinking, and the ability to construct a solid case for a point of view are some of the skills nurse managers need.[11] Nurse managers can evaluate their communication skills by observing staff response when information is presented. An important aspect of communication is perception. One cannot assume that the staff will always understand and follow through with the agenda communicated by the manager. Verbal communication should be followed up in writing when appropriate. Written staff meeting minutes dispensed to all staff members unable to attend deflect the excuse, "No one ever told me." Clear communication leaves no room for conjecture, and all have an understanding of the material presented. With some staff members, this may require that the nurse manager request immediate feedback to validate the communication. For an in-depth discussion about communication, refer to Chapter 4, "Communications."

Three other aspects of communication vital for the new nurse manager are (1) negotiation, (2) the effective use of positive feedback, and (3) conflict resolution skills. Negotiation can be useful as a tool to persuade even the most resistant staff member trying to exercise her/his power, which is a problem situation, directed towards the new manager. The new manager should assess whether this forcefulness results from insecurity of the staff person before using negotiation as a management tool. As an example, suppose a length of time has passed between managers, and this staff nurse has become an informal leader among the staff. This nurse probably needs some time to adjust to changing roles within the group. That power of the "de facto" leader can also be used to enable the staff as the new manager establishes her/his role.

THE IMPORTANCE OF POSITIVE FEEDBACK

If the new manager has evaluated the behavior and identifies it as insecurity, positive feedback may dispel any challenges to the manager's power. Positive feedback can be an icebreaker, is always necessary, and should be given sincerely in an atmosphere of team building. It can include any praise for any job well done:

- Strong assessment skills.
- Effective handling of an emergency.
- Working extra hours.
- Support during change.
- Support of another staff member—either emotional or physical.
- Handling a heavy assignment.
- Early detection of clinical signs requiring intervention.
- Working together as a team.
- Dealing with difficult physicians.
- Leadership skills demonstrated by staff.
- Dealing with supervisors.
- Maintaining consistency in management on a daily basis.

This list is by no means complete; please think of your own positive feedback and use it. At the end of each day, some managers thank staff members. Others get in the good habit of giving positive feedback daily. These are not empty words; they contribute positively to staff autonomy and self-esteem. For an in-depth discussion on communication, please see Chapter 4, "Communications."

Positive and negative feedback, negotiation, communication skills, and choice of leadership style are the responsibility of new nurse managers. The methodical evaluation, choice, and development of managerial style and characteristics is never time wasted. It is easier for the manager and the staff as a group when the manager selects and implements a style that matches the manager's best skills and begins the process of fostering growth and unity among staff. The long-term effectiveness and excellence with which the organizational goals are attained are worth the effort because then patients' needs are met and professional nursing careers are fulfilled.

THE NURSING PROCESS

Nursing management involves nursing, general business, and management theories. Nursing theories abound and must be studied at greater length than is possible here. Nursing theory can lay the groundwork for nursing standards in any specialty. As an example, Orem's self-care theory[12] is adaptable to community health. Orem's emphasis is on health promotion and states that health information given to the consumer causes change in those behaviors that are deemed unhealthy, which is also the basis of community health nursing. Behavior change used as a demonstrated patient outcome can then be formulated into nursing standards of care. Nursing theory can be used when updating or creating nursing standards.

Regulations are promulgated by federal (e.g., Medicare, OSHA, CLIA, CDCP) and state Medicaid agencies or accreditation organizations such as JCAHO or CHAP. A heightened emphasis is on patients' rights and responsibilities, customer service, cost-effective care, and outcome achievement. The ongoing review of standards is a part of the responsibility of the nurse manager.

The new manager can use another theory that is very familiar when called on to problem-solve, evaluate nursing compliance to standards, or assess quality assurance and quality improvement processes.

Remember the nursing process:

Assessment
Planning
Implementation
Evaluation

The nursing or scientific problem-solving process helps the manager track or organize any issue objectively. Once potential solutions are identified, they can be categorized, studied, and (when managers are democratic or participatory in management style) shared with staff for their input and ideas. The manager projects an implementation time frame. Once the time frame is met, the evaluation process begins (or is initiated). The evaluation must continue to remain objective. Thus the cycle is complete and the next problem or issue can be confronted. The nursing process is one tool managers can use among other nursing and management theories.

WRITTEN RECORDS

The dynamic aspect of the manager role entails that even while planning for future needs, the staff's past cannot be forgotten. This historic overview is sometimes helpful to new managers. The long, sometimes tedious process of change and growth must be documented accurately to ensure that the process was true to objectives. A dependable method, which is needed when the manager must provide facts to defend positions, is written communication. Written communication, as an adjunct to the spoken word, can be difficult to incorporate into a busy day, but it is essential that the new nurse manager do so. The practice of committing to memory observations about behavior, good or bad, without actual notations is no longer feasible and is not responsible to the staff. Those preceptors or individuals guiding new managers must foster the use of anecdotal recording on a regular or as-needed basis as a management tool and assist new managers to develop strategies to meet this goal.

During meetings with the staff on a group or individual basis, the discussion should be summarized orally and then the plan of action summarized in writing. Short notes kept on the staff's performance can make evaluation time objective and full of examples, positive and negative, on which manager and staff goals are designed. All that must be noted are (1) the topics of discussion and (2) the outcomes or goals for either or both parties. Then the next meeting will first address the progress or steps being taken to meet the goals.

A manager owes the staff a meaningful performance evaluation, citing examples of behavior being reviewed. An example could be a review of the staff members' clinical documentation and a comparison to the organization's written documentation standards. This helps the manager be more realistic and fair, without being influenced by personality or popularity attributes. Some incidents will be remembered without hesitation; times of high emotion and tragedy, personal losses, and the legions of patients for whose lives the staff fought are emblazoned on everyone's mind. Time passes quickly between events that nurses remember, so notation of regular activity is a management obligation.

A new manager should begin by writing thoughts when evaluating the staff's performance of patient care, keeping in mind the objectives of the organization. Such documentation can be helpful in other situations; for example, the new manager might record that the staff members need more equipment or training, listing specific examples. She/he could then discuss this subject with her/his manager. The documentation then makes important information quickly available when needed. The ability to rapidly provide specific rationales supporting the manager's point is a key to the manager's credibility and ultimate effectiveness in an organization.

NURSING MANAGEMENT BY OBJECTIVES

Anecdotal comments, and their use as a daily chronicle, are beneficial as practice for working with management by objectives (MBO). These anecdotal notes reduce assumption and provide a foundation for evaluating staff performance. MBO for nurses uses the setting and meeting of goals, usually behavioral, that cause improvement in patient care and other valued outcomes. MBO causes one to strive to attain further goals within a specific period, and goals are designed at the individual's pace. The use of MBO provides focus and direction to both managerial and institutional goals. An objective of a new manager might be, "Evaluate all RNs by observation of their work and documentation, among other factors, and conduct a personal review with each RN by June 30, 1999." This objective is measurable and has a specific time frame. Anecdotal documentation assists the manager in meeting this goal. MBO is for managers who want to create a new environment for progress and quality patient care. For the benefit of the new manager, MBO can be practiced whether or not the organization promotes it. Once the principles are understood, MBO can help in many ways as a step towards achievement of goals in any organization. Manager's Tip 2-2 presents MBO guidelines and characteristics.

MANAGER'S TIP 2-2

MBO GUIDELINES AND CHARACTERISTICS

Guidelines

All objectives must:

✔ Have a specific time frame.
✔ Be behaviorally stated.
✔ Be objectively evaluated.
✔ Identify positive rather than negative outcomes.
✔ Maintain and adhere to the organization's standards of practice and/or policies

Characteristics

A well-designed objective:

✔ Sets limits on the time for behavior to change.
✔ Uses negotiation.
✔ Is effective by making the point cumulatively.
✔ Is a clear and concise form of communication.
✔ Controls change.
✔ Can be used by any level of staff.
✔ Varies from the global to very specific.
✔ Documents problems beyond the manager's control.
✔ Aids analytic thinking.
✔ Encourages staff development.
✔ Improves skill in planning.

MBO identifies where you fit in, organizationally or within the smaller group you manage. Expectations are put out for discussion and direction for the manager and her/his group or the manager's meeting with the nursing executive. Clear expectations leave little room for misunderstanding, and individuals must improve or restate their objectives. The staff who do their best identify those who are not effective.

Observation of staff performance, evaluation of written documentation, patient satisfaction or customer service surveys, and manager and staff position descriptions can be steps toward identifying realistic goals. Another example of an objective might be, "By June 30, 1999, the nurse manager will:

1. Set up June—December in-service topics as prioritized by the staff.
2. Accomplish all staff performance evaluations by a specified deadline.
3. Perform documentation reviews in view of agency/institutional standards.
4. Evaluate staffing patterns and rotate once to each shift every _____.
5. Schedule all registered nurses to have a minimum of one week in charge every _____ (defined by manager)."

An MBO Example

Practice of MBO is advantageous to the new manager. Much new information can be categorized and relegated to a step outlined in an objective. This allows the new manager to spend time prioritizing where attention is required first. MBO also lends the novice manager more objectivity, rather than "gut feelings" when learning and being challenged. For example, specific effects on the group by a staff member's tardiness can have extensive ramifications. The nurse manager, on identifying this problem, may create this objective, "By Friday:

• Schedule and hold an individual meeting with the tardy staff member.
• Negotiate a contract to stop tardiness. Check personnel policies, procedure manuals, and staff member's file to assess need for verbal warning.
• List specific tasks done by others, in place of tardy nurse, and any other outcomes of the behavior (e.g., second report).
• Document the meeting and agreed-upon goals and objectives."

The new manager will be consistent with all team members using this method. Consistent behavior towards all staff members sends the message that criticism is constructive and fair. The manager's attitude should be positive, as much as possible.

Time can be spent on identified issues, improving operations, or patient care, as well as improving the staff's enjoyment of their work. Nurses can use objectives to require staff development in meeting individual and group goals. MBO encourages forward thinking by its use of setting objectives for the future.

The nurse manager can also use MBO to guide the staff towards larger, organizational targets. Dates for accomplishing objectives must be flexible, without negating the use of this tool. Thinking forward using goal-setting fosters continued personal growth and open communication.

MBO can be adapted to any work situation and, when gradually introduced, can be a positive growth experience for all. Control of growth by the staff can relieve some of the stressors of nursing in the 1990s. MBO for managers is an adjunct to improving:

- Interviewing.
- Negotiating.
- Delegating (and then leaving them alone!).
- Sharing power/authority.
- Performance evaluation.
- Managerial growth.
- Development of leadership qualities and management style.
- Budgetary responsibilities.
- Problem-solving.
- Building of credibility consistently.
- Decision-making.
- Listening.
- Other skills.

MANAGEMENT THEORIES

Management philosophy within the health care organization may encourage a specific style or theory utilization. Generally, if the organization values managers and encourages longevity, there is specific training directed towards leadership development and exposure to management theories. Several theories would be covered during the management's continuing education. The management philosophy of McGregor is a good beginning:

Theory X: The average human being has an inherent dislike of work and will avoid work where possible. This causes the need for direction and control in employee management.

Theory Y: Physical and mental effort is as natural as play or rest. If employees are committed to organizational objectives, they will be self-directed and need fewer controls.[13]

These motivational theories can be likened to transactional (Theory X) and transformational (Theory Y) leadership styles. Blending the leadership style with the management theory can help the new nurse manager focus behavior towards staff for the best results. Management theory was further developed by Ouchi in his Theory Z. Theory Z principles provided some of the basis for the concept of quality circles—a group process for improving quality through worker-management cooperation.[14]

An accepted concept being adopted as a management theory for organizations involves total quality management developed by Deming. Quality is achieved by:

- Fostering cooperation/collaboration among staff, rather than competition.
- Identifying the customer, be it the patient, staff member, or physician (dependent upon the encounter).
- Empowering the customer.
- Identifying flaws in the process or system rather than blaming staff.[15]

Increasingly, total quality management (TQM) is being adopted by institutions and organizations and is being woven into everyday operational practice. New nurse managers may have already been exposed to these principles during committee participation—whose mandate is to improve service delivery. TQM focuses on identifying problems within established systems and processes rather than with the people performing within the systems. Examples abound in the literature of the use of continuous quality improvement (CQI) to generate ideas for improved patient care services. Some of the many issues addressed utilizing CQI concepts include:

- Patient weights.
- Unusual occurrence reporting.
- Meal service in nursing homes.
- Emergency services
- Industrial accidents.
- Discharge planning.
- Postanesthesia care.
- Managed care in psychiatry.
- Cardiopulmonary rehabilitation.
- Intershift report.
- Infection surveillance.
- Nursing documentation.
- Medication error prevention.
- Pressure sore prevention.
- Childbirth education.

Participation as health care providers and consumers is key to improving health promotion behavior as well as systems and processes in care delivery for future viability and survival. Efforts to study systems within health care organizations must include the providers of care—the staff. Leaders in nursing management must establish trust between themselves and staff so that the processes to improve care and work situations will be followed. Participation in the education, support in allowing time for meeting attendance, and honest evaluation of results without repercussions will be beneficial in the long run for staff acceptance of TQM principles. These principles may be intertwined into patient teaching, since they are not just designed for the management of people or the evaluation of current systems.

The use of TQM principles has been increasing in health care and has achieved support from the JCAHO. However, Smith et al[16] and McConnell[17] warn that without organizational commitment, TQM may be much less successful. Initial training can be supported by time and managerial coaching; however, in the long term, education and guidance are considered most important. The sometimes tedious need to examine every step in a process or system to extract unnecessary steps can be directed towards improving the work culture. Managers must remember that staff are very important as customers, as well.

Ultimately, management philosophy determines the growth and level of staff fulfillment. Guidance and direction should be provided by administration for all managers, giving them the responsibility to make decisions and control their work environment. Managers work best when they develop staff in a consistent and supportive manner and enjoy the same approach from their superior or senior manager.

The management team works most effectively when the environment is collegial, respectful, and nurturing. New managers should elicit advice about the level of support and managerial development systems from both peers and bosses. Gradually increasing responsibility while new managers expand their skills and are groomed in the management philosophy generates strong, decisive, and successful managers. The new nurse manager provides leadership to the staff while learning administrative skills.

An immediate source of information and guidance for the new nurse manager is her/his supervisor. Initially, the new nurse manager should expect frequent meetings, weekly perhaps, and should use this time with the supervisor wisely. Assessments of staff abilities and needs made by the new nurse manager can be reviewed with the supervisor, with problems and solutions identified. Explanation of channels of communication, rules, and etiquette expected of administration may be covered.

The new nurse manager should evaluate the level of support available from administration. Observing discussions and reactions of upper management with their managers and peers can give the new nurse manager insight into the hierarchy of the organization. The new manager determines whether the organizational philosophy is compatible with her/his own values. Ideally, the manager feels wanted, being part of an organization that historically promotes from within and rewards the progress and development of employees.

New nurse managers are thrust into a fast-paced job and so must rapidly determine how much authority is part of the position. If too many decisions are made above the nurse manager's level, she/he may feel stifled. The nurse manager must then decide whether the organizational goals permit some control and thus make the situation workable, or whether it would be better to move on to a new professional experience.

More often, nurse managers are allowed flexibility in such key tasks as hiring and scheduling. Building on these tools, new nurse managers develop their own style of leadership within the management group.

The nurse manager should strive for certain outcomes in the new role. As the new nurse manager tries to achieve these outcomes, she/he develops an ability to analyze the power structure of the organization. Box 2-2 on p. 46 lists role outcomes.[18]

box 2-2

NEW NURSE MANAGER ROLE OUTCOMES

POST-ENTREPRENEURIAL STYLE

The ability to relinquish bureaucratic styles of leadership; more employee-centered with core characteristics of innovation, efficiency, and reward of outcomes; authority derived from expertise and experimentation

EMPOWERMENT

Ability to empower self and staff for quality patient outcomes; ability to influence organizational policy development as related to patient care

VISION

Ability to foresee the growth and development of nursing and managerial practice and strategically plan to assist these processes

ENHANCEMENT OF IMAGE

Ability to identify self as a professional nurse and manager, perceiving self as a leader and enhancing the profession of nursing in the community and organization

FLEXIBILITY

Ability to adapt to turbulence in the organization and practice environment; ability to assess outcomes; ability to design better and newer processes in patient care and management to achieve quality service

CLINICAL EXPERTISE

Ability to identify with those who are managed; staying close to the client and the practice environment to manage the delivery of health care effectively

ANALYTIC THINKING

Ability to problem-solve effectively using logic and decision support systems and models; ability to conduct research in nursing management

LEADERSHIP ROLE IDENTITY

Ability to see self as a leader, mentor, and nurse or patient advocate; ability to assist in meeting institutional goals and objectives through effective performance; ability to get things accomplished

AUTONOMY

Ability to practice nursing and management in a highly decentralized environment without alienation of executive leadership

MASTERY OF CHANGE

Ability to identify, cope with, introduce, and assimilate change successfully in the practice environment

Flarey DL: Redesigning management roles, *J Nurs Adm* 21:44, 1991.

ORGANIZATIONAL CHART

Each organization has a formal and an informal communication system, also called a table of organization, and a chain of command that reflects the manager's base of power. Unofficial personal relationships may command more authority than the organizational chart structure, and all new managers should ascertain allies and adversaries. This will take longer for new managers who have just joined an organization but can also create an opportunity for improved communication among managers and administration. The middle manager is working from both sides, between staff and upper management and, as such, is vital to any organization.

Concepts to evaluate when beginning as a nurse manager are, as noted by Gillies[19]:

- Role
- Power
- Status
- Authority
- Centrality
- Communication

Studying these aspects of organizational hierarchy and using communication to validate perception make up an important exercise for new managers.

There will be occasions that test new managers. This is particularly true when management delivers an edict to the new nurse manager that is contrary to her/his principles. There are no rules as to which side wins, and this situation can cause both personal and professional stress. Sometimes the new nurse manager's loyalties will be with staff and in conflict with administration or vice versa, and managers need to know with whom conversation is confidential. New managers need to have a sounding board to assist in formulating answers, especially when directives appear to be unfair to staff.

The level of decentralization present in the management structure determines the autonomy allowed. Decentralization permits control or delegation by the nurse manager and the chance to develop and empower the staff. Decentralization promotes manager-manager communications and meetings and avails the nurse manager to other nurse managers or committee chairs of quality assurance, utilization review, continuing education, and infection control. Acknowledgment that highly educated or knowledgeable workers can evaluate, design, and implement the complex care required by nurses can be the attitude of an effective decentralized nursing department. Committee memberships add further to the amount of opinions generated and policies implemented on various issues that help establish management styles.

As a middle manager in nursing, the novice needs patience, advice, and a confidante with whom to debate strategy and concerns, pros and cons. Whether or not the manager's supervisor becomes the resource, that relationship is important to cultivate as well. Sometimes staff members become important as allies to the nurse manager. Their support during day-to-day operations and in crises is the real concern of the nurse manager. The manager acts as a filter through which administrative goals are communicated to staff and change-directed. As it is possible to change a dressing differently, still using aseptic principles, the nurse manager can divert information not necessary for staff to know and still communicate necessary policy. Many times rationale is explained when change occurs. Administrative policies can be explained and practiced within the style of the nurse manager. As long as organizational principles are maintained, implementation can be staged by the manager.

Through autonomy, independence, and decentralization come accountability and performance. Efforts at group cohesion and quality must be a result of the manager's ability to motivate and develop staff that is fulfilled and productive. Survival in middle management means success, with respect from both upper management and subordinate staff.

MENTORING

Mentoring is a subject not covered with any depth in traditional nursing school curricula. It is seen as a subject for those in business and management. For nurses, mentoring is relegated to graduate school, a step too late for many nurses despite their leadership desires and goals.

A mentor should be an individual who:

- Inspires risk-taking and action.
- Constructively criticizes without overpowering.
- Allows freedom for growth.
- Assists with goal-setting.
- Provides guidance with problem-solving.
- Coaches the protégé through difficult situations (such as conflict resolution).
- Provides positive feedback.
- Serves as a role model.

Mentoring is an important skill to develop for those in management positions. Guiding a young or new nurse manager can be a growth experience for both the mentor and protégé. Seeking out a mentor-role model as support for the new nurse manager should be a high priority while identifying other tasks already discussed.

The mentor acts as a nurturer who listens and guides the new nurse manager through dilemmas, with each encounter ultimately requiring less input from the mentor. The mentor-protégé relationship must not be a power struggle but rather a nonjudgmental, comfortable association. The capacity to have honest discussions without consequences can be enriching. The mentor must remain loyal through all phases of the new manager's growth. The new nurse manager must utilize newly learned strategies consistently until they are mastered. The mentor-protégé relationship is a dynamic one that goes through both periods of relative stability and

Considerations for Home Care Managers

THE MANAGER'S ROLE: LEADING AND EMPOWERING

All of the tenets of this management chapter apply universally to the home care manager, with special emphasis on developing leadership skills to motivate, challenge, and direct a staff who are not usually physically present in the office environment on a daily basis. The autonomy of home care staff provides a distinct challenge to the home care manager, who needs to continually empower staff to make the best clinical decision while following appropriate organizational policies, procedures, and standards of care.

Home care has been in existence for a number of years; however, its rapid growth and expansion has generated a large hole in available, trained, and motivated leaders. In that respect, it is essential for home care managers to act responsibly and professionally, making a commitment to mentor staff nurses or other clinicians for professional growth into managerial positions.

times of higher need. A mentoring relationship may be the most important determinant for success in leadership roles.

According to Holloran in her study of mentoring among nurse executives, "there were consistent differences between those who had a mentor versus those who had not."[20] She also found different levels of mentoring, depending on a participant's definition of the term. Role models may be guiding forces without the more personal commitment of the mentor.

Mentoring is an interpersonal, nursing, and management tool to be used for decision-making, problem-solving, and planned change. Mentor connections may be long- or short-term but always should be gratifying and supportive. Confidence in one's abilities is a first step towards choosing to mentor new nurse managers or to develop the leadership potential of those we manage.

SUMMARY

The new nurse manager may feel overwhelmed after the "honeymoon" period and as the realities and constraints of daily group management are identified. Early adoption of a leadership style that is effective for both staff and manager provides order and security in a highly stressful atmosphere. Consistency and objectivity with the staff create an environment of stability that can foster further growth and a higher level of professionalism.

The test of managerial success in nursing is developing a comfortable and consistent managerial style that facilitates growth and satisfaction for both the manager and staff. Professionalism includes experienced nurses and managers mentoring new nurses and new managers. Nursing may not have promoted this concept as well as has been documented in the business world, and despite the popular notion of nurses as nurturers, nurses have not always been supportive of or encouraging development of each other's leadership qualities. Nurses have a very important role in the positive nurturing of new managers and new nurses. Mentoring, whether formal or informal, must be considered, as is continuing education, a professional responsibility.

References

1. McGregor D: *Leadership and motivation,* Cambridge, 1983, MIT Press.
2. Miller M, Babcock D: *Critical thinking applied to nursing,* St. Louis, 1996, Mosby.
3. Bethel S: *Making a difference: 12 qualities that make you a leader,* New York, 1990, GP Putman and Sons.
4. Dunham J, Fisher E: Nurse executive profile of excellent nursing leadership, *Nursing Administration Quarterly* 15:4, 1990.
5. Burns JM: *Leadership,* New York, 1978, Harper & Row.
6. Dunham J, Klafehn K: Transformational leadership and the nurse executive, *JONA* 20:28, 1990.
7. Barker A, Young C: Transformational leadership—the feminist connection in postmodern organizations, *Holistic Nursing Practice* 9:1, 1994.
8. Hersey P, Blanchard K: *Management of organizational behavior: utilizing human resources,* Englewood Cliffs, NJ, 1988, Prentice Hall.
9. Fiedler F, Chemers M: *Improving leadership effectiveness,* New York, 1984, John Wiley & Sons.
10. Tannenbaum R, Schmidt W: How to choose a leadership pattern, *Harvard Business Review* 51:164, 1973.
11. Stivers C: Why can't a woman be less like a man? *JONA* 21:51, 1991.
12. Orem D, *Nursing concepts of practice,* New York, 1971, McGraw-Hill.
13. McGregor D: *The human side of enterprise,* New York, 1960, McGraw-Hill.
14. Ouchi WG: *Theory Z—how American business can meet the Japanese challenge,* Reading, MA, 1981, Addison-Wesley.
15. Deming W: *Out of crisis,* Cambridge, MA, 1986, MIT Press.
16. Smith B, Discenza R, Piland N: Reflections on total quality management and health care, *Health care supervisor* Gaithersburg, MD, 1995, Aspen.
17. McConnell C: Total quality and the shifting management paradigm, *Health care supervisor* Gaithersburg, MD, 1995, Aspen.
18. Flarey D: Redesigning management roles, *JONA* 21:44, 1991.
19. Gillies DA: *Nursing management: a systems approach,* Philadelphia, 1989, WB Saunders.
20. Holloran S: Mentoring: the experience of nursing service executives, *JONA* 23:2, 1993.

For Further Reading

Blanchard K, Johnson S: *The one minute manager,* New York, 1982, William Morrow.

Blanchard KB, Lorber R: *Putting the one minute manager to work,* New York, 1987, William Morrow.

Clinical managers help agency staff cope with growth, stress, *Hospital Home Health* 9(8):108, 1982.

Davidhizer R: Managerial credibility, *Nurs Adm Q* 13(3):17, 1989.

Douglas L: *The effective nurse: leader and manager,* St Louis, 1984, Mosby.

Drucker PF: *Managing for results,* New York, 1984, Harper & Row.

Etzioni A: Humble decision making, *Harvard Bus Rev* 21(2):69, 1989.

Gillies DA: *Nursing management—a systems approach,* Philadelphia, 1982, WB Saunders.

Hackbarth DP, Androwich FM: Graduate nursing education for leadership in home care, *Caring* 8(2):6-8, 10-11, 1989.

Hood JN, Smith HL: Quality of worklife in home: the contribution of leaders personal concern for staff, *JONA* 24(1):40, 1994.

Kosowski M et al: An interactive model of leadership, *Nurs Adm Q* 15(1):36, 1990.

Lasater ME: Strategies for organizational change in home healthcare, *Home Health Care Nurse* 11(2):38, 1993.

Leuesque RF: Business planning in home health agencies: a guide to nurse executives, *Columbia University Teachers College,* 1991 ED.D.

Manthey M: The art of management: three simple rules, *Nurs Manage* 21(12):19, 1990.

Moloney M: *Leadership in nursing: theory, strategies, action,* St Louis, 1979, Mosby.

Noone C, Szekely L: Working with consultants to achieve home health agency goals, *JONA* 21(10):61, 1991.

Orth CD et al: The manager's role as coach and mentor, *JONA* 20(9):11, 1990.

Phifer L: Managerial leaders and their influence in nursing, *Pediatr Nurs* 16(3):222, 1990.

Rosener JB: Ways women lead, *Harvard Bus Rev,* 68(6):119, 1990.

Shoemake A: Solutions to the home health nursing shortage, *Home Health Care Nurse* 12(4):35, 1994.

Stachura LM, Hoff J: Toward achievement of mentoring for nurses, *Nurs Adm Q* 15(1):56, 1990.

Walton M: *The Deming management method,* New York, 1986, Dodd, Mead.

CHAPTER 3

HUMAN RESOURCE MANAGEMENT

T.M. MARRELLI

Personnel decisions and issues can be some of the most challenging episodes of any managerial career. Conversely, the effective use of human management skills can be the highlight of your professional career. With this in mind, this chapter emphasizes the latter. It is important to note that we all improve and grow through practice. This is especially true in personnel or human resource (HR) management functions. According to Patz and others,[1] a national survey of academic health chief nurse executives and nurse managers demonstrated that human management skills were considered the most important criterion of effectiveness. Flexibility, negotiation, and compromise were second.

WHAT IS HUMAN RESOURCE MANAGEMENT?

Simply put, HR management can be defined as effective interpersonal communications among all levels of employees and staff. (Manager's Tip 3-1 on p. 54 summarizes some key issues in human resources.) This chapter is organized into the format followed in the employment process. Therefore the discussion begins with the recruitment process and proceeds to interviewing, hiring, orienting, coaching, counseling, training, motivating, and evaluating performance.

STAFF RECRUITMENT

If all managers were able to recruit the right staff for the right positions, their jobs would be tremendously easier. However, that is not the case, primarily because of human nature and the inability to discern the small seed of discontent that the candidate has with the organization or position during the interview process. There are methods to eliminate as many of the variables as possible in the new manager's search for the right candidate.

MANAGER'S TIP 3-1

NINE VITAL HR POINTS

✔ Hiring and other personnel decisions are some of the most important decisions made as a manager.

✔ You make better, more informed decisions as you gain experience.

✔ HR issues must be addressed and dealt with effectively; usually they will not be solved without interpersonal action or intervention.

✔ You cannot communicate too often; convey unit and organizational goals, constructive or positive feedback (including a thank you for a job well done), or any issue affecting the staff's work.

✔ Remember that all work is done through the staff. This is the core of HR management.

✔ Familiarize yourself with your organization's policy and procedure manuals dealing with HR issues.

✔ Remember, you are not alone. The problems surfacing have occurred before and there is probably a standard procedure for you to follow. Integrate the knowledge from the manuals into daily practice.

✔ When making personnel decisions, particularly those involved with hiring, consider your needs (e.g., the organization, staffing patterns, care delivery system, types of patients or clients, shifts offered, benefit packages, tuition reimbursement for professional staff, and the type of nursing or administrative experience needed). Prioritize these needs.

✔ Use all resources and experts available to you for your growth as a manager in this important area. For example, if special HR department professionals or nurse recruiter professionals are available, use their services and expertise. This is especially true for areas where state or federal laws apply and you may not be aware or have the in-depth knowledge needed to interpret or implement these laws in your setting. Examples of these areas include equal opportunity employment concerns, workers' compensation questions, benefit compensation issues, and other areas of a specialized nature.

Recruitment in health care is a strong industry—it has been for the past 20 years. From the nursing, physical therapy, and pharmacist shortages of the 1970s and 1980s to the shortages of health care managers, recruitment has definitely been a major challenge to all levels of health care management. A needed trait for the new nurse manager is proactivity. Not waiting until a staff member's final week before beginning the replacement process is the sign of a proactive manager. Historic unit-patient census trends over a period of time and anticipated openings of new units, beds, or services should give a manager a general idea of the amount and types of staff needed and when. Management by objective planning should occur, with the manager "mapping" out a strategy to get the needed staff according to the unit timeline. If the position is a critical one and historically has been hard to fill, the manager must have plans B, C, and D ready should plan A prove unsuccessful in identifying potential candidates.

First of all, even though it sounds so simple, develop a detailed outline of what traits and skills are being sought in this search. Understand all the requirements of the position and determine what the organization needs in this individual. Loyalty to the organization's staff should be a major initiative for the manager. Always look within your ranks for the new potential manager or candidate for another prime position. If you have been mentoring and developing staff, there may be individuals looking for an opportunity to expand their career horizons and move up in the organization. However, this type of recruitment should be done carefully and the position requirements should never be forgotten in an effort to "fit the job to the person."

The most common avenues to pursue when initiating the recruitment process (once the position and the hiring ability have been approved per organizational policy) are as follows:

- Human resource department posting boards.
- Local colleges or technical schools.
- Local professional organizations.
- Professional contacts.
- Newspaper or professional journal classified sections.
- Job fairs.
- Specialty recruiting agencies (for the hard-to-place or specialty positions).
- Informal contacts/employee referrals (bonus programs).

Reviewing Applications and Resumes

After the search has produced a number of applicants for the position, review the applications/resumes and rank each accordingly:

1. Inappropriate (candidates lack the required education, experience, and/or salary requirements)
2. Possible (second-tier candidates—skills/experience/education not exactly as requested)
3. Most likely (these candidates should be invited for the first interview)

Remember not to depend too heavily on what is written on an application or resume. It is the interview and reference checking process where information is elicited about the skills a candidate will bring to the position. It is advisable to have at least five potential candidates to interview in the first round. As per organizational protocol, plan for the interview sessions.

INTERVIEWING

In planning the interview process, a succinct guide for the division of time has been developed by Donald Lombardi in his text, *Handbook for the Health Care Manager*. Lombardi divides the interview time into three sections, stressing that the candidate should do most of the talking (about 80% to 85%) during the main part of the interview; 90% to 95% is too much, not affording the interviewer the chance to ask the leading or needed questions. The following list describes the three sections, the time usually allotted, and the percentage of time normally allotted to each participant:

- Introduction/warm-up (3 to 5 minutes)
  Interviewer 75%
  Candidate   25%
- Interview conducted (15 to 25 minutes)
  Interviewer 15% to 20%
  Candidate   80% to 85%
- Interview questions and answers/wrap-up (4 to 5 minutes)
  Interviewer 75% to 80%
  Candidate   20% to 25%[2]

Manager's Tips 3-2 and 3-3 present some suggestions to help in preparing for and conducting an interview.

MANAGER'S TIP 3-2

PREPARING FOR A SUCCESSFUL INTERVIEW

✔ Read any organization manuals available on the process. There may be factors unique to your setting.

✔ Plan for the interview. This is vital to an effective interview for both the interviewer and the applicant. Clearly define goals and needs before the actual interview. The applicant who cannot understand your needs may make incorrect assumptions and accept the position but leave shortly thereafter, disillusioned and angry. Clearly defining your needs includes the answering of the following questions: Do you need a nurse who has been or wants to be cross-trained in a particular specialty area? Do you need an experienced hospice nurse with specialized symptom management expertise? Try to define succinctly what your patient area needs to function more effectively.

✔ Plan your discussion with the specific questions and topics to be addressed, especially outlining situational questions that test the applicant's ability to think on her/his feet.

✔ Use the same questions for all the candidates, so that the interview answers may be compared when making the hiring decision.

✔ Arrange to have your phone calls held and other interruptions deferred until the interview is complete. This demonstrates to applicants that you respect them and value their time.

✔ Schedule someone to be in charge during your interviews. This is particularly important if you schedule consecutive interviews.

MANAGER'S TIP 3-3

CONDUCTING A SUCCESSFUL INTERVIEW

In an effective interview the parties are allowed to clearly communicate and should be allotted enough uninterrupted time so that the interviewee is comfortable. Both parties should be allowed to meet their common objectives of exchanging information.

✔ Start on time. Do not keep the applicant waiting because this is not a sign of power, but of rudeness. If you are not punctual because of a unit emergency or other emergent concern, be professional and apologetic.

✔ Provide the applicant with a copy of the position description, if not already done.

✔ Describe the position to the applicant and delineate the responsibilities of the individual who will be chosen to fill the position.

✔ Remember how you felt when you were interviewed for your last position and what was said that put you at ease.

✔ Clearly outline at the onset the time allotted for the interview. For example, "I know personnel told you this interview would be approximately 1 hour. We need to cover the important information and wrap up by 2 PM because I have a meeting immediately following our interview."

✔ Have the applicant verbally verify what has been written on the application or resume.

✔ Protect yourself by avoiding statements or words that may lead to accusations of sex or other types of discrimination. Common examples, very well known to most female nurses, include *honey, sweetie,* and *dear.*

✔ Do not inquire about spouses, children (or plans for children), day-care situations, or other sensitive areas.

✔ Treat everyone with the same respect, consideration, and professionalism.

✔ Be professional, kind, and a good listener. The better your active listening skills, the more information you receive from the applicant.

✔ When possible, use open-ended questions to elicit an open response. Ask about common problem situations and how the applicant would resolve them.

✔ Use silence; this allows the applicant to share more information.

✔ Remember first impressions do count, so make it a good one. You may want this applicant to also want to work on your team.

✔ Be enthusiastic and talk about the good things happening in your health care setting.

✔ Give a walking tour of the clinical area and of the institution, when appropriate.

✔ Provide a brochure on your program or health setting. Use the information listed as general information to relax the applicant initially or as points of discussion during the interview.

✔ Outline the health care organization's mission statement or values statement and how this position helps to achieve those goals.

✔ Dress professionally and neatly. If the interview is in your office, remember your office reflects you and the organization.

✔ Talk about the orientation program for new staff.

✔ Discuss the day-to-day operational aspects of the position.

✔ Elicit from the applicant why she/he is applying for this job. Though this sounds simple, the responses are rarely as simple.

Continued.

✔ Ask the applicant to describe what her/his contribution would be to the department.

✔ Validate the applicant's understanding of the position.

✔ Repeat the applicant's response to make sure that what you understood to have been said is correct.

✔ Discuss the time frame in which you would like to fill the position.

✔ Have the applicant describe how her/his last manager and peers would describe her/his performance.

✔ Ask where the applicant would like to be in 5 years.

✔ Ask the applicant if she/he has any questions for you.

✔ Bring the applicant back for another interview if appropriate.

✔ Talk about the staff development program.

✔ Discuss the type of documentation used in your unit or area.

✔ Discuss the dress code requirements of the position.

✔ Summarize what will happen next at the conclusion. For example, "I have interviews scheduled through. . . . I hope to have the process completed by. . . ." (specify time frame or date).

✔ When appropriate, have the nurse recruiter or your staff interview your final candidate(s).

✔ For managerial candidates (e.g., assistant nurse manager), have members of your staff interview the final applicant(s).

HIRING A NEW TEAM MEMBER

Congratulations! You successfully sold yourself and your organization and you now have a new staff member. Hopefully, your staff members were involved in the process and welcome this new nurse. There are steps you can take to ensure a smooth transition for new staff members (see Manager's Tip 3-4).

Making a new staff member feel welcome and part of the group is the key to long-term employee satisfaction. The ideas in the above tip list are simple yet important in making your practice setting a place where new staff feel comfortable and grow professionally.

ORIENTATION FOR NEW STAFF MEMBERS

Orientation is the most important time frame for a new employee. Starting a new job is both frightening and exhilarating and the welcome and integration into the team is of prime concern. In nursing, orientation has not been given the respect and commitment that it deserves. This time period is useful in many ways:

- It provides the employee with an overall perspective of the goals/mission of the organization.

- It familiarizes the new employee with organizational and clinical area–specific policies and procedures.

- It allows the new employee to interact with staff on a less stressful basis.

- It allows the employer to verify the competency and skills of the new employee.

MANAGER'S TIP 3-4

WELCOMING A NEW STAFF MEMBER

✔ Show the new staff member her/his personal space. This can include the locker, mailbox, phone message slot, or other areas. Make sure to clearly mark her/his name, spelled correctly, on such items.

✔ Schedule the new staff member to have lunch with those members of your staff who can be positive role models.

✔ Have the new staff nurse's identification badge, access/parking sticker, and security card completed as soon as possible.

✔ Schedule a lunch with all other new professional nursing staff. This peer camaraderie leads to job satisfaction. It also teaches the new staff members about other aspects of your facility or setting.

✔ Schedule and lead a personalized walking tour for the new nurse.

✔ Introduce the new nurse to key personnel and others encountered during the tour.

✔ Discuss the organization's buddy, preceptor, or mentor system.

✔ Allot time in your schedule at least three times a week (even if for a few minutes) for the first few months to check on the new staff member's progress. Delegate this responsibility to a trusted nurse leader on your staff if you will be unavailable. This is also a good time to ask if what you said in the interview holds true in practice. This will help you tailor comments to future applicants.

✔ Write a welcome note to the new staff member and have other staff members sign the note.

✔ Hold a breakfast or lunch meeting so all staff members can meet the new nurse. This is particularly important in practice areas where the staff members are rarely together, such as a home health agency or a community-based hospice.

✔ Personally spend time with the new staff nurse, especially introducing her/him to other team members in the organization at all levels.

✔ Create a phone list for new staff members. Alphabetize the list by first names. (Everyone else can remember the new nurse's first and last names, but it is unrealistic to expect the new nurse to remember all other staff members' last names immediately.)

• It allows both parties time to determine if this hiring decision was correct. Manager's Tip 3-5 on p. 60 provides a checklist for use in orienting a new staff member.

Remember, you get out of people, or staff, only what you expect. Studies have shown that the manager's expectations are the key to the staff's behavior and development. Livingston,[3] who has studied this "Pygmalion" performance, states that, "The way managers treat their subordinates is subtly influenced by what they expect of them. If managers' expectations are high, productivity is likely to be excellent. If their expectations are low, productivity is likely to be poor. It is as though there were a law that caused subordinates' performance to rise or fall to meet managers' expectations."

MANAGER'S TIP 3-5

A NEW STAFF MEMBER ORIENTATION CHECKLIST

Professional nurses practice in so many settings that it is not possible to list all areas that must be covered with the new nurse. This list contains the most common themes. Some items mentioned are clearly specialized areas of practice.

✔ Benefit; compensation packages, including medical and dental policies (including when coverage begins); malpractice; licensure; professional in-service credits; physical, overtime, and compensation time policies; other benefits.

✔ Leave allotments, including vacation, sick days, holidays, educational leave, other leave.

✔ Frequency and schedule of paydays.

✔ Savings plans available (e.g., thrift or credit union).

✔ Position description.

✔ Description of other team members' roles in patient care planning process.

✔ Hours of shifts, specific time to report, check-in procedures, break times.

✔ Uniform requirements and any associated compensation, and name tag or access/security badge.

✔ Employee assistance program availability.

✔ Personalized orientation schedule, including clinical demonstrations, CPR, and other educational resources specific to clinical practice.

✔ An in-depth personalized tour.

✔ Availability and hours of organization's day-care facility and/or benefits, if applicable.

✔ Confidentiality policies.

✔ The health care facility's Nursing Plan for Care and philosophy.

✔ The state's Nurse Practice Act.

✔ The written standards of care.

✔ Schedule of probationary and ongoing performance appraisal evaluation(s).

✔ On-call schedule and compensation process for on-call.

✔ Supply acquisition and process for charging to patient or unit account.

✔ The committees that the unit or staff are represented on and the process for input into change.

✔ Clinical and administrative policies and procedures.

✔ The program mission statement and objectives.

✔ Safety or risk management policies—include security (both patient and staff), Occupational Safety and Health Administration (OSHA), Centers for Disease Control and Prevention (CDCP), or other safety concerns (e.g., fire or emergency preparedness plans, universal precautions, seat belt use for staff members driving in the community, violence in the workplace).

✔ Clinical documentation orientation, including forms, type and frequency of documentation required, paper flow, and an introduction to the nursing computer system.

✔ Quality improvement processes.

✔ Distribution and stocking of initial supplies for nurse bags in the community or other outreach setting (e.g., maps, resources available after office hours, report processes, use of pagers, car phones, and mileage reimbursement forms).

✔ Process review of how employee actions affect patient care and reimbursement systems.

With this information in mind, it is important to note that your enthusiasm (or apathy) is contagious, and work output is directly related to the level of managerial expectation. Use this important information to your advantage.

Nurse managers should make every effort to allow new employees the time to attend all elements of the orientation program—for both the unit and the organization—no matter how busy the patient area is. Allow new staff members to complete this process. They will respect you more as a manager and will be unable to claim that they were not exposed to needed information. It is very hard to catch up when these orientation programs are curtailed or deleted.

The clearer the instructions and direction provided in the orientation period, the fewer problems you will usually face in the future. Therefore the extra time you take in the beginning will pay off. You will not have to be continually clarifying rules. When you communicate rules or important information, use direct eye contact, be professional, and restate the specifics that need to be understood by both parties. There is nothing worse than a nurse saying, "I was never told that," when the subject relates to an important part of the job or could have caused a poor patient outcome. For this reason, another nurse whose judgment and skills you trust should be "a buddy" with the new nurse during the formal orientation period. In some settings this person is called a preceptor. This delegation accomplishes three things: it (1) behaviorally demonstrates your trust in your staff; (2) frees you up from day-to-day operational orientation; and (3) develops the managerial skills of the staff nurse to whom you have delegated the preceptor responsibility. This type of delegation of responsibility empowers your staff and helps them to achieve more personally and professionally.

There are two main methods of ongoing communication once the official orientation or probationary period is completed. They are (1) counseling or coaching and (2) staff development. Both processes are equally important in different ways. These two major communication methods are discussed below.

Coaching

It would be ideal to work in a setting where everyone, once adequately oriented, functioned smoothly as if on automatic pilot. Unfortunately, this is not realistic. However, with careful planning nurse managers have been able to choose, groom, and motivate a special group of nurses to work together, address issues, and reach consensus so effectively that it felt that way. This then can be a realistic goal.

Until that point is reached, ongoing training and reeducation must occur to attain professional and program goals. Counseling is often the vehicle used for this needed communication. Positive communication, such as that used in orientation and training sessions, is usually valued over corrective action, which is how counseling is sometimes perceived. Although it is often considered negative by some managers, counseling or coaching should be viewed as an opportunity for growth or to identify individual problem behaviors before they affect staff. Often, it is in the one-to-one encounters with staff members that the effective manager learns information informally that assists in unit or program planning. With this in mind, it is important that effective counseling skills be addressed (see Manager's Tip 3-6).

An example of coaching documentation using SOAP. The following is a common example of unacceptable behavior that a nurse manager may encounter; it would affect other staff members and the smooth operation of your unit. A new staff nurse, 2 months out of formal orientation, spends the first 20 minutes of most mornings trying to change the unit's patient care assignment. She usually confronts you in front of the entire change-of-shift staff and, it always seems, on the mornings following an evening-shift crisis that needs to be immediately documented by you. Her behavior negatively impacts your unit, setting the stage for a stressful day. Even though she is relatively new, her clinical skills are strong, and she has already assumed the role of informal leader in the group.

As an effective manager, you (1) identify a problem behavior, (2) address it early and when you are not angry, and (3) ask her privately to stop by your office in 10 minutes (delayed counseling only adds to her worry and may cause the employee to become defensive and upset). It is 7:40 AM and she comes into your office. The following is an example of the documentation that addresses what occurred in the meeting and the joint plan for resolution.

S(ubjective): Ms. Davis says, "I don't know why I do that every morning. I don't like my assignment. I still think though that Mrs. Smith should stay with Nurse Carter and I should get Mr. Jones, since he has cancer and you know I'm in school to become a clinical specialist in oncology."

O(bjective): 7:40 AM, 12/15/99, Ms. Davis is in my office after two previous informal *(list dates, when known)* discussions with her about the same topic: wanting to revamp the patient assignments totally. Today specifically there were two nurses upset because they told me they were still not sure what their assignments were—and this was after report. Ms. Davis was calm and clearly stated that she transferred 2 months ago to care primarily for cancer patients.

A(ssessment): Situation leaves the staff feeling unsettled and compromises patient care by the nonproductive time spent haggling over assignments. After an open discussion with Ms. Davis, she believes I am not respecting her area of expertise and that she had the understanding when she transferred to this unit that she would care primarily for oncologic and hospice patients.

P(lan): Ms. Davis verbally validated that she understands how this behavior is not conducive to a team effort in caring for patients and why some of the nurses have discussed the problem with me. The plan we agreed on is as follows: when possible, I will assign her cancer patients. However, she verbalizes understanding of changing staffing needs and will accept assignments without comment or further discussion starting tomorrow at morning report. In addition, she asked that I investigate the possibility of her being cross-trained to the organization's affiliated hospice program. She stated that she believes this

MANAGER'S TIP 3-6

SUGGESTIONS FOR EFFECTIVE COACHING OR COUNSELING

✔ Look at counseling as positive and as a challenge.
✔ Visualize yourself as being good at it.
✔ Remember, expect the best and chances are your staff will live up to your expectations.
✔ Know and abide by contractual guidelines of union agreements, if applicable.
✔ Always address an identified behavior problem sooner rather than later.
✔ Do not attempt to counsel or reprimand staff in front of other people.
✔ Respect the staff's right to disagree with your assessment of the situation.
✔ Be objective. When discussing an incident use the factual *who, what, when,* and *where* queries that reporters use.
✔ Try to not allow your feelings to color your input or behavior. If you are very angry or irritated, it is usually better to talk at a later time when you have calmed down and can think and speak objectively and rationally.
✔ Do not overreact. Talk to a peer manager or a mentor for input before the session and imagine and act how that calm and effective role model would react in the same situation.
✔ Use organizational mandated formats. Document objectionable behavior in a factual, concise manner, listing the desired behaviors, policy or procedural reference(s), and time frame for adherence to a written action plan. If this is a written counseling statement, make sure that the employee acknowledges receipt of the information, in writing. Date and countersign the employee's signature, as appropriate.
✔ Discuss all written statements with the human resource department manager or designee to clarify that all organizational procedures (e.g., union contractual guidelines) are being met. This discussion should occur before the employee session.
✔ Set a time limit on the discussion. For example, "Lisa, as I said at the start of our meeting we have 15 minutes, so now we need to wrap-up in 5 minutes."
✔ Use listening skills and silence after you ask the employee to detail for you the events or incidents in question.
✔ Summarize the discussion and the outcomes or plan of action clearly and succinctly.
✔ Try to schedule the session at a time and in an environment free of interruptions.
✔ Conversely, if this employee has a long-standing pattern of behavioral infractions and does not listen to time or other limits you set, control your environment by setting up planned interruptions (e.g., have someone page you). Do not reinforce the employee's behavior by putting up with it.
✔ Always keep employee comments focused on behaviors, not personality or another employee's actions. Bring an employee back to the conversation at hand by saying, for example, "...that may be true about John Doe, but today we are discussing your behavior and how it is impacting our unit's ability to accomplish our objectives."
✔ Treat all staff members the same; be consistent and thorough.
✔ Practice the skill of not being defensive and always try to see the other's point of view.
✔ Use the same documentation format for all staff members. Some health settings have their own counseling forms. Many use the SOAP format with very good results. (An example can be found on p. 62.)

Continued.

✔ Determine what infractions at your place of employment are cause for verbal or written warnings.

✔ Be a prudent nurse and document all coaching sessions. In addition, any written anecdotal notes or documentation of critical incidents will assist in your objective feedback and recall for performance appraisals. Use this written documentation as a reminder to yourself by keeping it in the staff member's personnel folder. Remember, awards, counseling, and other discussions are written objective reminders when it is performance evaluation time.

✔ Follow up counseling with another scheduled session as indicated in your disciplinary protocol. Hopefully, the problem is resolved and you will be giving positive feedback to the employee at the second meeting.

✔ Do not allow the employee to continue practicing unacceptable behavior. Instead, continue on to the next step in the disciplinary process. If you do *not,* the resultant problem behavior will only increase and other staff members will lose respect for your managerial abilities and/or act inappropriately themselves.

✔ Remember that effective employee counseling does modify behavior (but the employee has to want to modify her/his behavior).

✔ Managerial avoidance of counseling employees who do not abide by organizational policies and/or procedures can result in the employee being allowed to continue such behaviors, based on "past practice." At that point, it becomes very difficult to discipline the employee and it may also be demoralizing for other staff to work in such an environment.

✔ Always try to end these sessions on a positive note.

✔ Believe that all employees want to do a good job.

✔ Give feedback to all staff members on a regular, frequent basis.

would allow more flexibility and perhaps continuity of care for some of our unit's in-patients. We will meet next Tuesday at this time to follow up on our plan and to validate that the complaining sessions have stopped as demonstrated by timely acceptance of assignments delegated.

The documentation of employee performance demonstrated specific, objective behaviors that necessitated the meeting. As shown in this example, training needs are often identified through effective counseling. The outcome of these sessions should leave both parties feeling better; the manager, who will see a positive behavior change because of the information learned in the session, and the employee, who sees that the effective manager identified training needs that will help the organization as well as the nurse's professional goals. These training needs are best met in ongoing staff development or educational programs.

Staff Development

An effective staff development program and expert patient care clinicians are vital to patient care, staff growth, satisfaction, and a quality care environment. Orientation, planned services, and continuing education programs all support an effective staff development program. With the constant development of myriad clinical breakthroughs, new technology, legislation, and other factors, professional nurses must be kept up-to-date. These educational encounters help ensure nursing maintains recognized standards of practice. In addition, a well planned and executed staff development program is valued highly by staff. The effective new nurse manager recognizes that allowing staff specialization through continuing education is an adjunct to her/his role modeling and facilitates staff attendance, thus behaviorally reinforcing the value of ongoing education and training in professional practice.

The role of the staff development department is one of support to the patient care staff of the health care organization. Its department structure and reporting mechanism is as varied as the different health care organizations and mission/philosophy statements. It is becoming more common to see nursing education and/or staff development merged into the education departments serving the needs of other personnel in the facility in an effort to combine services and become more cost-efficient.

The nurse manager should have a basic understanding of the role of the staff development department and how each patient care unit interfaces with the department. Some of the more basic staff development responsibilities should include (but may not be limited to):

1. Competency-based orientation.
2. Competency program development and implementation.
3. Adjunct to health entity's improvement of organizational performance (IOP).
4. Planning, development, implementation, and evaluation of organizational education program.
5. Presentation of classes.
6. Maintenance of staff education records.
7. Community health education programs.
8. Consultative services to internal and external customers (department managers, local community health groups, others).

As employee monetary benefits start to plateau or decline, educational opportunities become more of a motivation and reward function. Continuing education classes, in addition to mandatory regulatory requirements, are always in demand by professional staff and positively reinforce the organization's commitment to staff growth and development.

COMPETENCY-BASED ACHIEVEMENT

Because of the very nature of health care services and the impact that one staff error can have on the well-being of a patient, competency-based achievement is extremely vital and important in the delivery of patient care. Over the past 20 years health care technology has progressed rapidly with new, complex treatment and diagnostic changes; new, more potent medications; and an increasing number of specialties within the nursing profession. The ability to keep abreast of all the new changes demands commitment on the part of nurses working with patients.

The viability of a health care setting depends on being able to accept patients for admission and care by having available and adequate staff. The nursing shortages of the past two decades forced health care institutions to recruit registered nursing staff whose competency was usually never questioned beyond the preemployment reference checks. Nurses were required to float from one patient care unit to another, no matter how the assessment and treatment needs of the patients differed. Nurses were uncomfortable with such practices and worked with their professional associations and unions to limit such practices in an effort to improve patient care.

Temporary nursing staffing services proliferated as the demands for licensed personnel increased. Unfortunately, not all nurses kept abreast of changes within their work environment and therefore may not have provided the highest quality service possible. In addition, as outcome-focused patient care becomes a reality, it is imperative for health care settings to establish standards of professional practice and institute protocols that will regulate how care is provided. It is a natural progression to have competency-based performance evaluation and achievement processes as indicators in the quest for the quantification of quality of care.

Competency assessment and evaluation should address the skills, knowledge, and abilities of staff required to promote safe, outcome-oriented patient care. Competency assessment can include educational programs, simulation of actual care practices, and review of documentation, as well as other methods. The validity of the testing apparatus should be evaluated by personnel knowledgeable in education and performance assessment criteria measurement.

All staff should be measured for competency at the time of hire (during orientation), when taking on a new role or job (e.g., promotion or cross-training), when performance expectations change (new equipment or operating standards), when there is evidence of performance deficiencies, and at the annual performance appraisal/review.[4] Competency testing is an integral part of the organization's plan for performance improvement and should include elements of validity and reliability in terms of assessment tools and evaluators.

It is the health care organization's responsibility to designate the individuals who will administer the competency evaluation. Their specialized skills should be maintained and enhanced as needed to ensure objective and up-to-date testing ability. Staff who have been in the same or similar jobs may have competency gauged through the following methods:
1. Achievement of clinical or service outcomes
2. Processes by which they deliver care or services
3. Resource utilization
4. Satisfaction with performance by others, including patients, physicians, managers, and other staff[5]

Through the establishment of quantifiable management goals and objectives that are derived from the organization's strategic plan, a manager's competency can be measured. Quality of care (as evidenced by successful accreditation), customer satisfaction (as documented through internal and external customer survey), and financial performance (as evidenced by successfully meeting or exceeding budgetary goals) indicators are all measures of a manager's competency.

Competency-based achievement also becomes a basis to quantify compensation and other monetary awards. Objective criteria lend themselves to fairness in evaluating managers from various departments with different goals and objectives.

Some examples of competencies that have been developed for nurses and incorporated into job descriptions and performance appraisals may include:

1. Orients to care environment with collaborative practice and safety and security
2. Provides nursing care to patients with alterations in pulmonary status
3. Provides nursing care to patients experiencing pain
4. Identifies priority of actions for admissions/discharge, transfers/transport
5. Provides nursing care based on a patient's developmental stage (pediatric)
6. Others

Performance criteria associated with item 5 may include the following (with an area for the new orientee to self-assess and for the preceptor or manager [deemed competent to evaluate others] to document competency demonstration):

a. Reviews growth and development theories during orientation
b. Accurately completes and documents developmental assessment on patient admission
c. Care interventions reflect nursing care based on patient's developmental stage

For an example of a criteria-based job description/performance evaluation, see Appendix 3-1 at the end of this chapter.

STAFF MOTIVATION AND RECOGNITION

Just as important as developing goals, objectives, and action plans for staff and your department is the attention a manager pays to staff, motivating and recognizing them for positive achievements and attainment of personal and unit goals. As mentioned earlier in this chapter, the rate of monetary gain for health service personnel will decrease in the future and the need to maintain a positive work environment, build team spirit, and motivate staff to continue to challenge and improve their performance will be more intense. Management texts have described many different theories of human motivation and outlined strategies to improve productivity and morale within teams and organizations.

The most basic element for new nurse managers is the ability to lead staff and then thank them for their participation in a unit success. The success reflects the employee's personal actions as well as the organization's achievements. People generally want to perform to the best of their ability; they want to believe that the work they are doing is necessary for a greater good. From the administrator of the hospital to the housekeeping or security staff, each individual contributes as much to the goal of providing the best patient care as does the registered nurse, pharmacist, or physician. The ability to be part of a team, with a larger goal in mind, is the foundation for well-motivated staff.

Staff members also appreciate the efforts of their manager to understand and empathize with the job that has to be performed. They want to be able to depend on their managers to assist them in a crisis and they respect and will be led by managers they believe will stand by them. It is important for the new nurse manager to understand that the power of the new position does not preclude the manager from ever having to "answer a patient light" or "make a home care visit" again. It is during those busy times that the manager truly exhibits the mission of the organization or the department by showing staff that patient care comes first and that management is there to support and lead the front-line, patient care staff.

Recognition needs to be regular, sincere, and from the "top down." Monthly recognition sessions lose their impact when staff members perceive the awards as shallow, insincere, and rotated among all staff regardless of actual input. On limited budgets, plan for special occasions, such as nurses' week, hospital day, or home care week, and recognize all appropriate staff. Make every effort to ensure that all staff who should be recognized are recognized! Printing the names of all the hospital nurses in a newspaper advertisement celebrating nurses' week and forgetting about the home care nurses or those working in the radiology department becomes a disaster. A rift widens between the staff themselves and the hospital that has publicly minimized their contribution. Also, the celebration of hospital week should include all staff, not just nursing, showing the staff that they are one team.

Examples of Recognition

Examples of positive and rewarding recognition can include:
1. Impact/on-the-spot awards (based on customer service/quality indicators).
2. Employee of the month/year (based on customer survey results).
3. Quality idea (based on contributions of staff that positively improve a process both qualitatively and quantitatively).

The awards could be monetary, gift certificates, points for future awards, choice parking, recognition at special functions, or as special and unique as you want to make them.

Team building can occur through both formal and informal efforts, from planned meetings and gatherings that effectively build consensus on your unit to informal, spontaneous potlucks or banding together during a crisis (e.g., keeping a unit open with 50% of the department out on sick leave).

TERMINATING OR LAYING OFF A STAFF MEMBER

Probably no management decision is as difficult to be involved in as the process of firing or laying off an employee. In most organizations, termination is the last resort.

In rare instances, this process has been in the works for some time, but the infractions were not documented correctly or personnel's policies were not effective until the new nurse manager arrived. Should such a serious and ongoing problem be given to you, share this responsibility with both your immediate supervisor and the personnel manager. There are legal concerns, staff ramifications, confidentiality issues, and other areas that should be addressed by those with the qualified expertise in your organization. In most settings, these situations occur only with the concurrence and involvement of the HR manager. In all cases, it is a difficult process for those involved. Because of this, you should not handle this process without adequate support and direction, particularly in a situation that has been ongoing for some time and began before your tenure.

EVALUATING PERFORMANCE

Generally, no area creates more feelings between manager and staff members than the performance evaluation or appraisal process. Because it is often tied to money and self-esteem, it may become the focus of some disagreement between supervisor and employee. An effective performance evaluation is beneficial to both the manager and the staff member being evaluated. In addition, the performance evaluation should be a written validation of what the manager and employee have been discussing and documenting throughout the period before the formal process. Sadly, this is not always the case and so the employee feels and has a right to complain that the manager did not communicate problems to the employee before the meeting.

Usually there is a formal structure for the process and a time frame for appraising performance. Most settings also have a standard format and criteria on which to base the evaluation. It is very important that you learn the organization's evaluation process. Various evaluation tools are available, and you need to familiarize yourself with them. The purpose of this section is to prepare you for your first employee performance evaluation or to reinforce information if you have previously administered evaluations.

What Is Performance Appraisal?

Performance appraisals occur to (1) give formal feedback on the current nursing performance and competency in the work setting and (2) determine the employee's development within the staff or other growth needs for the future. This is provided in a private discussion and can be a positive experience for both nurse manager and employee.

Though the process and time frames may vary, effective performance appraisals can accomplish several things:

- They provide needed recognition and structured feedback.
- They allow the manager and staff nurse time to reevaluate the bigger picture of organization, unit direction, or goals.
- They allow the nurse manager to clarify behavior or other expectations.

- They allow the staff nurse a reading on her/his defined or written priorities, goals, and objectives.
- They permit the nurse manager another opportunity to create an environment that fosters personal and professional growth of staff nurses in an open environment that encourages risk taking, where appropriate.
- They provide another time when the nurse manager can allow the exchange of creative ideas to accomplish work in a different or better way.
- They can provide the opportunity to coach the nurse employee to meet program or unit goals or objectives.
- Sometimes, they are the environment for addressing the core of why we choose to be nurses. For example, discussions of effectiveness, professionalism, client relations, clinical expertise, and other factors all determine the level of the performance appraisal. All nurses and employees want to do a good job—this is a unique opportunity to find out what is impeding the employee's attainment of goals and what you can do as the manager to facilitate goal achievement. This role as coach and mentor solidifies your working relationship with your staff.
- They allow the quality of the work performance to be evaluated against specific predetermined standards that are correlated with the employee position description.

Legal and Risk Management Issues

As with all of health care, human resources are also affected by risk management and legal concerns that can prove frustrating and demoralizing for the new nurse manager trying to effectively manage a department. The most important point to remember is that as a middle manager, you are not alone. There is the expertise of your senior manager, legal counsel (in-house or contracted services), and human resource department manager and staff. Strong policies, procedures, mission statements, and integrated values all add to a structure that protects both staff and management when making decisions that may be a potential for disagreement.

Some of the major human resource legal and risk management concerns affecting nurse managers today may include:

1. Delegation of patient care duties—from professional to unlicensed assistive staff.
2. Competency of staff.
3. Wrongful termination.
4. Unfair layoffs.
5. Substance abuse in the workplace.
6. Violence in the workplace.
7. Patient abuse by staff.
8. Nonreporting of child, adult, and elder abuse by patient care staff.

9. Pay practices (especially home care per visit pay and overtime issues).

10. Harassment.

Be aware of your institution's human resource policies and procedures and always adhere to them closely. Ask for input and support from your senior manager and human resource director when confronted with a nonfunctioning staff member who needs to begin the counseling process. Understand and abide by union contracts and work with the shop steward for your department in planning and implementing changes that affect staff. Always respect your staff. Never belittle or deride anyone in public. The best adage for a new manager is to *treat staff as you would like to be treated.*

VIOLENCE IN THE WORKPLACE

Reports of workplace violence have increased tremendously during the past few years, the violence being especially due to increased pressure to improve productivity, layoffs, disagreements between management and staff, and disturbed relationships. Special training programs have now been established to assist managers in assessing and defusing potentially volatile situations. According to the Northwestern National Life Insurance study on nonfatal workplace violence, over two million people were attacked on the job, six million were threatened with violence, 16 million suffered harassment, and 25% of all full-time workers were either harassed, threatened, or attacked on the job between July 1992 to July 1993.[6] Health care organizations have not been immune to violence. Emergency departments are prime areas for angry clients to express their hostility over the type or lack of treatment being afforded them or a significant other or, in most cases, the length of time waiting to be seen by a physician.

For the new manager, it is important to understand the build-up and progression of violent behavior. The checklists in Box 3-1 on p. 72 describe the various levels of violence and certain behaviors associated with them.

In defusing a volatile situation or responding to aggression, either from a patient or a staff member, all staff should be aware of the signals they are sending the aggressor. Develop the following behaviors:

- Always actively listen to and focus on the individual.
- Show respect and concern for her/his issues.
- Control your body language and emotions during the conversation.
- Think twice before responding in anger, accusation, or humor.
- Remain calm and exude your authority and control of the situation.

Having a program in place is the first line of defense in dealing with workplace violence:

1. Know the signs to look for in a potentially violent individual.

2. Utilize criminal checks in preemployment procedures.

box 3-1

LEVELS OF VIOLENCE AND ASSOCIATED BEHAVIORS

FIRST LEVEL

❑ Sexual comments
❑ Noncooperation with supervisor
❑ Spreads rumors and gossip
❑ Argues with co-workers
❑ Belligerent towards customers
❑ Swears at everyone

SECOND LEVEL

❑ Argues with everyone
❑ Refuses to obey policies/procedures
❑ Steals for revenge
❑ Sabotages equipment
❑ Writes sexual/violent notes
❑ Makes verbal threats
❑ Feels victimized
❑ Sexually harasses others

THIRD LEVEL

❑ Frequently displays intense anger
❑ Often threatens suicide
❑ Frequent physical fights
❑ Destroys property
❑ Uses weapons to hurt others
❑ Commits murder, rape, or arson[7]

Adapted from Gilham DS, Schweitzer SM: *Workplace violence prevention*, Texas Association for Home Care 26th Annual Meeting and Exhibition, Dallas, September 1995.

3. Have policies and procedures on:
   a. Acceptable employee behavior (no threats, violence).
   b. Possession of weapons.
   c. Duty of other employees to report suspicious behaviors.
4. Outline and use employee progressive discipline protocols.
5. Make sure that an Employee Assistance Program is available.
6. Have a plan for violence management (similar to a fire/emergency-preparedness plan).

In the event of a potentially violent situation, notify your supervisor and human resource manager for additional assistance in dealing with the crisis. Do not act alone; there are experts in human behavior at your institution or, if not, consultants who can be brought in to help defuse the situation.

Conflict Resolution

Effective managers try to maintain a calm, objective work environment; stress may exist and conflicts may arise, but overall there is a general understanding by staff members that they are respected, their opinions are important, and resolution will be attempted in an objective but firm manner. Conflict resolution has four major points:

1. Clarification—the issues and the parties involved in the conflict.
2. Performance—identify with the involved parties the potential outcomes from the behaviors exhibited.
3. Question—what were the behaviors that initiated this conflict and how best to avoid them in the future.
4. Expectations—describe in detail (in writing if necessary) what the manager's expectations are, based on policies and procedures, and what will happen if these behaviors continue (further disciplinary actions).

Organizations with clear, concise, and complete policies and procedures have less opportunities for potential conflicts between interdepartmental and intradepartmental staff. By having objective and fair policies in place for reference, managers are not put into the unenviable position of having to decide who is "right" and who is "wrong." Employee behaviors and performance are dictated by organization-wide protocols. As in all personnel issues, it is important to notify your supervisor and the human resource department manager, either for assistance or notification of the situation and a review of your proposed actions. (For further discussion of conflict, refer to Chapter 4, "Communications.")

Considerations for Home Care Managers

UNIQUE PERSONNEL ISSUES IN HOME CARE

Home care nurse managers face the same human resource management concerns as do their counterparts in other health care settings. However, similar to the listing in Chapter 1, the following is a compilation of personnel issues that need to be addressed by the home care manager:

1. Orientation and supervision of staff in the home setting.
2. Risk management issues surrounding patients and their belongings: privacy, respect, and security.
3. Staff safety in the home and commuting between visits and the office—driving and violence.
4. Staff development and growth opportunities as the industry changes.
5. Staff payment issues: per visit vs. salary vs. hourly pay and overtime hours.
6. Prompt counseling of staff after being apprised of questionable situations.

SUMMARY

The manager must effectively employ human management skills to achieve work objectives. The use of these skills, or their lack, is evident in any work environment. As the role model for the staff, it is imperative that the new nurse manager have an open attitude that creates a workplace where staff nurses can grow professionally. An effective workplace has the following qualities:

1. It is an environment open to new ideas.
2. Staff members feel they can safely take risks, when appropriate.
3. Planning occurs for short- and long-term activities and the staff is involved and apprised.
4. Both management and the staff are working towards the same goals.
5. All levels of staff value human management skills and treat everyone, including peers, patients, and visitors, with kindness and respect.

As a nurse manager, these are the elements to strive for in your setting. The important HR functions of interviewing, hiring, coaching, and evaluating performance are the hallmarks of the team's inception and structure.

Please see Chapter 4, "Communications," for a discussion of specific communication problems that may arise in HR management.

References

1. Patz JM, Biordi DL, Holm K: Middle Nurse Manager Effectiveness, *J Nurs Admin* 21:15, 1991.
2. Lombardi DN: *Handbook for the new health care manager,* Chicago, 1993, AHA Publisher, pg. 247.
3. Livingston J, Sterling HBR: Pygmalion in Management, *Harvard Bus Rev* 66:121, 1988.
4. Rodriguez L, et al: *Manual of staff development,* St Louis, 1996, Mosby, pg. 284.
5. Ibid, pg 281.
6. Gilham DS, Schweitzer SM: Workplace violence prevention *Texas Association for Home Care 26th Annual Meeting and Exhibition,* Dallas, September, 1995.
7. Ibid.

For Further Reading

Boyd C et al: Performance plan: a nursing management strategy to improve care delivery, *J Healthcare Educ Train* 5(3):12, 1991.

Davidhizar R, Giger J: When subordinates go over your head—the manipulative employee, *JONA* 20(9):29, 1990.

Del Bueno DJ, Walker DD: Developing prospective managers: a unique program, part I, *JONA* 14(4):7, 1984.

Donckers SW, Harris MD: Teleconferencing: home health administrators and educators enhance graduate education, *Journal of Nursing Administration* 22(10):38, 1992.

Family-friendly: hospitals begin to modernize their time-off policies. *Hospitals* January 20, 1992 p. 58.

Feldman R: Meeting the educational needs of home healthcare nurses, *Journal of Home Healthcare Practice* 5(4):12, 1994.

Fulghum R: *All I really need to know I learned in kindergarten,* Westminister, Md, 1988, Villiard Books, Random House.

Hefty LV, et al: A model skills list for orienting nurses to community health agencies, *Public Health Nursing* 9(4):228, 1992.

Hendricks W: *The manager's role as coach,* Shawnee Mission, KS, 1994, National Press Publications.

Hood JN, Smith HL: Quality of work life in home care: the contribution of leaders' personal concern for staff, *Journal of Nursing Administration* 24(1):40, 1994.

Huselid MA: The impact of human resource management practices on turnover, productivity, and corporate financial performance, *Academy of Management Journal* 58(3):635, 1995.

Janz M: Perception of knowledge: what administrators and assistants know, *Journal of Gerontological Nursing* 18(8):7, 1992.

King P: *Performance planning and appraisal: a how-to book for managers*, New York, 1984, McGraw-Hill.

Lachman VD: Increasing productivity through performance evaluation, *JONA* 14(12):7, 1984.

Lawler T: The objectives of performance appraisal or "where can we go from here?" *Nurs Manage* 19(3):82, 1988.

Livingston JS: Pygmalion in management, *Harvard Bus Rev* 66(5):121, 1988.

McAlvanah MF: Evaluations: an important managerial skill, *Pediatr Nurs* 14(1):75, 1988.

Ott MJ, et al: Peer interviewing: sharing the hiring process, *Nursing Management* 21(11):32, 1990.

Peters T: *Thriving on chaos: handbook for a management revolution*, New York, 1987, Harper & Row.

Shoemake A: Solutions to the home health-care nursing shortage, *Home Healthcare Nurse* 12(4):35, 1994.

Shugart EB: Using volunteer visitors in home care, *Journal of Nursing Administration* 22(4):42, 1992.

Simpson DB: The performance appraisal interview: putting it all together, *The Health Care Supervisor* 63-76, January 1985.

Trull S: Strategies of effective interviewing, *Harvard Business Review* 42(1):89, 1964.

Yochem B: Counseling: a "how-to" for new nurse managers, *Pediatric Nursing* 17(2): 201, 1991.

SAMPLE CRITERIA-BASED
POSITION DESCRIPTION/PERFORMANCE APPRAISAL

Position Description Data:

TITLE OF POSITION: TEAM SECRETARY	REPORTS TO: PATIENT TEAM MANAGER
Name of Staff Member:_____	Performance Reviewer:_____
Status of Position: FT/Nonexempt **Type of Review:** Probation ___ Annual ___ Other ___ Date of Review:_____	**Work Environment:** Noise level is usually moderate Employee may be required to assist in branch offices Employee must have vision capabilities to review and transcribe information from records to computer terminal and be able to work at CRT screen.
Position Description: Under the direction of the patient team manager, provides all administrative support to patient care teams by setting up, tracking, filing, and maintaining all patient care records, per agency policy and applicable regulation. Also responsible for the preparation and tracking of all statistics utilized in billing process and report generation and/or verification as required. Provides support to receptionist staff by answering telephone calls and routing as appropriate utilizing customer service techniques.	**Qualifications/Job Requirements:** High school graduate Graduate of medical technical school desired Familiarity with medical terminology Ability to type at least 60 wpm Data entry and word processing experience Organizational and time management skills Customer service orientation Ability to work as a team in a fast-paced environment Ability to lift up to 25 pounds

Performance Standards	Rating			
I. Maintains clinical record and billing information by accurately processing and filing all forms within specified deadline: a. Plan of treatment is mailed out to appropriate physician within 5 days of admission and is noted on physician order log	1	2	3	4
b. Verbal/supplemental orders are processed and mailed out to physicians within 48 hours of receipt.				
c. Completed clinical forms are processed and filed in the appropriate part of the clinical record within 5 days of receipt.				
d. Discharge summaries are processed and mailed out to physicians within 30 days of discharge date.				
e. Closed records are audited and completed within 30 days of discharge.				
f. Prebilling invoice is audited and compared to clinical record for accuracy of date, bill for service, and signed physician order is on file.				
ETC				

CHAPTER 4

COMMUNICATIONS

MARGARET SHARP WOODARD

T.M. MARRELLI

RECOGNIZING YOUR INHERENT INTERPERSONAL SKILLS

Managers can perform multitudes of tasks proficiently, effectively selecting and hiring staff, delegating appropriately, making sound decisions, and yet still not achieve maximal success. Strong, well developed interpersonal skills are key to all management functions and are a large element of the art and science of effective management. These skills are necessary in the development of trust and mutual respect between manager and staff members. This trust and respect foster staff development and retention and can minimize the effect of negative events such as times of high stress or change.

Interpersonal skills can be learned. yet we all have "inherent" interpersonal abilities that affect our success as managers. Elements of personality and style are unique to each individual. Successful use of interpersonal skills is varied and adapted to the specific situation. Reading, noting instances of effective communication, and seeking feedback from supervisors and the staff are all methods nurse managers can use to analyze the impact and effectiveness of their "inherent" qualities.

Through thoughtful self-examination, it is possible to temper or emphasize personal characteristics to enhance your success and meet management goals. Some nurse managers naturally exhibit warmth and inspire liking and trust. Some have an innate ability to excite and inspire the staff and others to do well. Although these gifts assist managers, the gifts must be accompanied by learned interpersonal skills and sound managerial skills and abilities. We all have probably known ineffective managers with great charm.

Conversely, many of us do not have a personality or style that gives us rapid acceptance or strong impact. It is important to remember that long-term effectiveness need not be diminished in this situation. Fairness, good judgment, accomplishment, and communication will eventually establish a true foundation of the trust and respect needed by all nurse managers to succeed.

The analysis of personal skills and abilities allows one to use them to her/his advantage, develop complementary skills, and compensate for weaker areas. An example of this analysis and compensation was an experienced nurse manager with great organizational and systems skills who appeared cold and directive. In previous jobs, she had discovered that her perceived personality tended to shut her off from the staff. It took her years to win their trust, since she often experienced knee-jerk resistance to and suspicion of new ideas or recommendations. Over time, though, this behavior decreased as staff began to recognize the benefits and results of her abilities. In her next job she proactively compensated for such a reception by initially telling staff that she realized she was often perceived as difficult to approach and lacking in warmth. She asked them to look past this initial impression and give her time to demonstrate caring and open-mindedness through her actions and work. She worked hard to consistently reward those who approached her. She also hired an assistant head nurse with a warmer, more open attitude. These actions worked towards decreasing the negative impact her natural manner tended to create.

While recognizing the importance of building rapport, trust, and a support base, the nurse manager must realize that her/his goal is not to be universally liked or popular.

There are learnable techniques of communication, leadership, development, and motivation of staff that are components of interpersonal skills. These techniques are discussed in the remainder of the chapter.

HOW TO GET WHAT YOU WANT

Interpersonal skills help you get what you want in order to achieve organizational work. This occurs directly, through clear communication, and indirectly, by creating an environment or unit culture that fosters open, trusting communication.

Know What You Want: Goals and Values

To get your desired outcome you and your staff must know specifically what you want. The first step is to establish clear, mutually accepted values. In most nursing settings, the focus of these values is directed towards providing quality patient care. It can be extremely useful to discuss and clarify with staff members what is valued and how those values are supported and demonstrated. A good place to begin this process is by reviewing your organization's mission statement or vision and values and philosophy. These should be frequently reviewed, even after consensus and clarity have been obtained. Most nurses are stimulated by this type of discussion. It causes them to remember why they became nurses and to examine their practice, work habits, and routines in a new light.

After values are clearly defined, future decisions and discussions of goals, standards, and performance should be guided by these values. Clearly stated goals for patient care, unit function, and individual staff members must be established. The goals should be behaviorally valued, measurable, and achievable. They should be developed using organizational, departmental, and regulatory guidelines, policies, and objectives. Staff members should always have ongoing input. Although goals should be achievable and realistic, they should also be challenging. Much productivity and pride in achievement is lost when goals are set at a low level. Relating unit goals to values concerning patient care is important. It is easier to set and strive for high-level goals when the effect on patients, if goals are not achieved, is clear and demonstrable.

The Nurse Manager Role

As the manager, your role in defining values and setting goals includes the following:
- Initiating and facilitating discussion to elicit clarification of values.
- Recording written value statements, seeking staff feedback, and incorporating revisions into the organizational review process.
- Initiating discussion of goals at the unit and individual levels with the staff you directly supervise.
- Bringing pertinent directives, regulations, accreditation standards, or other factors needing consideration to the discussion.
- Recording written goals and action plans for achieving them.
- Maintaining momentum of progress towards goals, giving positive and constructive feedback to promote progress towards meeting deadlines.
- Communicating to staff the progress towards goals through the use of Pareto charts or other visual tools.

DEVELOPING RESOURCES

Clear goals and values assist the nurse manager and nursing staff in finding direction and setting priorities. To reach these goals, the nurse manager must develop, maintain, conserve, and wisely use both personnel and material resources. The development and retention of employees involve important interpersonal skills in any setting and time. They are crucial in nursing and any other health profession. Advanced, more complex practice requires experienced nurses. The demands for efficiency can only be met with a complement of staff members who are familiar with unit and ancillary systems. Nurses continue to be in high demand, and the turnover created as they seek new opportunities is expensive in dollars, productivity, and training.

Each staff member on any unit is a resource to be highly valued. The nurse manager must have individual knowledge of every employee directly supervised and ongoing communication with those indirectly supervised. There are several purposes of this communication and knowledge.

The first purpose is to identify the skill level and learning needs of the staff. Psychomotor skills, critical and evaluative thinking, and the ability to plan and deliver care should be assessed. Knowledge of individual learning styles should be incorporated into planning for the development of each individual. Professional staff members should be involved in developing their own plan and take responsibility for their continued learning.

THE IMPORTANCE OF JOB SATISFACTION

Another key reason for the nurse manager to develop relationships with and knowledge of each staff member is that this increases the ability to maximize staff job satisfaction. Although the nurse manager must balance unit function against individual needs, there are many opportunities to assist staff in enjoying their work. Most nurses today balance family and individual demands against those of their career. A person who enjoy her/his work and workplace can be energized rather than drained by that work (on most days!). This allows the career person to carry energy rather than fatigue out of the workplace. It also leads to valuing that particular job setting enough to be less likely to leave it for other than serious career opportunities.

Mark Twain is reported to have defined the successful person as one who gets up in the morning and is excited to meet each day. When a job contributes to that feeling, one is not likely to move on. Many nurses today indicate that they leave their jobs because of boredom, poor work conditions, lack of opportunity, inability to advance, interpersonal conflicts, as well as conflict with personal needs.

THE NURSE MANAGER'S ROLE IN STAFF RETENTION

The nurse manager must understand the factors that satisfy or dissatisfy staff members in order to retain effective team members. Five examples of using this knowledge to retain your staff and create a healthier workplace follow.

Example One

An assistant head nurse approached the nurse manager about a trio of staff members. She was concerned because they tended to work together and adjust their assignments and schedules to accommodate this goal. She was worried that this might adversely affect productivity. The three were skilled, competent, and experienced nurses. One historically had a problem with absenteeism and another was previously a loner. On further discussion with the manager, it became clear that these nurses were completing assignments, were not disruptive to others, were not cliquish, and were enjoying working together. They functioned as an effective, cooperative team. Their patients had good outcomes. The assistant head nurse was worried because of vague feelings that sociability at work should be limited and sensed some loss of control. She was encouraged by the manager to examine this situation for actual, objective, negative results and could identify none. They then explored possible positive effects such as increased collaboration, support, and affiliation.

After further discussion, the assistant head nurse approached the three and remarked on their pattern. She verbalized appreciation of practice and collaboration, and support for its benefits (see Box 4-1). She encouraged them to continue, but discussed concerns about productivity. All agreed that patient care was the priority. Over time several benefits were seen: (1) the nurse with an absenteeism problem rarely called in sick because she did not want to let her friends down; (2) the three became very involved in unit orientation, and their skills and warmth were excellent for assimilating new staff members; and (3) the group also became a nucleus for social activities, as well as special projects—they worked so well together that they had very good ideas to share with others.

Example Two

A nurse manager met with an excellent RN who had been with the unit for 2 years. The nurse was clinically skilled but not very involved in unit issues outside of completing her work in a given shift. Historically, 2 years was the average turnover time for this particular unit. The manager and nurse explored the nurse's goals. The nurse liked the patient care setting but was in need of new stimulation and growth. They both agreed that she was not ready for a management position, nor was one available. After discussion, the nurse accepted an assignment to develop and implement patient teaching protocols for her area of clinical expertise. The manager met with her regularly to review progress, offer support, and assist her in obtaining needed resources (see Box 4-2). The nurse was later selected for a hospital-wide committee, which furthered her growth and development. She became very active on the unit by sharing her new skills and acting as a resource to peers.

---

box 4-1

SKILLS USED BY THE NURSE MANAGER

- Recognized staff and what motivates them
- Reinforced positive behaviors
- Verbalized appreciation of practice and collaboration

---

box 4-2

SKILLS USED BY THE NURSE MANAGER

- Identified staff member's goals
- Listened and created an environment that allowed the nurse to grow professionally
- Scheduled regular meetings to review progress, offer support, and assist in obtaining resources

Example Three

The nurse manager met with a staff member who was going to school to advance from LPN to RN. She worked full-time. They discussed ways to accommodate her class schedule without disrupting the staff schedule. She was given time frames for discussing scheduling needs in advance. At one point, it became clear that she would be 30 minutes late 2 days a week on the evening shift. She and the manager discussed options (see Box 4-3). As report was one-to-one on this unit, she was encouraged to approach others who might swap an hour during the week to be relieved 1 hour early on the weekend. This plan was successful for the nurse, the nurse manager, and the entire unit.

Example Four

The charge nurse on a step-down unit approached her nurse manager to discuss advancing her own critical care skills. The manager arranged for her to have access to an ICU preceptor. The charge nurse scheduled herself to spend time in the ICU when her shift was covered. She and the manager regularly discussed her progress and use of time (see Box 4-4). At the end of 6 months, the charge nurse in-serviced other staff on new procedures and began scheduling them for similar off-unit development.

Example Five

While meeting with a staff member, a manager discovered that an important part of her life was attending a Tuesday evening meeting. Without inconveniencing other staff, but with some effort on adjusting the schedule, the manager thereafter sched-

---

box 4-3

SKILLS USED BY THE NURSE MANAGER

- Behaviorally supported a staff member's professional growth
- Listened and implemented a plan based on staff member's goal
- Discussed option for scheduling

---

box 4-4

SKILLS USED BY THE NURSE MANAGER

- Supported professional autonomy by having the nurse schedule herself
- Arranged access for the staff member to the ICU preceptor
- Discussed regularly progress and time use

uled this nurse off on that evening whenever possible (see Box 4-5). The manager later discovered that of many more difficult tasks she performed on behalf of her staff this was one of the most appreciated.

In the above examples the managers were successful in developing and retaining staff. The key to these simple but successful examples is that the managers' responses were individualized to the specific circumstances and individuals. Some management situations do not lend themselves to a single strategy and require ongoing evaluation and support for successful resolution. Most importantly, development and retention of staff can occur consistently only in an environment where each individual is valued and appreciated. This is demonstrated through action and verbalization by the effective nurse manager.

USING RESOURCES: MOTIVATION

We know that clarifying values, setting clear goals, and developing resources are important in a successful operation. Nurse managers must also use resources effectively. In the case of personnel resources, this requires motivation coupled with effective leadership. Remember, all work is done by the staff.

Lancaster[1] defines motivation as internal and unique to each employee. In other words, managers cannot motivate employees—they must be motivated from within, and what inspires motivation in one may not in another. Lancaster states that all employees are motivated, but those who appear to lack motivation are actually motivated in a direction different, or towards other outcomes, than a manager may desire. Because managers cannot directly motivate staff, they must work indirectly by creating an environment that tends to cause individual motivation towards the desired goals.

We have discussed several activities that are part of a motivating environment. The suggestions presented in Manager's Tip 4-1 on p. 86 will help the nurse manager create a positive environment.

THE WORK ENVIRONMENT

A healthy work environment, put simply, is one where all employees, managers and staff members alike, work towards common goals, receive feedback and communications on an ongoing basis, and meet the needs of their customers.

---

box 4-5

SKILLS USED BY THE NURSE MANAGER

- Listened to and heard the staff nurse's need
- Altered the schedule to support the nurse's request
- Respected the staff member by implementing this change

MANAGER'S TIP 4-1

CREATING A MOTIVATING ENVIRONMENT

✔ Involve your staff through their participation and agreement on values and goals established.

✔ Get to know each staff member well enough to learn what assistance they need to achieve a goal and what constitutes a positive reward for them.

✔ Clarify, discuss, and reinforce the goals and what is expected with staff.

The presence or absence of some of the characteristics described above in an environment does not, in itself, determine a "good" or "bad" setting (see Box 4-6). Some organizations may exhibit a blend of both in some situations, depending on times and areas observed. However, in a recent study of nurses and the culture of excellence in their hospitals, as defined by the attributes of excellence identified by Peters and Waterman in an article by Kramer and Schmalenberg,[2] it was determined that "the presence of these attributes of excellence correlated with high job satisfaction and high self-esteem among the nurses."[2] In addition, when the authors looked at the data on the attributes of excellence, they saw "many more magnet hospital nurses indicated that their nursing leaders have power; that they're visionary; that they communicate and implement ideas, values, and goals; and that they function as a team."[3]

ABOUT FEEDBACK

The nurse manager should provide ongoing feedback and reinforcement concerning performance and achievement. Although feedback and reinforcement can be both positive and negative, Lancaster[1] suggests avoiding using threats and punishment as the predominating mode. Positive rewards and depersonalized, anticipated disciplinary action are more effective. Positive rewards should be individualized and can include raises, recognition, opportunities to participate in special activities, educational experiences, committee selection, and scheduling choices. Disciplinary action should be expected (i.e., a specific reaction to a specific behavior, consistent, timely, and focused on the behavior, not the person). It is important to remember that even discipline can occur in an atmosphere of approval and support.

COMMUNICATION PATTERNS

In any organization, both motivation and effectiveness are driven by the quality achieved in and patterns of communication. Without sound communication skills, the manager can be isolated and uninformed. Managers need to send and receive

box 4-6

ENVIRONMENT CHARACTERISTICS

CHARACTERISTICS OF A HEALTHY AND MOTIVATING ENVIRONMENT

Some work environments are healthier than others. The following list outlines common elements of healthy work environments:

- People feel part of a team.
- There is ongoing clear communication up and down the organization hierarchy.
- Everyone is aware of and works towards defined goals.
- Good behavior is valued and reinforced.
- Staff development is ongoing.
- Employees have the authority to complete their work.
- The work and the people are respected.
- The staff feels generally positive about the work and other staff.

CHARACTERISTICS OF AN UNHEALTHY ENVIRONMENT

Similarly, unhealthy work environments share some common characteristics. They are listed below.

- Divisiveness is apparent among the staff, as in a dysfunctional family ("we versus they").
- People complain continually or do not communicate at all.
- People do not want to come to work.
- New members may feel isolated.
- "Top down" communication is rare or nonexistent.
- An open-door policy is espoused but in reality is rarely practiced.
- There are continually identified problems without attempts at resolution.
- Paralysis through continual analysis is apparent, and no or very little effective action is taken.

clear, well understood messages. Communication patterns that affect their ability to do this are discussed below. Manager's Tip 4-2 on p. 88 presents some suggestions for effective communication.

The Communication Climate

In his book, Swansburg[3] discusses the importance of the overall tone of the environment in supporting clear communication, effective teamwork, and productivity. The supportive versus the defensive climate is discussed. The supportive climate is the goal of the manager who wants to encourage involvement and participation of staff at all levels. The manager must be open to disagreement, discussion, and input and use them constructively. Employees must feel they will be rewarded for speaking up, asking questions, and identifying problems. Individuality and spontaneity must be valued. Conflict should be seen as an opportunity for growth and learning. Empathy and support for and among staff should be evident. The only qualifier to these activities is that all should use them constructively to work towards unit goals.

MANAGER'S TIP 4-2

BASIC TIPS FOR COMMUNICATING EFFECTIVELY

✔ Sharpen and use your listening skills to hear also the tone and intent of what is being communicated.

✔ Use appropriate eye contact during your conversations with staff.

✔ Validate what you thought you understood or heard by repeating the message in your own words, when necessary.

✔ If you find yourself in a situation where you know you are too busy to listen and address an issue, schedule time with the staff member to focus on the concern.

✔ Create an environment where the only dumb questions are the ones that do not get asked.

✔ Encourage feedback, recommendations, and "ways to make things better."

✔ Understand and effectively use the personality differences between your staff and the group you will be actively communicating with:

> *"Talker"*: Do not give this individual continual openings by making eye contact. Defer to others in the group for a response to her/his comments.

> *"Recluse"*: Draw this individual out by asking for opinions, comments, or questions on discussion at hand. Support this person by making environment as risk-free as possible.

> *"Arguer"*: Do not act defensive when this individual questions or argues with each statement made. Respond to remarks with questions to clarify what is being said and steer or focus discussion back to desired areas.

> *"Expert"*: Avoid having this individual monopolize discussion by directing conversation and having staff respond to comments with their impressions and interpretations.

✔ Smile when speaking with staff members whenever possible and appropriate.

✔ Summarize the conversation or discussion when finished.

✔ Ask for and thank staff and other team members for their ideas, input, and time.

✔ Be courteous and respectful of staff ideas and recommendations, even when they do not work out once implemented.

IMPEDIMENTS TO EFFECTIVE COMMUNICATION

Because of interference and noise, messages sent are frequently distorted before reception. Miscommunications can be caused by the sender, the listener, intermediaries, or the environment. The sender may clearly understand the message because of having had previous discussions and thoughts about the topic. The message may be poorly understood by the listener, who does not have the sender's frame of reference. The listener may produce interference simply by thinking about her/his response or another issue instead of listening carefully. A common example of intermediary interference is the parlor game where a phrase is whispered from person to person and the first and final messages are compared. In the game, the disparity between the first and final messages can be very amusing, but in a work

Manager's Tip 4-3

FOUR EXAMPLES OF WAYS TO AVOID MISCOMMUNICATIONS

✔ Communicate directly to groups.
✔ Hold meetings in a quiet setting.
✔ Encourage discussion of information given.
✔ Include a feedback loop in communication channels. After one-to-one, group, or written messages, the manager needs to ensure the message was understood as intended.

setting it is a serious problem. The nurse manager must consider possible sources of communications interference in advance and eliminate as many as possible (see Manager's Tip 4-3).

VERBAL VERSUS NONVERBAL COMMUNICATION

How something is said can be as important as what is said. Tone of voice, gestures, and posture greatly affect the listener. The nurse manager needs to appear assured, modify her/his feelings before speaking (or acknowledge rather than deny them), and maintain an open, attentive posture. The manager must also note body language in staff members that appears to be blocking communication. If an employee is turning away, or making a dismissive gesture, the manager must investigate or intervene at the appropriate time.

The nurse manager must always be aware of being a role model to the staff. The manager's example and behaviors must be consistent and professional. Communications should follow the formal chain of command. Nurse managers should be clear about the organization's expectations for intradepartmental and interdepartmental communications. They should make staff aware of these and their own expectations.

Inappropriate and negative forms of communication that the nurse manager should discourage in staff members, and must never personally demonstrate, include:

- Profanity, crudity, and personal criticisms. Professionals should express themselves professionally and demonstrate respect for others.
- Rumors and rumor spreading. Rumors can be destructive, divisive, and counterproductive.

The nurse manager serves as the vital link between the staff and the organization at large. The manager must accurately receive and transmit messages in both directions. Staff concerns, patient care issues, and system needs must be taken to administration or ancillary services. Imperatives, directives, objectives, procedures, and policies must be brought to staff. The manager uses writing, verbal, and listening skills to fulfill these linking functions. The nurse manager should review the institution's organizational chart with both supervisor and staff. The organizational chart delineates the chain of command and communication. It assists in clarifying direct, indirect, and collaborative relationships. Analysis of the chart can assist the nurse manager in ensuring that appropriate sources of information are fully used and that written and verbal communications are properly directed.

LISTENING SKILLS

It is important to remember that listening is an active process. It involves focusing, questioning, and validating, as well as allowing time to process the information gained. The listener who is judging the message or messenger, distracted, preparing a response, or not attentive cannot be listening effectively or gaining what is possible. Through meetings, nurse managers and their staffs maintain and work towards improving the function of their units. The new nurse manager needs to understand what information is important and must be noted and the process for recording such information. She/he needs to know how to obtain follow-up details and clarification, when needed. This clear, correct, timely information will then be communicated to all staff members. For an in-depth discussion of staff meetings, please refer to Chapter Five, "Day-to-Day Operations."

VERBAL SKILLS

Nurse managers must always be prepared to represent or speak on behalf of their clinical areas. Although one does not want to be perceived as a squeaky wheel in an era of constrained resources, the unprepared and nonverbal may lose out. The successful manager can clearly articulate problems and quantify them, as well as suggest solutions. The manager should consult with supervisors, resource persons, and peers to develop the ability to speak in the language style understood and appreciated by administrators. The economic and patient outcome issues of a problem should be clearly defined. Knowing when to speak and being able to defer an answer are other important considerations. The manager does not want to be recognized for noise but for valued input. The points listed in Manager's Tip 4-4 are concepts to consider.

COMMUNICATING EFFECTIVELY ACROSS AN INTEGRATED NETWORK

Just as important as communicating up and down a chain of command in a hospital or other health care setting is the need for effective communication when actively involved in an integrated network. With the fast mergers and affiliations of

MANAGER'S TIP 4-4

GUIDELINES TO CONSIDER WHEN REPRESENTING YOURSELF OR YOUR CLINICAL AREA

✔ If you do not have a complete answer for superiors or staff, say so, and commit to follow-up.

✔ Know your listener. Some people prefer a time-saving, "bottom-line" response backed up by written reinforcement or discussion. Others need a progression of thought and time.

✔ Say less. If you are clear and concise, you need not say more except to be certain you were understood. Do not dilute the message by wandering or defending. Stay on the topic if a discussion ensues.

✔ If you are not sure that you have been understood, ask your listener for feedback.

✔ Be positive and constructive. Problems can be presented in terms of needs, goals, and possible solutions. Disagreement can be presented as an alternative view while acknowledging others and encouraging comparison.

large health systems, it is common to see a lack of organization and focus until the communication lines are well-established and goals and objectives become aligned under strong leadership.

It is essential for the nurse manager of a patient care unit to understand the lines of communication and reporting mechanisms of the many departments on an organizational chart. The effectiveness of patient care planning needs to be emphasized from one setting to the next, and the relationship between each setting and the department that holds the groups together must ensure that the patient does not get lost in the system. In many instances, case management is the department that acts as the interface between different departments and different settings.

Regular written communication is needed between management and staff to enhance rumor control and keep staff informed of all appropriate changes. Management teams need to schedule, and keep, standing appointments with subordinates for discussions of ongoing happenings and the plans for upcoming events and projects. Many senior managers schedule routine meetings with their subordinate groups following their senior manager meetings. Department managers then follow suit and schedule departmental staff meetings within the next 24 hours to apprise staff of important items. This system is a viable adjunct to monthly department manager and divisional meetings. It keeps information fresh and timely and is a good deterrent to the rumor mill. One of the most frustrating, potentially volatile situations is when staff learn about events or happenings that will affect them from the media, such as television, radio, and newspapers.

ELECTRONIC MAIL (E-MAIL) AND THE INTERNET

Most large organizations with numerous departments or branch offices have established a form of communication called e-mail, in an effort to promote paperless communication. In most cases, e-mail can successfully replace the written memorandum because the sender can keep a written or saved copy on file, and the recipient can produce a written copy for personal files. Most e-mail systems also verify to the sender when the recipient actually pulled the transmission up for reading, proof of receipt.

Basically, electronic mail allows computers and their users to "speak" with each other as long as they are all on the same network or are interfaced with the communication network. Besides providing a medium for written communications to be sent instantaneously (without getting up and faxing a typed document), e-mail allows for quick notification of one or more parties who have been assigned stations or addresses on the system of official business.

E-mail allows a person to type a document once and send it on its way via modem. However, as with all computerized communications, there needs to be strict confidentiality and security precautions. There are few computerized communications systems that are impervious to hackers. Recent news stories have recounted the ability of international hackers, usually college students, to successfully breach government defense system computer networks and get access to top secret files. With that in mind, it is important to educate users to potential security breaches and what the organizational policies are in relation to confidentiality and the use of electronic mail.

The Internet is the latest tool in computer technology to make the world a smaller, more intimate place. With the appropriate computer hardware, software, server, and modem support, an individual can log into a multitude of web sites that span a wide range of nations, lifestyles, businesses, and recreational activities. The controversial downside to this vast "information highway" is the ability to disseminate different types of information found to be morally or legally offensive. However, technology is being developed and implemented that will allow users better control of their systems, with more accountability and responsibility being forced on those traveling on this vast highway.

Currently, the Internet offers nurses and other managers access to on-line clinical and administrative management information, as well as the ability to "chat" with other managers for collaborative problem-solving without the expense of traveling and long distance conversations. Bulletin boards exist in various nursing sites that allow the interchange of information between professionals. These sites become more specialized as they grow, targeting the interests and needs of their subscribers.

WRITTEN COMMUNICATION

The nurse manager cannot rely solely on verbal communication. Written communication provides important verification of verbal communication and discussion;

access to those unavailable for meetings; documentation of standards, policies, issues, and goals; and timesaving transmittal of details and facts.

When communicating with administration and ancillary services, the manager should write a short, concise memo clearly stating the issue at hand. A memo is not the place to slowly build a case; there is too much risk of losing the reader's attention. Back-up data and explanations can be attached and referenced. The manager's supervisor should receive a copy of important memos and should be consulted about forwarding them to others.

Memo Example

In the example in Box 4-7, a specialty care unit was hampered by delayed transportation of patients. This had been discussed in many meetings, and both the manager's supervisor and the Director of Transportation were aware of the issues. The Transportation Supervisor had assured the nurse manager that problems were now corrected and insisted service was adequate. The manager and her supervisor agreed that the Director of Transportation should receive a copy of the memo, but that the Transportation Supervisor should review it with the Director of Nursing.

··· box 4-7 ···

MEMORANDUM

DATE: November 13, 1999
TO: Alice Johnson
          Transportation Supervisor
FROM: Jean Brown, Nurse Manager
          Cardiac Catheterization Laboratory
RE: Transportation of patients for cardiac catheterization

Since our last meeting on October 12, I have carefully monitored transportation data to assess its effect on our patient care services. During the past month, 30 of 50 patients were delivered to the unit more than 30 minutes late, and 22 were held on the unit for longer than 45 minutes awaiting transportation after the procedure was completed.

This caused six cancellations of procedures because of lost time slots and a significant amount of overtime paid to staff to stay beyond scheduled shifts.

Patient safety was maintained, but they were quite frustrated by long waits and especially by cancellations.

Although I appreciate your efforts to improve services and also the constraints on your department, I feel we must further consider alternatives if we are to meet our goals of quality patient care. Please contact me in the next week to arrange a meeting.

Thank you.
jbw
cc: Jane Sessoms, Assistant Director
   Bill Elam, Director of Transportation

For an in-depth discussion of memos in daily practice, please refer to Chapter 5, "Day-to-Day Operations."

Other Written Products

Staff meeting minutes, recording of unit and individual goals, and performance evaluations and feedback also require written skills. Goals and evaluations are usually recorded in an institution-wide format. The manager should work with her/his supervisor and employees to ensure goals and evaluations are measurable, accurate, constructive, and clear. Ongoing meetings with the staff to discuss goals and progress should occur. Documentation of these meetings should reflect achievement, need for growth, and plans (in specific terms) to meet goals. This documentation will then support and verify the formal evaluation.

Staff meeting minutes are recorded to (1) ensure verbal information was heard, (2) document that all staff members received consistent information, and (3) supply detail that need not be discussed. In addition to recording attendance, minutes should be placed in a communication book or other device and signed by those staff who were unable to attend the meeting and have read the written minutes of the meeting. Memos, new policies and procedures, and written announcements introduced in meetings should be referred to in the minutes and placed in the book for sign-off. The manager should ensure this feedback loop is completed by all staff members by periodically reviewing for completion and giving feedback and direction as needed. These meeting minutes can also be helpful when orienting new team members.

PROBLEM COMMUNICATIONS

The new nurse manager must bring or develop a wide range of skills needed for her/his new role. As any staff nurse or nurse manager knows, conflicts with physicians, other team members, or difficult patients and families can present their own unique problems and resolutions. Historically, nurses have been subordinate to physicians. In addition, because nursing is a predominately female profession and medicine is a predominately male profession, gender differences can contribute to physician-nurse problems. As the numbers of female physicians and male nurses increase, physician-nurse relationships may improve. But traditional male physician domination still sometimes sets the stage for power and control games between physicians and nurses. Because of these factors, you may need your supervisor's support in the management of these conflicts. Some systems are openly addressing these concerns by establishing nurse-physician committees. The JCAHO or other standards for multidisciplinary care can be the catalyst for needed changes in the relationships between health care professionals that would affect patient care positively and support increased nursing professionalism.

Communication problems are often heightened by the need for some reporting mechanism when a patient is placed at risk, for example, when a procedure is done incorrectly. A staff nurse describes the situation, "The hospital administration wants us to tell them anytime a physician contaminates a subclavian catheter during insertion. The physician knows when he's done a procedure incorrectly, and it's not my responsibility to monitor him." In this example the nurse is incorrect in her assertion. The law, including today's courts' interpretation of it, requires the nurse to pursue affirmative actions for patients and to safeguard them against incompetent health care providers. Such affirmative action—according to the courts—would, as a minimum, include monitoring the physician, even to the extent of confrontation. Otherwise, the nurse would be considered negligent.[4]

These examples and others like them bring home this difficult but ongoing problem. Like any other area in conflict resolution, the individuals involved in such a problem can usually identify and work out the most effective solutions. This is where your tact and communication skills can be put to the test. However, in those instances where the patient is jeopardized, there is only one solution. A nurse's primary duty is to the welfare of the patient, and the physician must be reported. Of course, the nurse must go through the appropriate channels in the chain of command to ensure protection of self and the patient. This is the level where the nurse manager most often becomes involved. Beyond you, the usual route is your nursing supervisor through to an administrative representative. Many times the nurse manager will clarify the situation with the physician directly. By asking the physician to explain and by getting input from others and following facility policies, particularly on the completion of incident reports, the nurse manager can follow up on known episodes where the patient was at risk.

It is important to note that some studies have demonstrated that positive professional relationships are reflected in lower patient mortality rates. Those who have been in nursing for some years know intuitively that this would be true. This concept is further explored later in this chapter.

There are positive, proactive steps the effective nurse manager can take to facilitate and maintain ongoing open communications between staff nurses and physicians. In addition, the collaboration between nurses and physicians is increasing. According to the National Joint Practice Commission,[5] "Collaborative or joint practice in hospitals is nurses and physicians collaborating as colleagues to provide patient care." Some of the ways to increase cooperation are listed in Manager's Tip 4-5 on p. 96.

There is no question that increased collaboration of physicians and nurses as well as other clinicians will become the standard in all health settings. This era of doing more with less resources ensures that we all must work effectively together to meet patient needs. Respect must be valued and mutual for communications to be effective among all team members. We know that increased morale and "making a dif-

TECHNIQUES FOR IMPROVING NURSE-PHYSICIAN COOPERATION

✔ Establish a collaborative practice model.
✔ Provide assertiveness training for your staff, with an emphasis on clear communication skills.
✔ Be supportive by being an active listener for the nurses.
✔ Put the nursing or care philosophy and mission statement on the physician's bulletin board. This can help ensure that all are working towards the same goals.
✔ Develop and implement a buddy system to achieve these goals. Assign one nurse to one new resident or physician staff member. This will help increase the new physician's comfort level and ensure a complete orientation to your unit and to "how things are done." Most new physicians will welcome the opportunity for education rather than having to face learning by trial and error. In addition, such activities assist in the achievement of mutual respect and effective communications.
✔ Hear and understand both the physicians' and nurses' positions and roles.
✔ Develop and implement an integrated documentation system (if not currently available).
✔ Establish a physician-nurse committee for (1) collaboration (patient care review); (2) problem resolution, where indicated; and (3) continuing education.
✔ Provide ongoing education for nurses to ensure clinical expertise in care of patients. This promotes the nurses' self-esteem and is vital to effective communications or discussions with physicians about patient care.
✔ Schedule and maintain ongoing joint clinical care rounds for nurses and physicians. These are particularly important for planning care after discharge from your setting or program, considering increases in patient acuity, decreased lengths of stay, and increased patient turnover.
✔ Develop a communication process to keep physicians apprised of events, systems, or changes that affect patient care or their routines in your environment. For example, when you read your staff meeting minutes, look for these types of items. Then communicate them to the physician staff. Post a physicians' bulletin board on the unit. Information to post could include (1) new products selected and available for use; (2) staff changes and promotions; (3) QA/QI issues that affect your unit; (4) any research occurring; and (5) anything else that would give information to the physician that would facilitate being a part of the team.
✔ Involve physicians in new practice model development or in the planning of clinical pathways or other care protocols.
✔ Distribute communications about or from your area to physicians. It will help you and your staff by informing the physicians you work with in the facility. For example, accredited home health agencies or hospices are required to inform physicians of their responsibilities in the home care process. This is usually done at the time of first referral, by distributing a packet of agency information to respective physicians. This can include a welcome letter, signed jointly by the nursing and medical directors; the philosophy; the patient admission criteria; the types of patients that would be appropriate; an example of the referral form; and a brochure on the program. Follow-up could also

Continued.

be arranged to personalize this interaction or to address any questions that may have been raised by the information sent.

✔ Provide ongoing physician-and-nurse educational sessions. For example, the hospice medical director, the pharmacist, and the hospice/home care nurse could provide a seminar on "effective pain relief." These clinical conferences are useful to both nurses and physicians and, as such, are important to patient care collaboration. Some other areas could be ethical dilemmas, available resources for discharge planning, and clinical updates. Be sure to evaluate these sessions to ensure that nurse and physician needs are being met. In addition, ask physicians what topics they would like addressed in the future.

✔ Post the next scheduled session and specific information on the bulletin board. Some hospitals host Grand Rounds and have well-known clinicians speak on a particular topic. They invite all physicians, nurse managers, and staff members and may have an evening meeting over dinner.

✔ Be a role model to your staff in your communications and interactions with physicians. This is particularly helpful with "difficult" physicians.

✔ Host get-togethers on a regular basis for new residents or staff physicians and nurses to begin this pattern of effective communication and role definition from the onset.

ference" are important in nurse satisfaction and retention. The effective nurse manager can be successful as the catalyst to create this environment.

Coordination of Care Across the Continuum

One of the positive outcomes of the managed care revolution has been the need to improve patient care coordination across the continuum. Not only is it beneficial for a patient to have her/his care coordinated and discussed at the different sites of care, it is also more cost-efficient in terms of resource utilization to make sure that all the health care practitioners involved in a plan of care are "speaking the same language."

In recent years, collaboration has increased between the different professional clinicians involved in a plan of care, from the acute to subacute to rehabilitation to home care to outpatient through to community services. This collaboration is necessary because of the need to standardize elements of the care process. In so doing, we are able to measure accurately the outcomes of care and compare that data from one site or patient to another. It is necessary to clarify terms and establish a consistent frame of reference between all parties planning the care. Definitions of terms between health care providers are not always the same and may cause confusion that negatively affects the patient and the planning process. For example, if a nurse defines functional status in purely nursing terms and a physical therapist uses another definition, miscommunication and poor planning may occur. It is essential that care be planned, coordinated, implemented, and evaluated and that a common language is maintained.

In an effort to improve communication and standardize patient care protocols within existing professional standards of care, many agencies and health care systems have instituted clinical paths on certain patient care medical diagnoses and conditions. According to Marrelli and Hilliard in their text, *Home Care and Clinical Paths—Effective Care Planning Across the Continuum,* to make clinical pathways more effective, all the providers on the care continuum need to be involved in the development or adaptation of the care protocols. Besides the departmental representatives from the acute care setting, all the alternate site settings need to be represented so that effective planning can occur and problem areas addressed before implementation. This involvement also helps to ensure buy-in from staff at the alternate site settings. It is interesting to discover how little staff from one setting understand the role of staff from another setting and how more cost-effectively one setting can accomplish the same goals as another. This collaboration and planning is definitely an example of performance improvement.[6]

Nurse managers again are the only professionals who can span the different sites and can be the advocates for both the patient and the institution. They need to include all appropriate setting representatives as needed on the planning committees, so that time and efforts can be maximized.

Managed care has also focused on the benefits of patient care provided at settings other than the acute care hospital. Ideally, patients are treated at the lowest level of care needed, and will only utilize expensive, complex care settings as necessary. Home health care, subacute and skilled nursing facility care, and other forms of ambulatory and community care are becoming more involved in the patient care process. The hospital, no longer the only area where important care can be rendered, is simply another setting on the health care continuum.

THE WORK CULTURE

All work settings have a culture, which is the unique environment of the workplace. This culture includes the physical setting and layout, the management philosophy, and the written and unwritten rules for conduct and other activities. In nursing, the work of managing in this culture occurs in ongoing communications, usually with small groups, teams, or individual employees. A team is a group of people who perform the work of an organization to achieve that organization's goals.

Effective Team Building

Effective teams are the key to the accomplishment of all work. By the year 2000, it is projected that most organizations will be more decentralized and workers will be broken up into special work units, where they will have responsibility for all functions relating to their work.

These small teams will be autonomous for work products, including outcomes and even budget accountability. The cultures of some progressive companies are already structuring their work environments to facilitate this goal.

The Nurse Manager's Role With the Team

You manage a nursing unit where all work is accomplished by your team. Your team-building role provides a unique opportunity to develop staff, problem-solve, and meet the care needs of patients. The leader of any team determines the style of the team. Your most important and ongoing roles are communicator and being a role model. This is ensured through the activities in Manager's Tip 4-6 on p. 100.

Managers can create a motivating environment that empowers their nursing staffs. An environment where communications are open, where the manager listens, and where staff believe they have input and influence in decisions enables nurses to be committed. The team leader or manager must be trustworthy, honest, have good active listening skills, and communicate with the staff frequently about the achievement of the unit's and department's goals.

THE TEAM MEMBERS

Numerous categories have been used in labeling types of team members. Examples include natural leaders, initiators, motivators, loyalists, and other various types that contribute to a team's make up. In fact, labeling team members as types may be counterproductive. However, each of us may exhibit these characteristics in different situations.

The best groups function effectively when they have input into the methods to be used in reaching the defined goal. It has been said that the true test of effective management is how well the group functions when the manager is not present. Therefore use your staff's natural skills and abilities. We all do best in tasks that we enjoy. So, when possible, let staff members choose assignments or tasks they want to perform. These roles can be clear at the onset. For example, delegate organizational responsibilities to a particularly well organized staff member, someone who can remind you of the time, take minutes of meetings, or reorganize an ineffective process through to resolution with input from other involved peer nurses.

Team Problems

All teams or staffs can have problems at one time or another. These problems can range in scope and significance and can affect the functioning of the unit as a whole. These problems can include the following symptoms:

- Cliques.
- Increased errors or mistakes.
- Isolation of new staff members.
- Increased complaints.
- "We" versus "they" feelings.
- Scapegoating of specific staff member(s).
- Negative comments from peers or your manager.
- Decreased productivity.
- Silence.
- Failure to share needed information among team members.

MANAGER'S TIP 4-6

MANAGING A SUCCESSFUL TEAM

- ✔ Manage in a way that demonstrates respect to staff, peers, and others.
- ✔ Remind staff of the task at hand.
- ✔ Respect the team for their professional skills and knowledge.
- ✔ Project self-confidence.
- ✔ Show enthusiasm.
- ✔ Listen and problem-solve.
- ✔ Be flexible.
- ✔ Act as a role model.
- ✔ Provide support.
- ✔ Be organized.
- ✔ Continually use your human relation skills.
- ✔ Create an atmosphere of cooperation and collaboration.
- ✔ Keep the team on track and focused.
- ✔ Recognize staff.
- ✔ Give feedback.
- ✔ Share common goals.
- ✔ Give staff accountability and responsibility.
- ✔ Delegate effectively.
- ✔ Manage with a clear vision of where you are going; share it often.
- ✔ Allow staff to take risks.
- ✔ Provide encouragement and feedback.
- ✔ Clarify assignments when needed.
- ✔ Pilot staff-recommended changes.
- ✔ Listen to alternative solutions to daily challenges.
- ✔ Reward staff for work well done.
- ✔ Create and nurture rapport.
- ✔ Follow up on problems.
- ✔ Empower staff.
- ✔ Write about your team and their accomplishments in memos, newsletters, professional journals, and local papers.
- ✔ Be there to provide help when needed.
- ✔ Lead a well-balanced life.
- ✔ Create an ego-enhancing environment.
- ✔ Foster a cooperative environment.
- ✔ Demonstrate retention-directed management skills.
- ✔ Choose new team members effectively.
- ✔ Keep lines of communication open.
- ✔ Recognize individual nurses' contributions.
- ✔ Communicate to your supervisor the work accomplished by your team.
- ✔ Maintain and use your sense of humor.
- ✔ Share patient evaluation feedback with staff.
- ✔ Remove obstacles to work completion.
- ✔ Let go of owning all problems and solutions once you have delegated the work.
- ✔ Ask for suggestions on better ways to do things.
- ✔ Ask "What can I do to help you get your work done more effectively?"

When problem trends are identified, self-evaluation is indicated. Is the manager doing anything to increase the conflict? An example could be a reward system that reinforces undesirable behaviors. Does the staff feel or perceive that there are favorites who get better assignments or more staff education days than do others? For example, if one staff member goes to lunch with you, rotate this opportunity with all your staff. Certain behaviors or personalities can sometimes lead to conflict. The effective resolution of conflict is one of the responsibilities of all managers.

CONFLICT

It is important that the nurse manager remember that not all conflict needs management intervention. Welcome the existence of differences in your work setting. Much has been written on conflict management and individual styles for conflict resolution. It is thought that we all use different styles in different situations, though we may have a favorite style. Use the presence of conflict as a possible indicator of the need for change or problem-solving. Conflict can be a strong motivator for change or growth.

Your Role in Conflict Resolution Between Staff Team Members

The suggestions shown in Manager's Tips 4-7 and 4-8 can help facilitate effective conflict resolution. Two traits are needed for effective conflict resolution—trust and rationality.

MANAGER'S TIP 4-7

RESOLVING CONFLICTS

- ✔ Know that conflict is inevitable and not all conflict is destructive.
- ✔ Always work towards helping staff members settle differences themselves.
- ✔ View yourself not as a parent but as an objective observer only.
- ✔ Validate that you will not take sides.
- ✔ Be objective.
- ✔ Support harmony and resolution.
- ✔ Verbalize that staff members need to talk to each other and that you trust their problem-solving skills.
- ✔ Listen with understanding, not judgment.
- ✔ Clarify the issue only when necessary.
- ✔ Do not criticize or deny feelings such as anger or fear.
- ✔ Focus on maintaining the relationship between the conflicting parties.
- ✔ Create a problem-solving atmosphere.
- ✔ Offer your office space for a limited time for this discussion, when appropriate.
- ✔ Be able to identify a chronically complaining employee. This is important because such behavior can contribute to a depressing tone for the entire work environment.

MANAGER'S TIP 4-8

WHAT TO DO WHEN RESOLVING COMPLAINTS

✔ Listen to the complaint but set limits if it continues.
✔ Ask for the recommended solutions to the listed complaint.
✔ Work on the development of problem-solving skills for the staff members involved.

Considerations for Home Care Managers

THE IMPORTANCE OF EFFECTIVE COMMUNICATION

In home care, as in other health care delivery sites, effective communication is very important, both when working with clinical team members and when teaching patients and their families how to provide effective care at home. Due to the unique environment of home care, in which staff are in patients' homes most of the work day and available to office staff only by beeper and telephone, communication becomes more involved as well as more important.

All patient care managers need to understand how and what to communicate to the audience they are trying to reach:

- Peers (want to be included):   Tactical communication
- Subordinates (need to be instructed): Technical communication
- Supervisor (expects to be informed):   Strategic communication

Home care managers are also faced with regulatory and accrediting agency standards that focus on the effective communication and coordination of care across many professional disciplines, as well as between different providers of care (e.g., the home parenteral infusion pharmacy with an intermittent nursing visit agency, and home medical equipment company). Effective communication and timely documentation of communications between the service vendors and the patient care team led by the ordering or attending physician are needed both to achieve positive patient outcomes and to meet regulatory standards.

Case coordination, or team conferencing as it is frequently called in home care, is essential to effective care communication. It should occur at least twice a month, with all care providers attending, including the home health aide. Goals or outcomes of care that have been established need to be reviewed and revised based on the patient's progress, revised assessments, and identified new problems. The input of all team members should be respected and included in the planning process. The effectiveness of the care and the appropriateness of ordered services (or those services that should be ordered) need to be reviewed. Home care managers must ascertain that team conferences are productive and involve all team members. One or two problem patients and/or staff should not be

Continued.

Considerations for Home Care Managers

allowed to monopolize the discussion, and efforts should be made to adhere to an established agenda and include all staff.

Home care communication relies greatly on policies and procedures regarding staff members' notifying the office about patient care schedules, new admissions or changed assessments, and new or revised orders. A major problem in home care involves the timely documentation and submission of supplemental orders. Clinicians are required to update the physician on any significant changes in patient status and note new orders. The ability of the home care nurse or therapist to reach the physician on the first call is limited, and the exchange of telephone messages is common. Agency staff should be made aware of potential physician calls so that appropriate staff can react knowledgeably and accept any orders that might be given. Many agencies utilize staff voice mail/beeper communication systems so that clinicians can leave messages and receive direct answers that they can access from the field.

With the emergence of laptop computer documentation systems, modems, and cellular phones, communication has become more technologically complex but also more streamlined, making staff more accessible. However, confidentiality remains a major concern, especially for the staff member who receives or returns a call to the physician or office regarding another patient. The potential for confidentiality breach is enormous and the home care manager must ensure that the policies and procedures are present to cover these occurrences and staff are adequately oriented, trained, and supervised to minimize the chance of these breaches occurring.

SUMMARY

In conclusion, interpersonal skills important to the nurse manager include a variety of overlapping traits, activities, and attitudes.

The successful manager is open and supportive of staff, truly seeing them behaviorally as valuable resources. Constant communication, which is well planned, executed, and validated, combined with real caring and investment in staff creates an environment that fosters motivation, retention, and success.

The successful use of problem-solving skills ensures that the feelings and energy generated by conflict is directed towards creative resolution. This approach welcomes the uniqueness of all individuals and is potentially growth enhancing for individuals and teams.

References

1. Lancaster J: Creating a climate for excellence, *J Nurs Adm* pp 16, January 1985.
2. Kramer M, Schmalenberg C: Job satisfaction and retention, *Nurs 91* 21:51, 1991.
3. Swansburg RC: *Management and leadership for nurse managers,* Boston, 1990, Jones & Bartlett.
4. Horsley J: When to tattle on physician's misconduct, *RN* 4(12):17, 1978. In Luquire

R: Nursing risk management, *Nurs Manage* 20:56, 1989.
5. The National Joint Practice Commission: *The definition of joint or collaborative practice,* statement 4, September 1977.
6. Marrelli TM, Hilliard LS: *Home care and clinical paths—effective care planning across the continuum,* St. Louis, 1995, Mosby.

For Further Reading

Barr and Barr: *Leadership development—maturity and power,* Austin, TX, 1994, Eakin Press.
Covey SR: *The 7 habits of highly effective people,* New York, 1989, Simon and Schuster.
Donckers SW, Harris MD: Teleconferencing: home health administrators and educators enhance graduate education, *Journal of Nursing Administration* 22(10):38, 1992.

Drucker P: *The effective executive,* New York, 1967, Harper & Row.
Lombardi DM: *Handbook for the new health care manager,* Chicago, 1993, AHA Press.
Mackenzie A: *The time trap,* New York, 1990, Amacom.
Taylor MW: Listening a key management tool, *Pediatric Nursing* 17(4):390, 1991.

CHAPTER 5

DAY-TO-DAY OPERATIONS

LYNDA S. HILLIARD

T.M. MARRELLI

I t has been said that "managing makes a manager." However, it does help to have some information about the nurse manager's day-to-day duties and responsibilities before being faced with carrying them out.

Supporting effective day-to-day operations is the core of the nurse manager's activities. Staffing and scheduling personnel, delivering patient care through an appropriate nursing care delivery model, and meetings (e.g., leading staff meetings, organizational planning meetings, supporting patient care conferences) are all activities vital to the day-to-day functioning of a patient care unit or area. Information about these subjects, as well as others relating to the day-to-day operations of a nursing unit or area, is discussed in this chapter.

Intertwined with these subjects are strategies for their implementation, as well as the quest for cost-effective quality patient outcomes, with a focus on customer service. These are considered while working to promote the professionalism and satisfaction of the patient care staff.

CONTINUOUS QUALITY IMPROVEMENT: THE FOUNDATION FOR EFFECTIVE DAILY MANAGEMENT OF OPERATIONS

In the first edition of this book, quality assurance and improvement were discussed in a separate chapter outlining the program that would be developed and implemented to determine the effectiveness of patient care and services. However, as understanding of the continuous quality improvement (CQI) process evolved, it became more apparent that CQI was not an independent process, but one that must be intertwined in the daily operations of a department, as well as throughout the entire system. We have attempted to incorporate the elements of CQI throughout this book and will focus briefly on improving organizational performance (IOP) and its relationship to operational management.

Quality

Quality is a very difficult term to define, especially in health care. However, for the new nurse manager it is important to understand and integrate quality management and the elements of measurement, assessment, and improvement into daily routine, as well as to understand how each area's performance is aggregated into a total organizational view of quality for internal and external customers. In the late 1980s, the National Association of Quality Assurance (NAQA) Professionals defined quality as, ". . . levels of excellence produced and documented in the process of patient care based upon the best knowledge available and achievable at a particular facility."[1] The definition of quality in health care has grown to include the documentation of those structures, processes, and outcomes necessary to replicate quality of care. Quality of care is predicated on positive outcomes, customer satisfaction, best practices, and cost-efficiency.

Each health care system has the opportunity to develop its own philosophy of patient care delivery, based on its mission statement, values, and the accepted standards of practice for medical, nursing, and other health care providers. The Joint Commission on Accreditation of Healthcare Organizations (JCAHO), in an effort to help health care organizations systematically improve organizational performance, has restructured its standards to focus on the functions involved in patient care delivery, for all those settings that have the opportunity to be accredited (see Box 5-1).[2] The integration of the functions into the planning, delivery, evaluation, and revision process, all the while measuring outcomes against established benchmarks, is what constitutes an effective CQI program.

---

box 5-1

IMPORTANT FUNCTIONS ON WHICH JCAHO STANDARDS FOCUS

PATIENT-FOCUSED FUNCTIONS

1. Patient rights and organizational ethics.
2. Assessment of patients.
3. Care of patients.
4. Education.
5. Continuum of care.

ORGANIZATIONAL FUNCTIONS

6. Improving organizational performance.
7. Leadership.
8. Management of the environment of care.
9. Management of human resources.
10. Management of information.
11. Surveillance, prevention, and control of infection.

Adapted from *1995 Accreditation Manual for Home Care*, JCAHO, Oakbrook Terrace, IL, 1994.

Effective managers are never satisfied with the status quo, especially if there are methods to improve the products or service that their department produces. Those health care managers who "rest on their laurels" or maintain the same clinical practice or administrative operations because of a fear of change will not survive. Administrative and clinical functioning of a patient care department should continually be reviewed for appropriateness and efficiency, with all staff involved in reviewing what is done, for what reasons, and whether it is being done "right the first time." Managers must also think strategically and plan for the inevitability of change. Continuing education seminars, networking, and literature review of pertinent subject matter are all important for a manager to both maintain a general view of the marketplace and enhance the knowledge base to plan for the future. Box 5-2 outlines ten steps to help achieve and improve quality.[3]

---

box 5-2

TEN STEPS TO QUALITY TRANSFORMATION

- A quality organization begins by delighting customers and giving them more than they imagined possible.
- Remain close to your customer by knowing how customers use your products and services and any concerns or problems they have. Listen to customers and help them identify their needs.
- Lead customers into the future by anticipating their needs. Keep up-to-date on technologic advances that might prove useful to them.
- A flawless organizational system gives customers what they want, when they want it, with efficiency, precision, and consistency.
- The vision, values, and systems and process must be consistent with, and complementary to, each other. The vision answers the question, "What business are we in?" Values describe "how we conduct our business." Systems and processes are the sequence of activities by which all work gets done.
- Teamwork must pervade the organization and be based on commitment to customers and constant improvement. Teamwork results from a common understanding of the organization's vision and values, a dedication to delighting customers, and a shared commitment to the understanding and ongoing improvement of systems and processes.
- Everyone must know her/his job. This level of understanding requires both continuous education and regular feedback from each employee's customers. Employees must know how their work relates to the final product and ultimate user or consumer.
- Data and a scientific approach are used to plan work, solve problems, make decisions, and pursue improvement. All types of initiatives and activities are monitored to see how well they are working or can be improved.
- Select reputable companies from which to buy products or subcontract services, and develop working partnerships with these suppliers.
- Support and nourish improvement efforts of every group and individual in the company. Establish and maintain a spirit based on closeness with the customer, precise data, teamwork, constant improvement, and pride of work.

Adapted from Garland C, *Emporium Medical Supply*, Fullerton, CA.

Nursing Care Delivery Systems

New nurse managers need to understand the various types of nursing care delivery systems (NCDSs), the strengths and weaknesses of each, and their unique value in their own setting. In fact, Manthey[4] believes that of all areas of technical knowledge required to understand unit functions, NCDS operations, including work structure, make up the most important area to know.

An NCDS is the way in which nursing care is provided to the patient or, according to Wake,[5] is "an interacting set of structural elements which control the way care is provided." Manthey[4] says that a delivery system has to answer five questions:

1. Who is responsible for making decisions about patient care?
2. How long do that person's decisions remain in effect?
3. How is the work distributed among staff members—by task or by patient?
4. How is patient care communication handled?
5. How is the whole unit managed?

Team Nursing

Team nursing is an NCDS that uses an RN as a team leader to lead a group of nursing staff, which may include other RNs, LPNs, and nursing or patient care assistants, to care for a group of patients together. Sherman[6] identifies a basic belief of team nursing—team members of varying skill levels can contribute to patient-centered nursing care if their activities are coordinated by a professional nurse.

The team leader is responsible for assessing the patients' needs, planning the care, and delegating tasks to the other members of the team based on their skills and abilities in relation to the assessed needs of the patients and within the scope of their job description. In addition, the team leader evaluates the care given and revises the plan of care as necessary.

The key to successful team nursing is communication among team members and with the patient and family. This is usually facilitated with the patient care conference or team conference, which is held to coordinate care and to gain input from all the team members. Care can be evaluated from everyone's perspective and care plans developed and modified if necessary.

Proposed strengths of the team nursing system are efficiency and lower costs as compared with the total patient care and primary nursing systems, as well as making use of varying levels of nursing personnel. Theoretically, an esprit de corps develops among team members as they work together.

Negatives include a lack of accountability (because everyone is accountable) and the costs associated with the need for daily conference time. From the patient's point of view, several caregivers are involved with care rather than just one person. This results in a task-orientation versus total patient care approach, which may increase fragmentation of care.

Total Patient Care

Total patient care is an NCDS in which the RN or LPN is given the assignment of planning, organizing, and providing care to a group of patients. The RN supervising the LPN may perform some assessment and planning activities on the LPN's assigned patients, but generally most care is performed by the nurse assigned.

Strengths of the total patient care system are fewer caregivers for the patient and theoretically a better knowledge of the patient by the assigned nurse because the numbers of assigned patients are less than with team nursing.

Weaknesses of the system are a greater cost as compared with the team nursing system, a possible lack of continuity, and care coordination and accountability, and some aspects of care for the patient may be overlooked or neglected.

Primary Nursing

Primary nursing is an NCDS in which the RN, called a primary nurse, is given an assignment of planning and organizing all care for a group of patients for the total hospitalization of those patients, 24 hours a day. The primary nurse may also give the care but may delegate particular aspects. When the primary nurse is not on duty, an associate nurse cares for patients using the plan set forth by the primary nurse.

Primary nursing provides a nurse who has accountability for outcomes of care and care planning and documentation. Usually there is high patient satisfaction, continuity of care, and care of a high quality. Of course primary nursing is only as good as the primary nurse, and it is considered more costly than team or functional nursing because it usually relies on a larger number of RNs.

Modular Nursing

Modular nursing is an NCDS in which an RN is assigned the nursing care for a group of patients, generally grouped geographically, along with another caregiver (either an LPN or an unlicensed staff member). It is a form of team nursing in principle but uses smaller teams. it provides closer monitoring of care than does team nursing and uses fewer RNs than the primary nursing system. It is less costly than primary nursing and can use other types of caregivers. It is, however, less efficient and costs more than team nursing.

Functional Nursing

Functional nursing is an NCDS in which each caregiver is given a task to perform within the scope of her/his abilities and job description for all the patients on a unit. The patient thus sees a number of caregivers, each an expert in her/his particular task (similar to an assembly line). One nurse gives medications and another gives treatments, an aide changes linen, and so on.

It is considered the most efficient and least costly form of care, requiring fewer RNs. It takes advantage of differing skill levels.

However, from the patient's perspective, functional nursing focuses more on tasks rather than meeting the patient's needs with multiple caregivers, who may not see the patient as a whole. From the staff's point of view, boredom may result from performing repetitious activities.

Case Management

Case management is a form of primary nursing whereby the RN who is the case manager is responsible for managing the nursing care of a group of patients across all units during that hospitalization. Protocols are developed by the health care team to achieve clinical outcomes within prescribed time frames.

The case management NCDS has all the advantages of primary nursing. Although primary nursing is considered costly, the emphasis on protocols and meeting outcomes within defined time frames may help to save money in the long run because of reduction in lengths of stay. It also promotes nursing professionalism and collegiality with other disciplines.

NCDS Considerations

Organizations across the country have adopted one or more of the NCDSs described. Most have modified the original system as proposed and tailored it to meet the needs of their settings and the availability of staff. Keep in mind that any NCDS can be used with any skill level and mix of staff. Factors that influence which model is chosen include:

- The values and philosophy of the organization, especially those of the nursing department.
- The numbers and quality of available nursing personnel.
- Consumer demands.
- Competition in the marketplace.
- The retention status of staff members.
- Financial status of the system or how much money is available to spend on salaries for staff members.

In 1989, a survey was done by Wake[5] that asked for the status of, among other things, patient assignment in 1986 and 1989 and projections for 1992. Results showed that although team nursing and primary nursing NCDSs increased from 1986 to 1989, the case management system was projected by far to be the NCDS of choice by 1992. In fact, the case management system is not yet the NCDS of choice, but it undoubtedly will be in the near future. Obviously, we see that the models of nursing care delivery are continually evolving.

Professionally Advanced Care Team Model

Several NCDSs have been successfully implemented that may be of some interest. The Professionally Advanced Care Team model (ProACT) was developed through the work redesign process. This NCDS delineates two RN roles, the primary nurse and the clinical care manager. The primary nurse manages primary patients and delegates care giving to LPNs, associate nurses, and nursing assistants. The clinical care manager manages the entire hospital stay of a caseload of patients and ensures outcomes are met, much like the case manager. In addition, this model features unit-based nonclinical support personnel who function to relieve the nursing staff of non-nursing duties.

Partners in Practice

A form of primary nursing (or modular nursing) is partners in practice, which uses nurse extenders coupled with an RN to form a "partnership" to care for a group of patients together. The RN and nurse helper work the same schedule on the same shift to give care to patients. The RN assesses and plans care and delegates selected activities to the nurse extender.

Coprimary Nursing

Coprimary nursing is an NCDS whereby two nurses function together as one to be the primary nurse. They work the same shift on differing days to provide continuity. This system was developed originally in the critical care setting to help deal with the fragmentation of 12-hour shifts.

Patient-Centered Care

Many hospitals across the country have begun to restructure delivery systems to become more patient-oriented as opposed to hospital-oriented. Services are being organized around meeting the individual needs of the patient. This change in focus involves an analysis and redefinition of all activities involved with patients, a work redesign. It involves all departments that deal with the patient, including the nursing department, and is truly multidisciplinary in approach.

After work redesign is implemented, often "multipurpose" roles are created to perform ancillary tasks and procedures for patients that were formerly done in other departments, such as the admission registration process in admissions, a phlebotomy in the laboratory, or an electrocardiogram (ECG) in the cardiology department. Often these activities are all carried out in the patient's room by one person, who may be teamed with an RN. Many systems have the nurse manager or staff nurses supervising these individuals.

Forces driving the restructuring efforts are customer service concerns and consumer demands, quality and efficiency needs, and the need to reduce costs.

As more and more institutions are restructuring care, we are likely to see other innovations in NCDSs emerge.

Home Care Patient-Centered Care Teams

Patient care delivery models in home care have traditionally surrounded the case management of a patient by a registered nurse or physical therapist coordinating the care throughout the home care service, working with internal or external care providers such as the home health aide, parenteral therapy staff from a pharmaceutical agency, and possibly, home medical equipment providers. However, in many home care organizations case management was not truly implemented and care was not truly coordinated. A case manager may have been assigned, but nurses and other clinicians were assigned on a daily basis, based on scheduled availability of geographically assigned staff, as opposed to the assessed needs of the patient or an attempt to limit the number of different staff visiting a patient.

Home care organizations have received recommendations for improvement from the JCAHO if it was found that care was being provided by a large number of nurses and not being coordinated by either a case manager or patient care coordinator. In an effort to improve patient outcomes, standardize some of the elements of the care process, and provide more cost-efficient care, patient-centered care teams have emerged in home care as well. Many different models exist; however, the core element of each includes one case manager who is responsible for developing, coordinating, assigning, and communicating with the care team (including the ordering physician) to make sure the patient is following an individualized care plan or clinical path meeting the goals as established, based upon assessed needs.

This type of model is becoming more of a necessity as managed care practices impact the productivity of home care staff in different ways. It is not uncommon for the number of visits per patient to decrease dramatically under managed care plans (both Medicare-risk and general populations), as opposed to the current Medicare fee-for-service program. Physicians' groups or managed care case managers control and limit the types of services and number of visits a patient may receive from a home care organization. It is the responsibility of the home care case manager to communicate regularly with the authorizing staff to update the patient's condition and request more visits or other types of supplies or services. Traditionally, the case manager has worked with the physician in developing the frequency and duration of a plan of care based on assessed patient needs and communication focused on changes in the patient condition, not daily arguing or pleading for more services.

The typical home care patient-centered team may include a registered nurse/clinical specialist case manager to admit and regularly assess the patient and, dependent on caseload size, additional RN and LPN team members (e.g., revisit nurses, home health care aides, therapists and appropriately-credentialed assistant staff, and medical social workers). The case manager's productivity standards are less than the revisit nurses, since she/he is responsible for all the coordination and communication between managed care staff, physicians, and other team members, as well as the more labor-intense admission and recertification visits.

Evaluation of the Nursing Care Delivery System

One role of the new nurse manager is to analyze the current NCDS for adequacy. The following questions should be posed:

- Are patient outcomes being achieved in a timely, cost-effective manner?
- Are patients and families satisfied with care?
- Are physicians and other health team members satisfied with the care?

Information on how to conduct an in-depth analysis of an NCDS is available in *Nursing Assignment Patterns User's Manual* by Munson et al.[7] Piltz-Kirkby[8] discusses her experience using the tool on a rehabilitation unit. How to gather information on patient characteristics, nursing resources, and organizational support is described, as well as a way to analyze the data gathered. An informed decision can then be made to keep or change the NCDS.

Accreditation standards do not specifically dictate which type of NCDS a facility should adopt, but focus on care coordination, assessment, skills of the clinician matching the needs of the patient, and other facets of care delivery.

PROFESSIONAL PRACTICE MODELS

Although the NCDSs previously described address assignment of patients and roles of nursing personnel, they do not identify underlying professional practice issues such as autonomy in professional decision-making, budgeting of time for care activities, and nursing practice growth and development. Professional practice models do address these issues.

Shared Governance

Many facilities have adopted some sort of shared governance model within nursing. Shared governance is an organizational model that gives staff the authority for decisions, autonomy to make those decisions, and control over the implementation and outcomes of the decisions. Authority and accountability are shared between and among all the staff and the organization as partners.[9] Various models are in practice, but generally councils or cabinets of staff nurses are developed, with staff members serving in leadership roles and management advising and supporting. Bylaws are developed that guide the function of the nursing department. Nursing practice is defined by the staff through their council, and they, not the nurse manager, are accountable for the level of that practice. Likewise, staff members are accountable for all quality improvement and related activities. Continuing development and competency are determined by the staff council as well.

PRACTICE STANDARDS AND PROTOCOLS

As outcomes management becomes more integrated into the daily operations of all health care settings, the need for reliable and valid data is essential. In order for data to be reliable and valid there needs to be uniformity in how the data are collected and what criteria are utilized in collecting the data. In health care, it is important to keep a focus on the patient as a person and not just as an element of data. However, in order to analyze outcomes and how they were achieved, as well as to try to quantify the cost of care in terms of monetary values, core standardization has to occur. Chapter 7, "Resource Management and Budgeting Basics," discusses the financial implications of practice protocols.

Each health care setting has the ability to generate clinical practice standards or protocols based on acceptable medical, nursing, or other health care–related research data and standards of care. As mentioned in Chapter 7, the Agency for Health Care Policy and Research (AHCPR), a unit of the Department of Health and Human Services (DHHS), has developed a number of practice guidelines for various health conditions that are gaining much acceptance as the core foundation for development of specific practice parameters. Managed care organizations, as well as professional health care organizations, are accepting the validity of such practice standards, which, it is hoped, can decrease the legal liability of utilizing practice standards, once they are widely recognized and accepted by appropriate professional groups.

In the process of developing clinical pathways or protocols, planning staff need to be aware of the current scopes of practice of all licensed/credentialed staff, current regional or national published practice standards, and the desired outcomes of care. Many professional organizations have documented standards of practice for their individual profession outlining the scope of care that can be safely provided by competent, credentialed staff. However, as in all human-related endeavors, flexibility and the ability to apply appropriate medical, nursing, or other clinical judgment into practice standards or protocols are needed in any development and implementation of a prescribed plan of care based upon diagnoses and patient acuity levels. It is important to note that sound clinical judgment does not take the place of protocols as the health care industry moves towards standardization of care and care processes.

Compensation Innovation

Other concepts that have been integrated into some professional practice models are changes in compensation. Salaried nursing staff[9] and gain sharing[10] have been successfully implemented. The idea of "group-practices" has emerged; it is similar to the physician model. A group of nurses contracts to care for a group of patients for a specified period.[11]

The role of the nurse manager in the new practice models changes dramatically from the traditional one of "supervisor." The manager role is one of support and facilitation, ensuring that proper resources are available to the staff of her/his unit or area so they can do their jobs. Although it takes time to change philosophy, the result is a staff who have control over their practice, practice in a professional manner, and are more fulfilled and satisfied.

PATIENT CLASSIFICATION

A comprehensive staffing system comprises a patient classification system or acuity system, a master staffing plan, a scheduling plan, a position control plan, a budget, and reports that provide feedback to the manager on all components.

Patient classification is defined as "the categorization or grouping of patients according to an assessment of their nursing care requirements over a specified period of time."[12] It is seen as an objective and structured process to use in determining and allocating staff for patient care. In other words, patients are classified based on the projected number of nursing hours required to provide care. It can also be used as a measure of productivity and to help achieve compliance with accreditation standards. With increasing concerns about scarce resources, cost, and efficiency, patient classification systems can assist with appropriate allocation of resources to meet patient needs and provide justification as necessary for the decisions made. These standards imply the use of some type of patient classification system.[13] Patient classification can also be used to determine the cost of and bill for nursing services.

The patient classification process generally has two parts: (1) the actual classification procedure itself (using a tool), and (2) the quantification of the hours needed for the nursing care or staffing standards determined for each care category. In other words, for each category of care needed, from those patients needing the least amounts of nursing care to those requiring the most, an average number of nursing care hours is determined. Usually the tools are transferrable among facilities with similar groups of patients, but the staffing standards are not because of variations such as strength of support services, environmental factors such as unit or area layout, differences in philosophy including type of NCDS, differences in medical treatment, and levels and experience of nursing staff. Either work-sampling studies measuring indirect and direct care time or estimation procedures through trial and error can be performed to establish staffing standards for a tool borrowed from another facility.

Literally hundreds of patient classification systems are in use across the country. Some were developed specifically for a particular institution, and others were purchased from vendors. In a recent study, Nagaprasanna[14] found that a patient classification system is applicable to all types of nursing delivery systems. He also noted that internally developed systems were the most frequent type used, with four categories of patient acuity being the most common number of categories. Most facilities classify patients daily, and most systems are computerized, not manual. He found that the ease of classification is the highest rated factor in selecting a patient classification system.

The new nurse manager should become thoroughly familiar with the organization's system. Usually the system is managed by a person in the organization who assisted with its development and implementation; this is the person to seek out to explain the system. Questions to ask are outlined in Manager's Tip 5-1.

Two final points must be made concerning patient classification. First, the manager should understand that a high activity level in the unit or area and the acuity level of patients are not necessarily one and the same. Other causes exist that influence activity levels besides higher acuity levels, including factors such as experience and competency of the staff and presence and quality of support services at the unit level. Second, patient classification data are used as *supports* for decision-making. They never take the place of nurse manager judgment, nor should they ever be taken as facts not to be questioned. Despite millions of dollars expended to find the perfect system, no such thing exists. Keep that in mind.

MANAGER'S TIP 5-1

QUESTIONS TO ASK ABOUT CLASSIFICATION SYSTEMS

✔ **Is the patient classification tool based on prototype evaluation or on factor-analysis evaluation?** Prototypes are broad descriptions of three or four levels, and the patient is compared to the levels and placed in the one that most closely matches her/his description. Factor-analysis is based on a list of critical indicators that, when summed up, indicate a patient category.

✔ **What is the process by which the tool is used by the nursing staff?** It is essential to know each and every step. As issues arise, an awareness of where "things can go wrong" is helpful in solving problems with the system.

✔ **How is the system maintained and monitored? What is the role of the manager?** You need to know what orientation and ongoing educational programs for staff are available as relates to the system. Reliability checks are usually built into the system. Reliability means consistency between raters. Achieving agreement of at least 90% is generally considered acceptable. Validity monitoring refers to whether the system actually measures what it is supposed to measure. Sometimes surveys of the staff are done or actual time-motion studies are conducted to reaffirm the system.

✔ **How are data generated by the system interpreted? What should be done with data once they are interpreted?** Obviously the manager must understand what the data mean and then how they can be used as *aids* to staff the unit. Most systems compile and report an acuity number that is the sum of all patients' levels. They then predict the numbers of staff needed on the following shifts.

✔ **What exactly is patient classification used for in the organization?** Only for staffing on a daily basis? For the yearly budget? For productivity? For assignments? For placement of patients on units? For determining cost of patient services?

✔ **What are the current problems with the system?** The nurse manager should also ask this question of the staff. Sometimes there are problems with "acuity creep," or gradually rising acuity levels. Usually it is a managerial responsibility to identify and work at resolving problems related to the system.

SCHEDULING AND STAFFING

One of the activities that consumes the most time available to managers is scheduling and staffing. In a 1990 survey of nurse managers by the American Organization of Nurse Executives (AONE),[15] it was found that 11.1% of their time was spent on this activity. Not only time but concern and worry also are often hallmarks of this activity because the manager is ultimately responsible to see that the facility is staffed appropriately. There can be legal ramifications if staffing is not appropriate.

Nursing staff are very concerned about scheduling and staffing. In fact, the American Journal of Nursing[16] conducted a survey of its readers in 1987 and found that a "desired work schedule" was number one of the ten most important items that influenced decisions on whether to stay in nursing. Another top item was "having an adequate nurse/patient ratio," which again relates to scheduling and staffing. Clearly these two areas affect nurse retention, so sensibly, the new manager should be aware of scheduling and staffing practices and options.

As important as making sure that staff are scheduled and shifts or patient loads covered is the managerial responsibility of assigning patients to staff based on assessed patient needs, acuity levels, and the abilities and competencies of the staff members. Many hospitals and other types of health care settings have developed "cross-training" programs that assist in maintaining a stable staffing pool. Emergency department and critical care staff may be cross-trained, as may neonatal, labor and delivery, and pediatric nurses. With the emergence of more outpatient or ambulatory care areas, many nurses are cross-trained as "procedure" nurses to work in cardiac catheterization laboratories or the radiology departments for specialized angiography services. The core of a cross-training program lies in the regular testing of staff competencies to assess their abilities to work in those areas that they frequent less than their primary assignment.

Scheduling Patterns and Options

In the past 20 years, various types of scheduling practices and options have been developed over and above the traditional 8-hour-a-day, 5-day-a-week schedule. Several of the most prevalent patterns are noted in Table 5-1.

Almost every conceivable combination of shifts and days has been tried somewhere in the quest to find schedules that fit into every nurse's lifestyle, still meet patient care needs, and yet fit within the personnel budget and unit staffing model.

Cyclical schedules lend a degree of predictability to a staff member's schedule by using a pattern that is repeated consistently over a certain number of weeks.

Rotating shifts or permanent shifts for staff members are often an issue. Rotating shifts helps to share the burden of the less popular shifts and increases cooperation between shifts, but it does cause stress, depending on how often the rotation is done. Permanent shifts better meet staff members' needs, but a problem usually arises because most nurses want the popular daytime shift. In that case, seniority often determines who gets which shift. Rifts between shifts may happen with greater frequency with permanent shifts than with rotation shifts.

Control of staffing can be highly centralized, which may be more efficient and fair, or it can be decentralized, to the manager level or even down to the staff level, better meeting staff members' own individual needs.

Centralized scheduling can apply facility staffing and scheduling policies fairly throughout nursing, so no one individual or group gets preferential treatment. It is easier to use float or per diem staff to fill in empty shift spots with centralization. Computerization can be used with centralized scheduling. Data are entered on staff members' preferences and on facility policies and procedures regarding staffing and scheduling. Unit staffing patterns are identified, and patient classification data is entered. No doubt the advantages of computer scheduling include an easy-to-read schedule, fairness and consistency, and less time spent by the manager doing the schedule. However, centralized scheduling does set up a "we" versus "they" situation. Staff members may not feel any obligation to solve problems in the process of staffing and scheduling because it is not their job, but the job of the central staffing and scheduling office. They may feel that centralized scheduling lacks individual attention and also feel that the schedule does not meet their needs.

Decentralized scheduling can be done by the manager or the staff. If the nurse manager does the schedule, she often becomes an expert very quickly. She best knows the needs of the unit and of the staff, if the staff communicate with her. It does take the manager large amounts of time to produce a schedule, especially if a variety of scheduling options are available to the staff. One significant problem with the manager creating the schedule is that some staff members may perceive that others get favored treatment. Although this may not be true, it is very easy for the manager to misguidedly use scheduling as a reward-and-punishment system.

TABLE 5-1
Types of Scheduling Patterns

Pattern	Comments
8-hour/5-day week	Still the predominant pattern. Allows for a 30-minute meal break and a 30-minute overlap time if used for 24 hours.
10-hour/4-day week	Gives an opportunity for longer overlaps during activity times, meetings, or educational sessions. Allows the staff an extra day off each week.
10-hour/7-day week	Staff works 7 days on and has 7 days off. Gives better continuity and periods of time off, but fatigue has been reported by the end of the work week.
Baylor plan	Staff member works only on weekends and either works 2 days with 12-hour shifts and is paid for 36 hours, or 2 nights and is paid for 40 hours.
12-hour/3-day week	Gives better continuity over the course of the shift but not over the week. Allows staff 4 days off during week.

Self-scheduling by staff is being adopted by more and more facilities. Ringl and Dotson[17] describe it as a "process by which nurses collectively develop and implement the monthly work schedule." Criteria are mutually agreed on by the work group and applied. Peers can negotiate and trade within the guidelines. Often an individual staff nurse or scheduling committee oversees the process, a position that may be rotated among every member of the work group. The manager usually works with the group, especially when beginning the process. Although implementation of self-scheduling is not without problems, the process usually goes more smoothly the longer it is in place. Most staff members do not want to give it up once they have worked with it. It is said to increase job satisfaction, increase autonomy and control, and decrease turnover and absenteeism.[17]

Staffing

Despite the best scheduling efforts, staffing disasters do occur. Nurse managers should be aware of the options available to deal with these crises and of the fact that everyone has them at one time or another, to a greater or lesser extent.

Sick calls are notorious for causing the manager headaches. They can be handled in a variety of ways, depending on the options available in your facility. Manager's Tip 5-2 outlines some of the methods that may be used.

There are pros and cons with each method used. One point to make about the final option is that new managers particularly often work the shift themselves because it is the easiest solution. Although it may initially solve the problem, working as a staff member by necessity leaves other parts of the job undone and may set a precedent for what to do in a "crunch"—call the nurse manager. This may ultimately hurt the staff more than it helps them. It is up to the manager to help the staff learn that each member has a job to do that is valuable and to get them to feel a responsibility to help with staffing as much as does the manager.

MANAGER'S TIP 5-2

HANDLING A SHIFT THAT IS NOT COVERED

✔ Use a float, per diem, or agency nurse assistance.
✔ Ask a part-time staff member to work the extra shift.
✔ Ask a staff member to work for the person who is ill and cancel a subsequent shift later in the week.
✔ Ask a staff member of the previous shift to stay over for either part of the shift or the whole shift.
✔ Ask a staff member on the shift following the shift in question to come in for the whole shift or part of the shift.
✔ Substitute one type of job classification for another, such as an LPN for an RN.
✔ Do without anyone.
✔ Work the shift yourself.

Sometimes, if the supply of staff cannot be obtained, the manager can meet the need by working from the other side of the equation; that is, by reducing the need for staffing by transferring patients, screening types of patients that enter the system and thereby lowering acuity, or by "closing" beds.

Particularly during periods of nursing shortages, the manager might experience high vacancies on the unit. Although the solutions identified in Manager's Tip 5-2 for sick calls might help on an occasional basis, staff burnout will occur if they are used for prolonged periods. Using agency or traveling nurses has helped many facilities cope with vacancies until positions could be filled permanently. Closing, or "holding," beds also helps the situation. This practice, however, may decrease revenue for the facility if the patient goes elsewhere. The reasons for the vacancies and/or why positions cannot be filled should be thoroughly investigated and the causes fixed.

A master staffing plan (i.e., the guideline or plan by which the area is usually staffed) is usually developed for each area or unit. It is important for the manager to secure a copy of the plan and understand its components backwards and forwards. The components are the staffing pattern that gives the numbers and types of staff members to schedule on each shift and the numbers and types of staff members to hire to fulfill the pattern.

The design of the staffing pattern is based on a standard or statistic determined by the facility. That statistic will vary from facility to facility and might include factors such as patient acuity level and associated required hours of nursing care, census, numbers of procedures, and so on. Table 5-2 displays a staffing pattern for a 33-bed general surgical unit. The statistics that determined this pattern were patient acuity with associated hours of nursing care and patient census. Remember that this pattern is built on *averages*, usually identified from historic data. As you know, anything can happen, in which case deviations will occur from the pattern.

The pattern displayed indicates the number and type of staff members that should be routinely scheduled based on an average daily census and acuity score, which dictates the hours of nursing care desired. Decisions were made about the distribution of staff members by job category based on patient needs and work requirements.

The pattern should be reviewed periodically to see if staffing practices need to be changed based on statistical increases or decreases or on other factors such as the strength of support departments or changes in patient mix or flow.

From such staffing pattern is built a full-time equivalent (FTE) budget to which nonproductive hours are added, such as vacation, holiday, and sick hours and staff development time. An FTE is equal to 2080 hours worked per year (i.e., what a person would work if 40 hours a week, 52 weeks a year were spent working). The budget is then translated into positions that are designated full-time or part-time, and it is used as a basis to hire personnel.

It is a good idea to share the staffing pattern with staff members so they understand how it was developed and can assist in supporting it.

TABLE 5-2
Example of Master Staffing Pattern

33-bed capacity	Su	M	Tu	W	Th	F	Sa	
DAY SHIFT								
RN	4	5	5	6	6	5	4	35
LPN	1	2	2	2	2	2	1	12
AIDE	2	2	3	3	3	3	2	18
TOTAL	7	9	10	11	11	10	7	65
EVENING SHIFT								
RN	4	5	5	5	5	5	4	33
LPN	1	1	1	1	1	1	1	7
AIDE	1	1	1	1	1	1	1	7
TOTAL	6	7	7	7	7	7	6	47
NIGHT SHIFT								
RN	3	4	4	4	4	4	3	26
LPN	0	0	0	0	0	0	0	0
AIDE	1	1	1	1	1	1	1	7
TOTAL	4	5	5	5	5	5	4	33
TOTAL NURSING HRS	136	168	176	184	184	176	136	165.7 (average)
AVERAGE CENSUS	25	30.5	32	32.8	32.8	32	25	29.9 (average)
HOURS OF CARE	5.40	5.50	5.50	5.60	5.60	5.50	5.40	5.54 (average)
AVERAGE ACUITY	2.20	2.30	2.40	2.45	2.45	2.40	2.30	2.37 (average)

LIABILITY CONCERNED WITH STAFFING

On a daily basis, the nurse manager often faces the problem of trying to staff the area or unit with dwindling resources while still maintaining a standard of nursing care. Indeed, the manager's job description usually states something like, "is accountable for staffing the unit on a 24-hour basis." Questions may arise as to the liability of the nurse manager in relation to unsafe staffing levels; to float, registry, or agency nurse errors; to staff refusal to accept a unit or float assignment; and possibly to nurses walking off the job. As background for addressing these issues, the nurse manager should become familiar with the facility's rules, regulations, policies, and procedures concerned with staffing, floating, and overtime. They will help direct decisions that must be made when problems arise. If the day comes when all options to cover an unsafe staffing situation have been tried to no avail, the next step is to communicate the inadequate staffing situation to the supervisor.[18] The guiding principle is that of reasonableness. If the nurse manager has done everything possible to solve the problem and has communicated that fact to the appropriate persons, then she/he is most likely absolved of liability for the situation. The situation should be documented in a report, dated and signed, and sent to the manager's supervisor. The write-up should be factual and describe what effect the situation may have on patient care.

The use of float, registry, or agency nurses is one way some facilities are coping with the nursing shortage in general or with occasional staffing deficiencies. Is the nurse manager liable for their actions? According to Fiesta,[19] the manager may be placed in secondary liability for these nurses. These nurses must be screened and oriented as are the regular staff. Baillie et al,[20] regarding float nurses, said, "Regardless, before floating any nurse, supervisors should determine her level of knowledge, the skills necessary, and functions required in the new assignment and provide adequate orientation."

With agency nurses, the manager should try to assign them to low-risk situations and ensure that the patients realize the nurse is an agency nurse. If any question arises as to competency, the manager has a duty to report that, in writing, back to the agency. Of course, the nurse manager should follow the facility's standard operating procedures regarding communication with the agency.

What if a staff nurse refuses an assignment or threatens to walk off the job? It is wise not to react too quickly to the situation. Often the refusal or threat results from fear or feeling unprepared. The manager should sit down and unemotionally discuss the situation with the nurse. Find out what would make the nurse accept the situation and then attempt to remedy the problem if it seems reasonable. If it does not seem reasonable and if, after talking, the situation is not resolved, the manager should be sure the nurse has been given a clear and direct order that is not misinterpreted as a suggestion or request or as advice. The nurse should be queried as to whether the order is understood and is clear and whether she/he is refusing to do the order. The manager may want to forewarn the nurse of possible consequences if the order is refused. These consequences could be disciplinary action and perhaps even being fired, depending on the facility's personnel policies and practices.

Delegation of Nursing Tasks

Delegation of nursing tasks has been a growing controversy during the past few years, as hospitals instituted nursing care models that included unlicensed assistive personnel, initially as a measure to meet the demands of the nursing shortage and then as a measure to control or cut the cost of providing primary care when nursing salaries rose and reimbursement dropped. With factors such as increasingly "sicker" patients being hospitalized for shorter lengths of time, the increased demand to cut the number of nurses at the patient's bedside and replace them with unlicensed personnel, and the downsizing or closing of acute care hospital beds, the loss of registered nursing positions has caused major rifts in patient care philosophy between nursing staff and nursing management in many areas of the country.

The new nurse manager must realize that there are different health care providers who can safely and effectively provide care to patients if they function within the constraints of their state or national scope of practice and protocols of care. The change from primary to patient-centered team nursing advocates using unlicensed personnel to assist with those elements of patient care (e.g., bed baths, feeding, venipuncture) that had been accomplished by nursing assistants in the past. The important elements for both nursing staff and management are the training and credentialing of the unlicensed staff member. These staff members, similar to the home health aide in home care, are integral and useful and can bring new perspectives to the care planning process. However, their practice needs to be structured, supervised, and delegated appropriately.

Delegation has been described as the ability to assign work to a subordinate. However, the most important element in delegation is the ability to assign to another the responsibility and authority to complete a task with the knowledge that the individual has the capability to accomplish the task successfully. According to nurse attorney Kathleen Flynn Peterson, ". . . the judgment one uses in the act of delegation, not one's accountability for the act performed, is essentially the issue."[21] All nurses, but especially the nurse manager, need to be aware of and trust the competencies of the staff members with whom they are working. The risk management of such a situation lies in whether the nurse making the assignment or delegating authority had reasonable knowledge that the delegatee had the competent ability to carry out the task. What better way to establish trust between team members than to have standardized protocols and competency levels that must be met by all staff members in particular job categories? Those competencies should be extended to all staff who either float or are hired temporarily from registries to provide safe, competent care on fast-paced patient care units.

Finally, nurses need to rid themselves of the widely held belief that they are the only ones who can provide the best care. They need to learn to view themselves as the *leaders* of the work group, rather than the work group itself, and focus on what they do best: assessing, planning, and evaluating the care that a patient receives. We cannot do it all alone—especially when caring for sick patients across the care continuum.

CREDENTIALING AND COMPETENCY

Credentialing continues to be a major issue for all professional and licensed or certified staff. Credentialing encompasses licensure, accreditation, certification, and academic degrees.[22] The nurse manager plays a major role in ensuring that the process is implemented and that the staff practicing in her/his area are competent to care for the assessed needs of the unit's patients. Credentialing came about because it benefits and protects the patient by ensuring that the nurse has certain minimum skills and abilities. A professional license may ensure skills and abilities on entry into practice, but it *does not guarantee ongoing competency.* With medical and nursing practice changing so rapidly, additional credentialing activities must be added to licensure to ensure ongoing competency.

During the interview, the nurse manager discusses degrees and experience with the potential new employee. Licensure is checked, and a copy is made (based on state law) and inserted into the personnel file if the nurse is hired. Other information on courses attended may be obtained.

Usually during an orientation period, performance standards are met by the orientee. A skills inventory is completed after satisfactory demonstration of skills such as patient assessment, care planning, or medication administration, and this is maintained in the personnel record of an individual nurse. This inventory needs to be dated and signed. The skills inventory, or orientation checklist, provides legal documentation of professional skills competency. Additional specialty courses may be completed and tests taken that show mastery of the material (e.g., fetal monitoring or group therapy facilitation). The nurse manager's role is to ensure that this process happens through to filing the results. Often the skills inventory will be distributed, explained, and even completed, but never make it to the personnel record. (For an in-depth discussion, please refer to Chapter 4, "Communications.")

Remedial study may need to be undertaken if deficiencies are identified through critical incidents. It may be up to the manager to see that a plan is formulated with the individual nurse to correct deficiencies and attain the necessary skills and knowledge to improve performance. As discussed in Chapter 3, "Human Resource Management," competency evaluation is an important tool in the CQI process. An ongoing program of education and evaluation of both the general and the specialized skills of staff is needed to ensure quality outcomes.

It is important that the nursing staff understand why their competence is being checked and that they participate in the determination and development of the plan for ensuring competency.

Another aspect of credentialing is external certification. Almost every nursing specialty organization has a mechanism for certification. A test is taken and, in some cases, proof is required for a certain amount and type of clinical experience. Attainment of certification ensures a certain level of knowledge. For more information on certification, please refer to Chapter 12, "Where to from Here?"

Many facilities promote external certification by reimbursing nurses or by making it part of the requirements for a higher level within a clinical ladder system. Review courses associated with particular tests may be given in the facility. Manager support of external certification helps the staff pursue this additional level of professional expertise.

MEETINGS

All organizations hold meetings of one type or another, health care systems being no exception. Indeed, because the nature of the business usually encompasses 24 hours a day, 7 days a week, with a multitude of various departments and disciplines participating, the need for meetings may be even higher than in the industrial or general business sector.

New nurse managers must acquire the skills for either leading or helping others to lead meetings if the managers are to function at an optimum level in today's modern health care organizations. Gone are the days when a manager issued a dictum without consulting others in the work group. Group problem-solving activities and planning for change with group consensus are common practices, and leaders are needed to make the meeting processes efficient and help ensure the best outcomes.

STAFF MEETINGS

In general, the most common meeting a new nurse manager will lead is the group staff meeting. Purposes of a staff meeting vary depending on the situation for which the meeting is called (Table 5-3). Identifying the purpose is important because that assists group members in knowing what is desired of them and gives the nurse manager some guidance on what leadership techniques to use.

Meetings are expensive when the salaries of all involved are analyzed. Thus some techniques can be used to make a meeting efficient and get its purpose accomplished. Box 5-3 on p. 126 describes behaviors for leading an effective meeting.

Attendees at the group staff meeting are usually chosen according to the philosophy of the organization and past practice. Options include meeting with just the members of a particular position (i.e., RNs or nursing assistants); all staff members from a particular shift; or the total staff. There are pros and cons for each grouping. Small groups of 4 to 12 people seem to work best together. However, it is best to allow the group as a whole to decide who should attend the staff meetings. They should also determine the frequency, time of the day, day of the week, and length of the meeting.

TABLE 5-3
Purposes of Staff Meetings and Leadership Techniques to Use

Purpose	Techniques
Giving information (manager to group)	• Be sure the group understands what has been told to them by soliciting questions, approval, criticism, and so on.
Receiving information (group to manager)	• Ask clear questions and listen. • Use a "round robin" technique to solicit information from less verbal group members.
Interactional (group and manager) Problem-solving/decision-making	• Combination of above. • Help group identify real problem. • Use brain-storming techniques for alternatives. • Get consensus of solution. • Ensure actions are assigned.

---

box 5-3

TWELVE BEHAVIORS FOR LEADING EFFECTIVE MEETINGS

1. Prepare by drawing up an agenda well before the meeting, posting it, and allowing addition of items by the staff. Identify the purpose of the meeting.
2. Be sure all agenda items are necessary. Some might be better addressed in a memo, a message posted on the bulletin board, or dealt with on a one-to-one basis.
3. Start and end promptly. Keep on schedule. Close the discussion if necessary but be prepared to readdress unfinished business later.
4. Clarify and summarize discussions and decisions so the group is clear on outcomes. Lend structure to the discussion.
5. Ask vocal members to allow others to contribute. Encourage the less vocal members to talk.
6. Keep a neutral, friendly, and respectful attitude while leading. Thank everyone for attending.
7. If necessary, request that arguments, criticisms, and side conversations be held until after the meeting.
8. Set up an environment conducive to the meeting, including adequate ventilation, room temperature, and seating. Interruptions should be kept to a minimum.
9. Have all hand-outs available, including agenda.
10. Assure that minutes are taken.
11. Know that there may be more agenda items than time to discuss them all.
12. Prioritize agenda items and adhere to prepared agenda.

It is through documentation of the staff meetings (minutes) that evidence can be found that accreditation standards are being met. Thus it is vitally important for the staff meeting minutes to be accurate, specific, and detailed as to discussions, decisions, action plans, and so on.

Minutes should be retained on the unit for at least 3 years. However, the facility record retention policy should be followed in any case. The suggestions listed in Manager's Tip 5-3 describe important points to document in staff meeting minutes.

Two issues frequently arise in relation to staff meetings that the new nurse manager must often address: (1) the lack of attendance at staff meetings and (2) pay for attendance. In the former case, this is a problem the staff itself should address to determine the cause(s) and the solution. Absenteeism may be related to inconvenient times, inefficiently run meetings, or several other problems. Some organizations annually evaluate meeting structure to assist in meeting staff needs. Regarding the latter issue, most organizations have pay policies that outline whether staff members are paid for time spent at staff meetings when coming in on their own time. If not, a different policy would need to be developed by HR and/or Nursing Administration personnel because such a policy would affect the budget throughout the nursing department, if not the entire facility.

At times, the new nurse manager may lead other groups besides staff groups. These may include ad hoc groups formed to address issues or goals of the depart-

MANAGER'S TIP 5-3

IMPORTANT POINTS TO DOCUMENT IN STAFF MEETING MINUTES

✔ Who did attend and who did not attend.
✔ Issues discussed and decisions regarding the issues, with an emphasis on those related to patient care.
✔ Quality improvement monitoring results should be presented with conclusions identified, recommendations by the group noted, and action plans listed. The process for evaluation should be identified by the group, highlighting the group's involvement in the process. When problems are corrected, this should be identified in the minutes.
✔ Any issues relating to patient care standards, standards of practice, or patient care delivery systems should be detailed, along with the resultant decisions and actions. Reports by staff representatives on committees should be documented.

ment or facility. The same principles identified earlier can be applied to leading these groups as well.

CLINICAL CONFERENCES

In today's fast-paced, complex, highly regulated health care environment, it is essential that patient care be administered efficiently so patient outcomes can be achieved as rapidly as possible. Clinical conferences help in this process by assisting in the coordination of care for the patient among all the disciplines involved. Duplication of effort and unnecessary confusion and frustration for the patient, family, and health care team can often be eliminated by holding a clinical conference.

Although the primary nurse or the RN most closely associated with the patient usually leads the conference, the new nurse manager definitely has a role to play in the process. Mahan[23] believes that the nurse manager suggests, encourages, validates, role models, and educates and is a resource person and quality control agent.

Various members of the health care team may participate, including the physician, social worker, utilization review nurse, pastoral care staff, therapists, dietician, home health nurse, and any others deemed necessary.

Often the family and the patient participate in the conference as well. Once someone on the team, the patient, or the family decides a clinical conference is necessary, a leader is chosen, persons who should attend are identified, and a mutually accepted date and time are chosen. A conference room is procured. Arrangements may need to be made to cover the RN's assignment while she/he attends the conference. At the beginning of the conference, attendees are introduced, the purpose is highlighted, and the leader gives a brief overview of the patient's status, encouraging others to add additional data. Issues are identified, alternatives are discussed, and an action plan is formulated. Consensus is reached on follow-up and evaluation plans and the need for further meetings. The whole plan should be in the patient's record for easy access by all health care team members.

Documentation of the clinical conference should go beyond writing the action plan in the patient's record. Consistent documentation of attendees and the process and outcome of the conference will help demonstrate meeting these accreditation standards on care coordination.

ROUNDS IN THE CLINICAL AREA

Rounds made by the nurse manager in the areas where care is given can accomplish several things in a relatively short period. Making rounds gives information as to the performance of the staff because nursing care can be observed in practice and be compared with standards. Patient satisfaction with care received can be assessed by conversing with patients. Checks of the environment in regards to compliance with public health and safety standards can be done, and the area can be surveyed for aesthetic or other problems.

Although there is no hard-and-fast rule, daily rounds are suggested. Observations thus occur over a long period, and erroneous conclusions based on just a few observations can be avoided. Times of rounds during the day or night can be varied. Making notes as rounds are done assists in following up on issues that are identified. Staff members see the nurse manager as they work and may be more prone to bring up new issues when they see the manager. Stevens[24] feels that the presence of the manager on the nursing unit has the effect of decreasing the perceived distance between the employees and the manager. Also, the nursing staff feels that the manager knows what is going on, and this communicates authority.

Rather than putting patients on the spot with pointed questions concerning their perceptions of the quality of care, it is better to ask open-ended questions that might be less threatening, such as, "How is everything going?," "What is going on?," or "How are you doing?" If a patient's answer indicates the possibility of a problem, the manager can then focus the questioning further to get to the problem. Public health and safety standards should be reviewed by the manager by meeting with the person in the facility who is the most knowledgeable about them. One suggestion is to make a checklist from the standards that can be used during rounds to assess compliance. Aesthetic issues such as worn, broken, or tattered furnishings and building materials can be noted during rounds. The manager should view the unit or area as a patient or family might view it (similar to a hotel) and pass on a list of the deficiencies to the responsible department. Also, consider bringing in an objective person and asking for her/his aesthetic assessment and feedback for improvement.

Usually the list taken on rounds will have several items on it that the manager should plan to follow up on.

PRIORITIZING DUTIES AND TIME MANAGEMENT

A manager's work is never done, and there is never enough time to do it all. Those concepts are difficult for a new nurse manager to accept. By the end of the day, as a staff nurse, most likely all one's tasks were finished. The nature of a manager's work is longer-term, and projects and activities may take more than just a day—often months, and occasionally years—to complete. On a daily basis, managers must decide what activity or project takes precedence over another as they are faced with multiple and sometimes conflicting demands. How does the new manager prioritize her schedule? Manager's Tip 5-4 presents some suggestions to help manage tasks and time.

Patients are important to a staff nurse, and they still are to a manager. Issues surrounding patients should be addressed promptly, such as patient complaints, staffing issues, or concerns related to supporting patient care. Top priority should be those issues that meet human needs.[25] In other words, patients, families, and staff concerns take priority over preparing for a meeting or justifying a budget variance.

At the beginning of each day, a "to do" list should be made in descending order of priority. Unanticipated problems may occur throughout the day, so priorities will need to be reset. This is common and really no different from when the manager was a staff nurse.

One trap new nurse managers fall into is that of trying to solve everything for everybody. In their eagerness to prove themselves to their subordinates, they take on the world. This does nothing more than frustrate the manager, if not immediately, then in time. Be very careful of reverse delegation by your staff. It is wise to adopt a coaching attitude, assisting them in solving the problem and implementing the solution, rather

MANAGER'S TIP 5-4

DEALING WITH THE WORKLOAD

✔ Make a "to do" list.
✔ Organize your office by labeling file folders for each staff member, for staff meeting agenda items, and for issues to discuss with your supervisor.
✔ Place agendas and minutes of all meetings you attend in folders.
✔ Delegate activities to others when possible.
✔ Always question whether a problem or an issue is yours to own or whether it is better handled by another person.
✔ Organize communication with staff members by using bulletin boards and communication books.
✔ Always carry a calendar and write down standing meetings, lunch, and other appointments.
✔ Schedule time in your calendar for planning and organizing.

than ending up with all the problems heaped on your back. Solving problems can help the staff grow professionally as well as give them a different perspective.

Sooner or later the supervisor's priorities will clash with those of the manager. Rather than becoming frustrated, do not be afraid to negotiate a change in the project or the timeline.

DOCUMENTATION

Webster's New World Dictionary[26] defines documentation as "the supplying of documentary evidence . . . and the collecting, abstracting, and coding of printed or written information for future reference." This simple definition fits all of the varied and important roles that documentation, or the process of documenting and demonstrating delivery of patient care, assumes in health care. Nursing entries that appear in the medical or clinical record reflect the standard of nursing care, as well as the specific care provided to the patient. Other health care team members make decisions for further care based on the nursing entries. Also, today numerous third-party payers make legal and quality judgments, as well as administrative and payment decisions, based on the clinical record. Nurses have many responsibilities, all ultimately directed towards patient care. Because of these responsibilities, the actual task of documentation must sometimes be relegated to the end of the shift.

According to the AHA, patient charts now average 70 to 100 pages. This means that most midsized hospitals process 250,000 to 360,000 pieces of medical information each year.[27] The typical medical record may be read by a minimum of 10 persons during a patient's initial 24 hours in a health facility. These may include the admitting or attending physician, three nurses on different shifts, the utilization review specialist, several nurse aides, and a dietician. They may also include a surgeon, an anesthesiologist, and various technicians and therapists. With so many people depending on the medical record as a reliable and up-to-date source of patient information, the importance of the data contained in the record becomes evident. For an in-depth discussion of documentation, please see Marrelli's *Nursing Documentation Handbook* (St. Louis, 1996, Mosby).

THE PROFESSIONAL NURSE'S ROLE IN DOCUMENTATION

The professional nurse's entries in the patient's clinical record are recognized as a significant contribution documenting the standard of care provided to a patient. As the practice of nursing has become more complex, so too have the factors that influence the purposes of documentation. These factors include the requirements of regulatory agencies, health insurance payers, accreditation organizations, consumers of health care, and legal entities. The nurse must try to satisfy these various requirements all at once, often with precious few moments in which to accomplish this important task.

Any nurse writing a clinical entry today could be trying simultaneously to meet the standards of JCAHO, various insurers, state and federal laws and regulations, and other professional organizations. Fortunately, most hospitals have integrated many of these requirements, when possible, into hospital policy or procedure manuals.

The written clinical record is the professional nurse's best defense against litigation when malpractice or negligence is alleged. The increased specialization of health care providers and the complexity of patient problems and associated technology have contributed to multiple and varied services being provided to patients in a shortened time frame. The medical record is the only source of written communication, and sometimes the only source of any communication, for all team members. The members not only contribute their individual assessments of interventions and outcomes, but actually base their subsequent actions on the record of events provided by other team members. As such, the actual entries must be recorded as soon as possible after a change in the patient's condition is noted, an intervention occurs, or the response to a treatment is observed. Nurses can have their practice well represented and quality demonstrated through thorough, effective documentation. Manager's Tip 5-5 explains the importance of outcome criteria, process, and standards of care to such documentation.

MANAGER'S TIP 5-5

KEY TERMS RELATED TO DOCUMENTATION

✔ **Outcome criteria**—Outcome criteria are the desired results on completion or the objective (or demonstrable) evidence observed at the end of care (e.g., a patient's anticipated knowledge or activity level on discharge). In a specific case, a patient with diabetes mellitus returned to self-care status. Patient able to demonstrate all activities noted on the diabetes mellitus checklist on discharge and patient verbalized that initial complaints were resolved and needs met.

✔ **Process**—A process is specifically how the care is provided. An example would be a standard that requires that all patients receive a complete assessment within so many (specify) hours of admission. The specific parameters that must be included in the assessment would also be identified.

✔ **Standards of care**—There is a growing emphasis on the standardization of care, policies, and procedures. All patients or clients are entitled to a certain level, or standard, of care. As patients become more proactive consumers in the purchase of needed health care services, patient satisfaction with care provided becomes the key to the facility's reputation and ultimate survival. Nurses, because of their healing skills and other areas of proficiency, are pivotal in fostering patient satisfaction. The roles of the nurse as patient advocate, listener, and teacher have become widely accepted in recent years. With these roles comes the responsibility of maintaining the hallmarks of any profession. These include licensure, education, certification or other credentialing processes, and other ongoing educational requirements. Standards of care in nursing today are varied and include nursing specialty association standards and ANA national, state, and local standards that define the acceptable level of practice. These standards are vital to the professional nurse's ongoing education. For this reason, it is important that the nurse remain informed on all areas of practice that affect the provision of care.

FUNCTION OF THE MEDICAL/CLINICAL RECORD

Clear documentation in the medical/clinical record is highly important because this record is:

- The only written source that chronicles a patient's stay from admission through discharge.
- The primary source for reference and communication among members of the health care team.
- The only documentation that supports insurance coverage (payment) or denial.
- The only evidence of the basis on which patient care decisions were made.
- The only legal record.
- The foundation for evaluation of the care provided.
- The basis for staff education or other study.
- The objective source for the facility's licensing and accreditation review (e.g., JCAHO, the American Osteopathic Association Standards).

The above factors have contributed to an environment in which the nurse has increased responsibilities for documentation and a shortened time frame for producing such documentation because of the decrease in patient lengths of stay. This written record is the only account of a patient's stay. Many processes involve the CQI/clinical record for these reasons.

COMPUTERIZATION/MANAGEMENT OF INFORMATION

Patient-centered, cost-effective care has driven another industry to the forefront of health care: information services. Manual, paper-heavy documentation systems are unwieldy in terms of getting information to where it is needed—the site of patient care. From the acute care setting to the outpatient facility to the physician's office to the patient's home, information is needed quickly and accurately. Adding to this burden is the specter of health organizations merging, affiliating, and growing by leaps and bounds. The use of computers with patient care data bases is needed to move the patient safely and effectively along a care continuum, reducing unnecessary duplication of tasks and procedures, and quantifying appropriate outcomes and variance data in order to continually improve care processes.

Information systems for health care settings should include financial reporting as one element of the total product. Patient care planning and acuity systems, based on data generated and inputted from the patient assessment, will allow for more accurate scheduling and staffing systems. Data entry of physician orders (charge entry) should flow to all affected departments for appropriate service scheduling. As clinical protocols and outcome data are entered, appropriate variance collection and trending can be done, with resultant variance analysis as an integral part of a CQI system.

Health system information services staff and/or MIS vendors have developed, or are in the process of developing, interface capabilities between different computer

---

box 5-4

INFORMATION SYSTEM PLANNING/REVIEW CHECKLIST

- ☐ 1. Established goals, priorities, and outcomes of an information system—who will be end-users?
- ☐ 2. Budget guidelines
- ☐ 3. Timelines for implementation
- ☐ 4. Future capabilities of system to expand or interface with alternate care sites
- ☐ 5. Impact on documentation of staff
- ☐ 6. Reduction of documentation—not duplicating same information
- ☐ 7. Security/confidentiality features of system
- ☐ 8. Acuity, patient care planning, clinical paths or protocols integration
- ☐ 9. Support of vendor and information services staff
- ☐ 10. Training needs of staff or end-users
- ☐ 11. Commitment of resources for training and reinservicing of staff as needed
- ☐ 12. Ability to modify system for individual settings
- ☐ 13. Existence of ongoing information services committee and patient care staff involvement
- ☐ 14. Decrease in productivity (home visits) during implementation/learning phase.
- ☐ 15. Names of other users of this system to use as references for quality, support, and practicality of the system.

---

software that will allow for the quick and efficient passage of information from one secured system to another. Thus selected patient information from an acute care setting can be downloaded to a home care setting at a scheduled time, so that patient demographic and clinical information will be readily available to home care staff, as opposed to requestioning the patient and wasting valuable time.

As a nurse manager in any health care setting, you may be asked to assist in the assessment of information systems for your organization. The checklist in Box 5-4, which can be used in any setting, includes some of the issues you should want addressed or have information provided during these planning and review sessions.

SUMMARY

Knowledge of current NCDSs being practiced can help the new nurse manager in evaluating her/his own system. Knowledge of more recent concepts of restructured patient-centered care, shared governance, and professional practice models is essential as the nurse manager leads her staff in providing quality, cost-effective care to patients and families.

Understanding and using a patient classification system, together with a master staffing plan for the area, will help the new nurse manager to staff the area efficiently and effectively. There are always concerns about liability connected with staffing.

Text cont'd. on p. 135

Considerations for Home Care Managers

DAILY OPERATIONS IN HOME CARE

The daily operations of most nursing units, whether in the acute care or alternate patient care site area, are alike in many ways. The patient needs to be cared for, following physician orders and utilizing competent, oriented staff acting within their individual practice guidelines. Home care operations are unique in that the practice setting for the clinicians is the patient home, not an institution. The focus is, and always has been, on patient involvement and agreement on the plan of care.

Operationally, the home care manager must deal with the following issues:

1. Orientation and training of competent home care clinicians (generalist—Medicare visit staff vs. IV, maternal-child, pediatric home care competency)
2. Maintaining personnel requirements that are not always synchronous with acute care requirements (e.g., education records of home health aides [12 hours per year, physical examinations, etc.])
3. Assignment of patients based on patient needs and geographic location
4. Payment and scheduling of staff (per visit vs. hourly/salary staff)
5. Medicare Condition of Participation (COP) required team/case conferencing and staff meetings
6. Care coordination over a large geographic area and covering different vendors/providers of care
7. Physician orders need to be signed and on clinical records within specified time frame
8. Patient care records and security/confidentiality concerns (records taken out of office to patient homes)
9. Patient care delivery models that meet patient needs and regulatory requirements
10. Documentation requirements (more intense than other care settings)
11. Supervision of staff who are not visibly present in office
12. Medical emergencies in homes and staff member's "isolation" at those times
13. Need for collaboration with appropriate disciplines over patient care progress
14. Ongoing evaluation of staff safety driving to, and while in, patient homes
15. Administrative functions that encompass total patient length of stay:
    A. Admission process - rights and responsibilities
    B. Data entry of daily visits, supplies, and other billable services
    C. Verification of insurance, billing information
    D. Monthly (or other) billing routines to Medicare, other third party payers
    E. Accounts receivable management
    F. Computerization and financial management
    G. Discharge of patients
    H. Annual reports of total organizational functioning to governing body
16. Risk management issues (staff awareness of potentially volatile situations)

Issues concerning credentialing are important to learn, especially the issue of continued competency of the nursing staff.

Mastering the ability to lead efficient and effective meetings is of high priority, as is that of facilitating clinical conferences.

Learning to prioritize duties, including time management, is a necessity for the nurse manager, whose work never seems to be done. Making rounds in the patient area assists in maintaining visibility as well as in accomplishing many other managerial tasks.

Finally, internalizing accreditation standards helps the nurse manager in decision-making, which helps the unit achieve and maintain quality nursing care.

References

1. Kibbie PE, editor: *Quality assurance, utilization and risk management: a study guide,* National Association of Quality Assurance Professionals, 1986.
2. *1995 Accreditation Manual for Home Care* Oakbrook Terrace, Il. 1994, The Joint Commission on Accreditation of Healthcare Organization.
3. Garland C: *General Manager* - Emporium Medical Supply, Fullerton, CA, 1995.
4. Manthey M: Structuring work around patients, *Nurs Manage* 20(5):28, 1989.
5. Wake MM: Nursing care delivery systems: status and vision, *J Nurs Adm* 20(5):47, 1990.
6. Sherman RO: Team nursing revisited, *J Nurs Adm* 20(11):44, 1990.
7. Munson FC, et al: *Nursing assignment patterns user's manual,* Ann Arbor, Mich, 1980, AUPHA Press.
8. Piltz-Kirkby M: The nursing assignment pattern study in practice, *Nurs Manage* 22(5):96HH, 1991.
9. Porter-O'Grady T: Shared governance for nursing, *AORN J* 53(2):459, 1991.
10. Rose M, DiPasquale B: The Johns Hopkins professional practice model. In Mayer GG, Madden MJ, Lawrenz E, editors: *Patient care delivery models,* Rockville, Md, 1990, Aspen Publishers.
11. Lawrenz E, Mayer GG: Compensation for professional practice: an incentive model. In Mayer GG, Madden MJ, Lawrenz E, editors: *Patient care delivery models,* Rockville, Md, 1990, Aspen Publishers.
12. Perry L: Group practice model brings nursing unit's turnover to nil, *Mod Healthcare* 20:90, 1990.
13. Giovannetti P: *Patient classification for nurse staffing: criteria for selection and implementation,* Edmonton, Canada, 1983, Alberta Association of Registered Nurses.
14. Nagaprasanna BR: Patient classification systems: strategies for the 1990s, *Nurs Manage* 19(3):105, 1988.
15. Barrett S: *Executive summary of 1990 National Nurse Manager Study by American Organization of Nurse Executives,* Chicago, 1991, American Hospital Association.
16. Huey FL, Hartley S: What keeps nurses in nursing—3,500 nurses tell their stories, *Am J Nurs* 88(2):181, 1988.
17. Ringl KK, Dotson L: Self scheduling for professional nurses, *Nurs Manage* 20(2):42, 1989.
18. Fiesta J: The nursing shortage: whose liability problem, Part II, *Nurs Manage* 21(2):22, 1990.
19. Fiesta J: Agency nurses—whose liability? *Nurs Manage* 21(3):16, 1990.
20. Baillie VK, Trygstad L, Cordoni TI: *Effective nursing leadership—a practical guide,* Rockville, Md, 1989, Aspen Publishers.
21. Manthey M: Trust: essential for delegation, *Nursing Management* 21(11):28, 1990.
22. Lewis EM, Spicer JG: *Human resource management handbook—contemporary strategies for nursing managers,* Rockville, Md, 1987, Aspen Publishers.
23. Mahan F: Patient care conferences: a model, *Nurs Manage* 19(7):60, 1988.
24. Stevens BJ: *The nurse as executive,* ed 3,

Rockville, Md, 1985, Aspen Publishers.
25. Seven ways to sharpen your leadership skills, *Nursing '89* 19(10):130, 1989.
26. Guralnik DB, editor-in-chief: *Webster's new world dictionary,* ed 2, college, 1982, Simon & Schuster.

27. American Hospital Association: Medical records: increasing importance, heavier workload. In *Side-by-side profiles,* Chicago, 1990, The AHA.

For Further Reading

Adams C, Biggerstaff N: Reduced resource utilization through standardized outcome-focused care plans, *JONA,* October 25(10), 1995.

Arikian VL: Total quality management applications to nursing service, *JONA* 21(6):46, 1991.

Bailet H, et al: Use of outcomes studies by a managed care organization: valuing measured treatment effects, *Medical Care,* 33(4), 1995.

Batalden PB, Stolz P: A framework for the continual improvement of health care: building and applying professional and improvement knowledge to test changes in daily work, *Journal on Quality Improvement,* October, 19(10), 1993.

Bayley BK, et al: Measuring the success of treatment in patient terms, *Medical Care,* 33(4), 1995.

Bennett MK, Hylton JP: Modular nursing: partners in professional practice, *Nurs Manage* 21(3)20, 1990.

Beyers M: Quality: the banner of the 1980's, *Nurs Clin North Am* 23(3):617-623, 1988.

Bushy A: Quality assurance in rural hospitals, *JONA* 21(10):34, 1991.

Computers in home care *Caring Magazine* August 1995 (complete issues dedicated to computer issues in home care).

DeGroot HA: Patient classification system evaluation. I. Essential system elements, *JONA* 19(6):30, 1989.

DeGroot HA: Patient classification system evaluation. II. System selection and implementation, *JONA* 19(7):24, 1989.

Del Bueno D, Vincent PM: Organizational culture: how important is it? *JONA* 16(10):15, 1986.

Del Togno-Armanasco V, Olivas GS, Harter S: Developing an integrated nursing case management model, *Nurs Manage* 20(10):26, 1989.

Dieneman J: *Continuums Quality Improvement in Nursing,* Washington DC, 1992, ANA Publishing.

Dunn M, et al: Expert panel method for nurse staffing and resource management, *JONA* October 25(10), 1995.

Fletcher W: *Meetings, meetings: how to manipulate them and make them fun,* New York, 1984, William Morrow.

Gage M: The patient-driven interdisciplinary care plan, *JONA* April, 24(4), 1994.

Gillem TR: Deming's 14 points and hospital quality: responding to the consumer's demand for the best value health care, *J Nurs Qual Assur* 2(3):70, 1988.

Giovannetti P, Thiessen M: *Patient classification for nurse staffing: criteria for selection and implementation.* Edmonton, Alberta, Canada, 1983, Alberta Association of Registered Nurses.

Glazer SK, Gaintner JR: Hospital administrators: the challenge of living in a glass house, *The Journal on Quality Improvement* July, 1994 20(7).

Greer EG: The search for what works, *HealthCare Forum Journal* July/August 1992.

Guadagnoli E, McNeil B: Outcomes research: hope for the future or the latest rage? *Inquiry* Spring, 1994.

Hansten R, Washburn M: Delegation: how to deliver care through others, *American Journal of Nursing* March 1992.

Harbin RE: Practicing effective delegation, *Pediatric Nursing* January-February 1990 16(1).

Hengst WG: Outcomes—the cutting edge for improving care, *Advance/Rehabilitation* July/August 1994.

Home care automation report . . . *home health line* January 1996.

Hungate R: Purchase quality measures: progressing from wants to needs, *Journal on Quality Improvement* July, 1994 20(7).

Jencks S: The government's role in hospital accountability for quality of care, *Journal on Quality Improvement,* July, 1994 20(7).

Katz J, Green E: *Managing quality—a guide to monitoring and evaluating nursing services,* St Louis, 1992, Mosby.

Lewis BE: HMO outcomes research: lessons from the field, *Journal of Ambulatory Care Management* January, 1995, 18(1).

Manthey M: Primary practice partners: a nurse extender system, *Nurs Manage* 19(3):58, 1988.

Manthey M: Structuring work around patients, *Nurs Manage* 20(5):28, 1989.

Manthey M: Delivery systems and practice models: a dynamic balance, *Nurs Manage* 22(1):28, 1991.

Marchionno PM: Modified cyclical scheduling: a practical approach, *Nurs Manage* 18(10):60, 1987.

Mark BA: The black box of patient outcomes research, *Image: Journal of Nursing Scholarship* 1995 27(1).

Marrelli TM: *Nursing Documentation handbook,* St Louis, 1996, Mosby.

Marrelli TM: *The handbook of home health standards and documentation guidelines for reimbursement,* St Louis, 1994, Mosby.

Marrelli TM, Hilliard LS: *Home care and clinical pathways: effective care planning across the continuum,* St Louis, 1996, Mosby.

Marrelli TM, Whittier S: *HomeHealth Aide: Guidelines for care,* Annapolis, MD, 1996, Marrelli & Associates.

Marriner-Tomey A: *Guide to nursing management,* ed 4, St Louis, 1992, Mosby.

Mayer GG, Madden MJ, Lawrenz E, editors: *Patient care delivery models,* Rockville, Md, 1990, Aspen.

Michael A: Team nursing and primary nursing can coexist, *Nurs Manage* 19(4):99, 1988.

Morrissey J: Interface engines rev up, *Modern Healthcare* May 8, 1995.

Munson FC et al: *Nursing assignment patterns user's manual,* Ann Arbor, Mich, 1980, AUPHA Press.

Murray JA: Benchmarking: a tool for excellence in palliative care, *Journal of Palliative Care* 1992 8(4).

Nagaprasanna BR: Patient classification systems: strategies for the 1990s, *Nurs Manage* 19(3):105, 1988.

O'Dell C: Building on received wisdom, *Healthcare Forum Journal* January/February 1993.

Pace K: Data sets for home care organizations, *Caring Magazine* March 1995.

Patterson P, et al: Nurse information needs for efficient care continuity across patient units, *JONA* October 25(10), 1995.

Perry L: Group-practice model brings nursing unit's turnover to nil, *Mod Healthcare* 20(36):90, 1990.

Peters TJ: *Thriving on chaos,* New York, 1987, Alfred A Knopf.

Porter-O'Grady T: Shared governance for nursing, *AORN J* 53(2):458, 1991.

Porter-O'Grady T, Finnigan S: *Shared governance for nursing—a creative approach to professional accountability,* Rockville, Md, 1984, Aspen.

Price CA, Southerland A: Rethinking staffing patterns in critical care nursing, *Nurs Manage* 20(3):80Q, 1989.

Ringl KK, Dotson L: Self-scheduling for professional nurses, *Nurs Manage* 20(2):42, 1989.

Shaughnessy P, et al: Outcome-based quality improvement in home care, *Caring Magazine,* February, 1995.

Successful delegation multiplies achievement, *Home Health Executive Report* Introductory Issue, 1986.

Teeter D, Johnson R: The roadmap for clinical quality, *HMO Practice* March 8(1), 1994.

CHAPTER 6

EFFECTIVE TIME MANAGEMENT

T.M. MARRELLI

ffective time management is vital to accomplishing all work. Time management problems are easy to recognize; there is always too much pending work. The symptoms are papers piled high in baskets and stacks on your desk, notes attached to your office door, unread mail, and the inability to locate a specific piece of paper when you need it. The behavioral signs include thinking about the next project while discussing a current one, procrastinating about picking up the top piece of paper for fear of what's underneath, and forgetting appointments. These problems can be remedied. Effective time management, or habits that contribute to the effective use of this limited commodity, can be learned. More importantly, habits that are no longer efficient for you can be discarded. Working smarter, not harder, demands setting priorities, delegating effectively, and using other time management skills to achieve personal and organizational goals.

Effective time management has become even more important with the increased mergers, downsizing, and general increase of individual workloads over the past 5 years. In order to survive, management has had to restructure departments or job positions so that each middle manager may be wearing many different hats, picking up the job duties or managerial functions of individuals who have left or have been laid off. The important thing to remember during this stressful time is that one person may not be able to do it all or do it all as it has been done in the past.

Use your newfound skills as a manager to take stock of all the priorities and responsibilities of your position, work with your senior manager to define what needs to be done, delegate effectively, and do the best you can. As Chapter 10 will explain, balance is needed in everyone's life to prevent the negative outcomes related to increased pressure and stress.

THE THREE *P*S OF PROCRASTINATION

Three *P*s may especially impede competent nurse managers from accomplishing dreaded work. These are:

1. Procrastination
2. Perfectionism
3. Prioritizing

Procrastination is generally defined as habitually postponing performance of burdensome tasks. Symptoms may include multiple stacks of paper on your desk overflowing onto credenzas, unopened mail, or the feeling of not wanting to go to work for fear of not meeting a deadline on a project. The problem with procrastination is that it is a learned habit. Like all habits, it can be unlearned and replaced with more successful behaviors. Examples of procrastination are delaying finalizing the minutes of the last product selection committee until the night before the next meeting or delaying performance evaluations because they are time-consuming. When this occurs, the added stress and pressure become greater than if the minutes had been completed earlier or if one performance evaluation were completed every afternoon. All of a sudden, routine items take on immense importance and a dread of not meeting deadlines sets in.

It is interesting to note that in Webster's New World Dictionary,[1] the word deadline has its origins as a "line around a prison beyond which a prisoner could go only at the risk of being shot." It is no wonder that we take deadlines seriously and feel impending discomfort as they approach and we are not or perceive we are not ready. This feeling usually lasts until the work is accomplished, then tremendous relief is felt.

Also, while working, a realization usually is made—the task was not as bad as anticipated, or such a delay should not occur again because it takes too much energy. It is at this point that a conscious effort and decision must be made to change the habit of procrastination. Everyone endures certain job aspects that they do not enjoy. However, these dreaded duties grow in importance and cast a shadow on all other activities until completed. Just "doing it" results in incredible relief. In addition, it usually takes less time and energy than was anticipated. Most importantly, the feeling of accomplishment and satisfaction when done can reinforce the new just-do-it habit the next time. Therefore when you initially get these dreaded uncomfortable feelings, it usually means you should do this job first and stop procrastinating.

Perfectionism is known generally to mean that work is never perceived to be "good enough." Perfectionists usually procrastinate because at some level they believe that no product is better than a poor product. Although this is not true, we all have known successful, competent people who function with these beliefs. If this sounds familiar, it is important to realize that, generally, any work product is better than none, and you may never have the luxury of time or other resources to accomplish a given project in the manner you believe it should be accomplished. Trying to be perfect wastes time and is an unrealistic goal. This is perhaps one of the most frustrating aspects of being a manager; not only will your work product often be incorporated into your supervisor's project, but in the end it may not resemble the same product at all. In management, you must make it okay (to yourself) for your managers to "own" parts of your work and recognize that you cannot control your product once it is submitted to your manager.

Prioritizing is the decision-making process that results in a systematic order in which to accomplish identified tasks. Prioritizing leads to organization, which is vital to effective time management.

Prioritizing can be closely linked to perfectionism and procrastination in two ways: (1) putting off or delaying what you do not want to do (procrastination) can result in those tasks being relegated to the end of your list of priorities, and (2) avoidance of starting and completing a task moves other tasks towards the end of the priority list. As the dread of deadline looms, there are seemingly endless lists of newer items given higher priority. It is at this point that the perfectionist starts believing that it is just too late for an acceptable product to even be created.

Though it is hard, *do* the most difficult task first. Even a draft of the project will give you some sense of accomplishment and a feeling of control over your work environment. The difficult tasks we put off are what become bigger and cause stress in the workplace. Doing the dreaded task will give you a sense of relief, rejuvenation, and accomplishment.

THE RIGHT STUFF ATTITUDES

Kenneth Pelletier of the University of California San Francisco School of Medicine conducted an ongoing study of executives in the telecommunications industry, as reported by Olsen.[2] The telecommunications industry has been plagued by turmoil and changes. It was found through this study that the people who thrived on the continual fast-paced changes shared some common beliefs. Some of these lessons may be applicable to the health care setting because of the dynamic and ever-changing environment health care managers face. The suggestions for thriving on change in Manager's Tip 6-1 on p. 142 may help you be an effective manager in today's fast-paced health care environment.

If you believe that you are alone in struggling to effectively manage your time, consider this thought. Large[3] states, "More new information has been produced in the last 30 years than in the previous 5,000 . . . and the total of all printed knowledge doubles every 8 years." There is clearly too much information and not enough time to incorporate it. What is more, not all information received is relevant to the task at hand. The new term that has been created for this overwhelming amount of knowledge is *information anxiety.* In addition to this overload, you may have sales representatives and other vendors who wish to further increase your knowledge of the particular product or service they are selling. Finally, your life does not comprise only work (though in difficult times it can certainly *feel* that way), and you may receive additional information daily through your personal mail and phone.

MANAGER'S TIP 6-1

THRIVING ON CHANGE

✔ **Challenge**—Do not view change as a threat. Perceive it as a challenge and the chance or opportunity to do something new and innovative.
✔ **Control**—Believe that you can make an impact or a difference. This is probably the most important trait for thriving in a changing environment.
✔ **Commitment**—Get involved and active in the new ideas and change. Do not deny the reality of the changing situation.
✔ **Social support**—Use your friends, family, and colleagues for support. It helps to have a sense of working and pulling together. Your network does not have to be large, just established and used. Pelletier says, "It's enough that you have a supportive, trusting relationship with the person at the next desk."[2] (This reinforces the importance and need for peer support among nurse managers.)
✔ **Stress management**—Learn your own stress signals. Pelletier found that the healthiest executives all knew what to do when their stress levels got too high. He said methods for relief varied and the one chosen did not matter. For this group, methods included, among others, listening to music. Relieving stress is vital to reenergizing oneself.[2]

MANAGER'S TIP 6-2

FOUR WAYS TO HANDLE PAPER

✔ Act on it.
✔ File it.
✔ Discard it.
✔ Regardless of the chosen category, try to handle it only once.

The good news is anyone can become organized. Contrary to belief, your desk does not need to be neat and clean to be organized. Tidiness works for some, whereas others can locate any needed piece of paper on what appears to be a messy desk. You can be more organized and use your limited time more effectively. The skills and time management suggestions recommended in Manager's Tips 6-2, 6-3, and 6-4 can also be extended into your home.

Handling Paper

Act-on-it items include action items such as memos needing response, confirmation of meeting attendance, scheduling changes, and other situations where your immediate input is needed.

MANAGER'S TIP 6-3

23 WAYS TO HELP YOU MANAGE TIME

✔ Recognize that time is a scarce and nonrenewable resource.

✔ Remember that being organized is a key component of effective time management.

✔ Evaluate your own use of time. Keep a log for 2 weeks and note the activities and time allotted for them. Keep another log after implementing these suggestions to see if measurable improvements in your work output occur.

✔ Understand that everyone has her/his own organization style. You do not have to have a neat and spotless desk to be organized. Some very organized managers have messy desks but can put their hands on any piece of paper when needed.

✔ Know that successful, busy people usually have effective personal organizational skills.

✔ Schedule time to file or do paperwork *every* day. Start files for such ongoing business as leave requests, unit activity reports, or QA/QI minutes.

✔ Prioritize tasks on a daily basis.

✔ Schedule and meet deadlines.

✔ Formulate realistic goals and break them down into tasks by creating short-range goals. When all these tasks are completed, long-term objectives will have been achieved. Break down all large jobs into small pieces. Schedule time to do the small pieces.

✔ Maintain your flexibility. Reorder priorities whenever indicated based on organizational needs.

✔ Know that if something is not a priority or important, it may not need to be done.

✔ Visualize yourself learning to effectively cope with change, turmoil, and chaos. With this attitude, it will not unduly upset you when it happens.

✔ Managing your own time effectively will result in more efficient use of staff time as your actions are copied.

✔ Accept that your schedule may change based on many situations, such as your manager's needs, a clinical problem, or an unscheduled lengthy disaster drill on your unit.

✔ Maximize your use of time because this improves overall performance and contributes to cost containment goals.

✔ Know that planning and delegation are vital to organizational and personal goal achievement.

✔ Realize that an effective time manager gets more accomplished, has improved quality of work, meets deadlines and other commitments, and increases effectiveness overall.

✔ Make and use "to do" lists or planners whenever possible.

✔ Take the last few minutes of your work day to reflect on your accomplishments and to prioritize the tasks of the next day. Feel satisfied with those completed tasks and the job you are doing.

✔ You can have an open-door policy and attitude without the door always literally being open. Staff should have access, but you can control that access.

✔ Pick a regularly scheduled day (e.g., every third Tuesday) for clearing off your desk totally and reprioritizing big projects.

✔ Use the phone whenever possible—it may save you writing a memo and time-consuming communications.

✔ Check off tasks as completed—it feels great!

30 ACTIONS TO HELP YOU MANAGE YOUR ENVIRONMENT

✔ Hang a large calendar in an accessible area on which you and your staff can identify vacations, in-services, or scheduled absences. If feasible, it is particularly helpful if you are able to read this at a glance from you desk.

✔ Choose the style of "to do" list that works best for you. Try different ones until you decide which method suits you best.

✔ Identify your peak work time. Try to schedule the most intense or important tasks during this time.

✔ Concentrate on the task at hand by controlling distractions. It is okay to schedule time for you; close your office door.

✔ Leave the work area, when possible, for at least a few minutes a day. Take a lunch or other meal break, even if it means just shutting your door and eating an apple in peace.

✔ Place mailboxes for your staff in an easily accessible place for your use. Mailboxes can be used for scheduling, feedback, and delegated work.

✔ Schedule time for all routine duties; otherwise they probably will not get done. For example, schedule time to review performance evaluations and other ongoing unit activity tasks. If it is not scheduled, it is not respected as a priority.

✔ Learn to use a computer for all written products. The editing, spelling checkers, and thesaurus tools are an immense help when memos or reports are due. When you use a computer, organize your disks in a manner effective for you. Remember to keep the phone, scissors, or other magnetic material away from your computer and the disks because such items may erase hours of hard work.

✔ Practice speedreading or proofreading skills if your position uses those special skills.

✔ Organize your phone numbers in a systematic way. This method should be whatever works and is easiest for you. Have the most frequently called numbers accessible and placed near your phone.

✔ Control interruptions for certain periods of each day. The ability to do this effectively will vary based on the work setting and other factors.

✔ Refer to a thesaurus and a recent edition dictionary whenever creating written products.

✔ Maintain and update a desk calendar or other organizer to determine your planned daily, weekly, and monthly schedules.

✔ Create an office environment that promotes work completion while also reflecting your personality.

✔ Organize and update your business phone numbers and addresses on a regularly scheduled basis.

✔ Make your environment work for you. Sometimes it may be appropriate to go to the hospital library to research a project for presentation. Other times, just closing your office door may be sufficient.

✔ Remember that becoming and staying organized is a learned skill and that, with practice, good habits can replace bad ones.

✔ Believe that you cannot do everything for everyone else and still achieve your goals.

✔ Use your interpersonal skills to politely end conversations. When phoning people known to be long-winded, set up the conversation to be short. This can be achieved in a couple of ways: (1) "Dr. No, this is Nurse Manager, I have only a minute between meetings to return your call and tell you. . . .," or (2) "Well, I've got to go, I think my

Continued.

manager is on the other line" or "I have a call I've been expecting and have to go." Your pager can also be used for this purpose.

✔ Practice visualization daily, seeing yourself as a calm and effective manager.

✔ Begin every morning by taking 3 minutes to relax and focus on the day's tasks ahead. With practice, this exercise will keep you centered throughout the day on your priorities.

✔ Listen to *any* recommendations that have the possibility of being a more efficient and successful way of doing things. Stop yourself the moment your automatic response begins with, "But it's always been done this way." That alone is usually a good reason to reevaluate the way something is done.

✔ Learn to say "no" and mean it.

✔ Be flexible in the time parameters set in your schedule. If you overschedule your time and consistently run over, you will feel even more harried and hassled. Allot sufficient time between scheduled activities.

✔ Accept that there will *always* be interruptions. This is part of being a manager. The key is controlling and balancing them. Evaluate your office space: is the furniture in a configuration that is conducive to decreasing or minimizing interruptions?

✔ Teach your staff that whenever a problem is brought to your attention, you will hear it only if a recommended solution is attached.

✔ Visualize yourself as an innovative, creative thinker and problem-solver.

✔ Practice relaxation techniques and deep breathing exercises on a regular basis.

✔ Take breaks. These are very important. Take them, do not feel guilty, and savor them. The restorative power of a break leaves you with more energy while increasing your productivity.

✔ Take great care of yourself. Get a massage, have manicures, exercise, eat well, play golf, or whatever *you like to do*. Effective time management will allow more time for those activities.

File-it items include items that may need retrieval in the future (e.g., communications from your manager, HR issues, and other important documentation).

Discard-it items include advertisements for various services or products that are not appropriate for your area and memos sent to you as occupant nurse manager or confirmation memos that need no further action on your part.

Try to handle it only once, regardless of the chosen category.

The main difficulty in this process is deciding what to file and what to discard. You can learn a lot about the nurse manager who preceded you and the filing system that may be acceptable at your work setting by reviewing the remaining files. The core files may include HR files, copies of patient complaints that may or may not have been forwarded to the patient ombudsman and/or risk manager, clinical and management articles circulated to all managers from administration, and voluminous paper communications sent to or from the unit.

You do not have to keep every piece of paper to be an effective nurse manager. Ask your peers what information they keep and what they discard. Avoid the tendency to be a pack rat.

THE IMPORTANCE OF DELEGATION

It has been said that the effective use of time, or time management, is more about management than about time. With this in mind, you will find that your staff is vital to accomplishing all work. Delegation is the tool that transfers the work to your subordinates, giving the nursing staff responsibility, which contributes to a sense of belonging and accomplishment. Successful completion of the duties delegated empowers and develops the staff member to whom the work was delegated. In decentralized organizations, delegation is key to work accomplishment. The nurse manager must achieve organizational and unit goals, and the ordering of the priorities and the management of the time allotted in which to do them is of great importance. The more responsibilities a person assumes and the busier a person becomes, the more effective delegation becomes the essential tool to accomplish work and achieve goals (see Manager's Tip 6-5).

RESOURCES FOR TIME MANAGEMENT

There are ways to improve time management. It is important to be open to new ideas. The resources discussed below are those that should be considered where possible.

Technology and Nursing

The time management implications of information systems for nurses and nurse managers are currently being discussed in all health settings and in the literature. Automation in documentation should be fully explored because documentation continues to be an area of duplicative actions and inefficient use of the professional nurse's limited time. Computers are encouraging a shift towards standardized care plans and other automated data trends. This needs to occur given the following information. The American Hospital Association[4] (AHA) says that patient charts now average 70 to 100 pages. Medical records departments in most midsized hospitals process some 250,000 to 360,000 pieces of information each year. Because a patient's medical record may be reviewed as many as 30 times and stored for up to 30 years, more than 90% of hospitals have turned to computers to manage the information.

Computerized nursing documentation is becoming more common in health settings as applications for automation in nursing have increased. In some systems, the nurse can identify those actions or findings appropriate to a specific patient to facilitate the clinical entry. Computerization, particularly at the patient's bedside, assists in ensuring frequent, timely nursing entries. Computerizing the record and the nursing notes and other entries may ultimately save hospitals money and increase the quality of care provided. Studies have shown that nursing costs can account for 30% to 40% of a hospital's operational budget. It has been estimated that 2 to 3 hours of a nursing shift is spent performing administrative tasks.[5] Nursing computer systems

MANAGER'S TIP 6-5

14 SUGGESTIONS TO DELEGATE EFFECTIVELY

As discussed in Chapter 3, delegation of nursing tasks to LPN/LVNs and unlicensed assistive personnel is still a controversial subject and is an element of the delegation process.

✔ Believe it is *not* easier or quicker to do it yourself. (It is not!)

✔ Realize you must delegate to accomplish work.

✔ Learn to delegate wherever possible; it frees you up to manage and it develops your staff.

✔ Delegate by stating clearly the work and the product expected; specify deadlines, including a date on which you want a draft or the product; state that you be apprised of progress weekly and that you want immediate notification if a problem is impeding completion by the due date.

✔ Give feedback, positive wherever possible, on the progress and on the final product. Share comments from others on the work product where possible. For example, if your manager compliments the work and writes you a note about it, share the note with the staff member who created the product. It also is helpful to keep such notes in the staff member's personnel file on the unit so that during performance evaluation, you remember work products accomplished and the feedback received.

✔ Teach and direct your staff to use each other as resources. This creates an atmosphere of autonomy and professionalism that keeps nurses satisfied with their jobs.

✔ Delegate initially to those who are assertive or have told you that they want more responsibility. At first it may be truly difficult to delegate; but give this attitude up. Believe that your staff will do a good job. Resist the temptation to meddle in delegated projects.

✔ Expect the best from your staff and chances are you will get it.

✔ Remember that working in an environment where autonomy and independence are valued is considered an asset by nurses and assists in nurse retention. Make that the environment where you are the nurse manager.

✔ Staff members should know they can make mistakes and recommend solutions and improvements.

✔ Be professional. Do not denigrate your staff or their work to anyone; it comes back around and does not support an environment conducive to effective team-building.

✔ Remember the concepts of accountability, responsibility, and authority when delegating. Work may not be done the same way you would have done it, but it was completed and you did not have to do it personally.

✔ Offer a choice in the duties needing delegation when possible. This encourages staff growth and autonomy.

✔ Realize what should not be delegated. This may include HR issues, any confidential issues, delicate political problems with other departments or units, conflicts started by "he said/she said" scenarios, and complaints/communications with physicians or visitors that have risk management implications.

available today are integrating the different components of the chart. For example, once the assessment is completed, an individualized care plan is developed. From that point, a patient-specific flow chart can be generated, thus decreasing the documentation process by 40% to 50% per nurse per shift. Kardexes and other pieces of information can also be developed via a computer system. Computerizing nursing documentation may be the next step in decreasing repetitive and duplicative administrative tasks. The confidentiality issues of computerized entries and retrieval of needed information are important factors currently being addressed by both systems users and developers. The growing specialty of nursing informatics is one resource available to nurse managers that facilitates the move towards automation in the work setting.

Detail Management (or, When You Cannot See the Forest for the Trees)

Undoubtedly, it is easy to be overwhelmed and burdened with details. Minutiae can leave you exhausted before you even begin your first priority task. Details that belong to a bigger project should be written down and placed in the folder for that project. Other details should be judged as to whether they have true value or can be thrown away.

Delegate the resolution of some of these details back to the staff members who brought them to you. As with all duties delegated, give a deadline for when you want a report on the outcome. An example could be the completion of meeting minutes that both you and a staff member attended. The staff member can use both of your notes to effectively complete the assignment.

Considerations for Home Care Managers

TIME MANAGEMENT: A KEY SKILL

Time management skills are needed by all managers in the health care profession in order to accomplish the many goals of their jobs. Home care managers are not unique in that respect, as they are faced with a multitude of responsibilities to keep their agency running smoothly and effectively. In many home care organizations, the home care manager position encompasses all of the same responsibilities as that of a larger organization's CEO or administrator, except on a different scale.

The need to be able to work productively on a variety of different projects, to be flexible enough to change "hats," and to address obstacles and challenges as they arise is more pronounced in home care, where the manager may be the marketing and strategic planner, personnel expert, information systems planner, and clinician. By utilizing the general skills of effective management with emphasis on disciplined time management, the nurse manager should be able to meet the demands of the position.

SUMMARY

Effective time management results in quality work produced by set deadlines. It also develops staff initiative and personal growth through effective use of delegation by the nurse manager. The nurse manager who practices effective time management skills acts as a role model to both staff and peers. It has been said that, "Misuse of time seldom involves an isolated incident. It is usually part of a well-established pattern of behavior." These patterns of behavior, or habits, can be changed.[6]

Greater job satisfaction is achieved through work being accomplished; all work entails time management skills. The improvement of these key skills will increase productivity, which in turn reinforces sound habits of time management. The nurse manager sees increased quality of care and improved morale in an atmosphere that fosters staff growth and autonomy. Time management is vital to the successful operation of any health care setting and to the personal health and professional growth of a nurse manager.

References

1. *Webster's New World Dictionary of the American Language,* second college ed, New York, 1982, Simon and Schuster.
2. Olsen E: Beyond positive thinking, *J Nurs Adm* 20(5):11, 1990.
3. Large P: *The micro revolution revisited,* Totowa, NJ, 1984, Rowman & Allenheld.
4. American Hospital Association: *Side-by-side profiles,* Medical records: increasing importance, heavier workload, Chicago, 1990, The AHA.
5. Carter K: Computer technology advances will help hospitals to compete, *Modern Healthcare* 15(24):90, 1985.
6. Bliss EC: *Getting things done,* New York, 1978, Bantam Books.

For Further Reading

Covey S: *The 7 habits of highly effective people,* New York, 1990, Simon & Schuster.
Drucker P: *The effective executive,* New York, 1967, Harper & Row Management Library.
Mackenzie A: *The time trap,* New York, 1990, American Management Association Publishing.

CHAPTER 7

RESOURCE MANAGEMENT AND BUDGETING BASICS

LYNDA S. HILLIARD

With the continued conversion of health insurance plans from fee-for-service to capitated or managed care, health care delivery managers need to intensely scrutinize the relationship between clinical and financial outcomes of care, whether that care is provided in the inpatient, outpatient, or community care setting. This intense analysis is needed to determine the point of intersection between the most clinically proficient method and the most reasonable cost of practice for a preestablished patient population. Not only must the finance department understand this data, but nurse managers also need a thorough understanding of the budget and resource management process to provide more cost-efficient management.

This chapter will explore the basic concepts of financial management for the new nurse manager, with a specific focus on the budget process—capital, personnel, and operations. The inclusion of definitions of commonly used financial or resource management terms will assist the nurse manager to better communicate the needs of the unit or facilitate the unit requests from the finance office staff, peer managers, or other management team members.

TOTAL QUALITY MANAGEMENT/CONTINUOUS QUALITY IMPROVEMENT

CQI, with a basis in total quality management, consists of principles that have been derived from the business sector and applied to health care objectives. Competition, scarce economic resources, and societal demand for outcome-oriented quality care at a reasonable price are all factors forcing health care administrators to conserve limited resources by streamlining operations, while continuing to provide quality service to their customers. CQI is a process that focuses not only on fixing problems, but also on searching continually for methods to improve and make more cost-effective the delivery of services.[1]

This has provided the impetus for staff members from all segments of the health care environment to meet, prioritize goals, and cross traditional professional boundaries to develop and test methods for better serving their patients' needs in a shorter period of time. Examples of quality work improvement teams that address patient customer service or clinical needs are:

- Outpatient service area wait times
- Coordinating care across the health continuum
- Patient/family education
- Patient care delivery models

All of the above quality teams may have staff members from various departments investigate and research the relevant issues and leave their territorial concerns behind as they search for solutions that enhance and improve the delivery of patient care. Patient satisfaction will ultimately be achieved. Also, this continuous review of operations will eventually make the organization more cost-effective—a needed ingredient in the health care arena of the next century.

BENCHMARKING

In order to focus CQI efforts in a health care setting to make the process more efficient, a goal must be established. Sometimes these goals, and the processes leading to them, are difficult for staff to visualize. For example, an attempt to decrease outpatient waiting time from 90 minutes to 5 minutes might seem admirable; however, on closer evaluation, it is too cost-prohibitive and unworkable in the available care environment. Benchmarking allows realistic goal setting because it compares a successful organization's processes and structures to the organization desiring improvement.

Benchmarking can be defined as the structured process of taking practices of the best organizations anywhere in any industry, comparing those practices to your own, and adapting the best of them to your organization. As discussed by James Heidbreder, in *Looking for the Light—Not the Heat,* benchmarking is done ". . . to make a quantum improvement in your process effectiveness or efficiency. Appropriately practiced, benchmarking guards against jumping to quick conclusions or reaching for highly publicized results without understanding the driving forces behind those results."[2] It is important to understand the relationship between the process and the results and not to reach for unrealistic objectives—a clear frustration to staff, and clearly a detriment to the change process.

Data are not always readily available to groups wanting to initiate benchmarking. The health care industry has recognized the benefits of benchmarking after other major American industries have embraced it. The automobile industry, as well as other industries that have been tremendously affected by higher quality, cheaper imports, saw the need for a process to make itself more competitive. In order to identify correct data sources to successfully benchmark specific functions or processes, health care organizations must first understand *who they are, what they want, where they are going,* and *how to gauge when they get there.* It is a process that can be entered into only with commitment from the entire organization. There needs to be an identified need and a desired outcome. Nurse managers may recognize the problem-solving process that is applied to benchmarking: (1) planning; (2) collecting data; (3) analyzing data; and (4) adapting the practices.

CLINICAL PATHWAYS

An important element of resource management, especially in the health care setting, is the incorporation of practice protocols, case management, and clinical pathways into the care planning of a given patient population. It is important to note that clinical pathways or care protocols have financial implications, since they dictate the types and amounts of care given.

In *Home Care and Clinical Paths—Effective Care Planning Across the Continuum,* Marrelli and Hilliard, described clinical paths as ". . . clinical tools that organize, sequence, and time the major interventions of the nursing staff, physicians, . . . for a particular case type, condition, diagnostic category, or nursing diagnosis." They also explain that clinical paths ". . . may describe an institution's collective standard of practice, and are, in essence, a clinical 'budget' . . . they provide a direction and predictability to patient care and to the caregivers interacting in that case."[3] The Agency for Health Care Policy and Research (AHCPR), funded by the Department of Health and Human Services (DHHS), has done a tremendous amount of research in the development of nationally accepted protocols for care of certain disease conditions. These protocols may be used in the development of individual institutional care practices or clinical paths as the foundation for different clinicians from the various health professions to begin the discussion of standardization of the many facets of health care. With increased and improved standardization, outcomes of care can be studied and scrutinized to determine the practices that will best lead to positive outcomes for all parties involved.

As a direct link to the controlling of costs, clinical paths are also integral to improving care processes, since variances gleaned from clinical path implementation should be reviewed and analyzed so improvements can be made to the care process. As explained in *Home Care and Clinical Paths,* clinical paths are not for all patients or conditions and need to be adjusted for complexity and acuity of patients.[3] Paths are a tool in the arsenal of health care providers to standardize, control, and ultimately improve care through scrutiny of measured outcomes. For more information on this subject, please see Chapter 5, "Day-to-Day Operations."

DIAGNOSTIC-RELATED GROUPS

Nurse managers must understand the types and complexities of the resources needed to achieve patient care outcomes, and they also must be aware of the fiscal constraints placed on operations for the proper use of limited resources.

Diagnostic-related groups (DRGs) is a classification system that was developed in the 1980s and adapted by the Health Care Financing Administration (HCFA) to control the cost of health care to its Medicare beneficiaries by assigning a cost per diagnostic category to include all services provided.

Before the advent of DRGs, most nurse managers were not actively involved in the budget process. However, nurse managers must now be responsible for the development of their unit's budget and reducing or maintaining the cost of operations within the approved budget dependent on patient census.

Positive performance evaluations and career progression within the health care setting depend on a manager's fiscal knowledge and performance, as well as clinical expertise.

COST-BASED REIMBURSEMENT

With the advent of the Medicare program in 1967 and prior to the 1980s, hospitals were reimbursed by the federal government on a cost basis. Basically, cost-based reimbursement for the Medicare program classified the various costs of operating a health care facility, noted the number of patients served, determined the average cost per patient, and then reimbursed the entity for all Medicare patients.

This generous but inefficient system, combined with the impact of Hill-Burton legislation after World War II (to expand hospitals into smaller communities) and expansion of medical technology and pharmacology, allowed hospitals to grow at a record pace and provide a wide array of very expensive, often duplicative, services without any incentive to economize.

Today, nurse executives, chief executive officers, chief operations officers, and chief financial officers review and analyze daily the financial operations of their institutions. Operational decisions are made quickly to react to adverse conditions (e.g., negative payer mix, low census, or rising staffing costs not related to increased volumes) that may endanger the financial viability of a hospital or other health care entity.

The nurse manager must continually view the patient care unit as a viable business and be able to react to financial changes immediately. To do that, the effective nurse manager must understand the complexities and terminology of the fiscal process to be able to react quickly to change. A glossary of financial terms is available for review in Appendix 7-1.

FISCAL MANAGEMENT

Senior managerial staff are responsible to the governing body of a health care entity for the effective management of that institution. Proper financial management is just as important as the provision of quality patient care services. A hospital or other health program cannot survive in the twenty-first century without a fiscally astute management team. To understand fiscal management, a few basic concepts must be learned.

Fiscal or financial management is derived from basic accounting principles. According to Shillinglaw and Meyer,[4] "Accounting is the primary financial method of gathering, organizing and presenting information that can be utilized by management and outsiders in evaluating an organization." Manager's Tip 7-1 defines some fundamental accounting terms.

As with all professional disciplines, accounting uses methods or measurements that follow prescribed rules to provide standardized analysis when comparing one institution with another.[5]

Hospitals and alternative health care organizations follow the standards of the JCAHO to prove the quality of their services. Accounting practices are governed by the Financial Accounting Standards Board, which issues statements of financial accounting standards.

Nonprofit Versus Profit Status

In the health care industry, hospitals historically have been nonprofit institutions, making them tax-exempt. In years of efficient operations, hospitals list their excess revenues over expenses as a positive fund balance, or net worth.

In a for-profit business, a positive fund balance would be called profit and divided among stockholders in the form of a dividend, or it would be reinvested in the business. In a nonprofit hospital, excess money should thus be reinvested in the facility and/or in expanding services provided to the community it serves.

Capital Expansion or Reinvestment

Prudent business managers realize the need for a business to reinvest in its plant and facilities to maintain viable operations. Generally, health care institutions must re-

Manager's Tip 7-1

ASSETS, LIABILITIES, AND NET WORTH

The most fundamental accounting maxim is:

$$\text{Assets} = \text{Liabilities} + \text{Owner's equity (net worth)}$$

✔ An **asset** is any property (tangible or intangible) that is owned by the institution (e.g., cash, accounts receivable, and property).

✔ A **liability** is a debt that the institution owes to other businesses or individuals, such as accounts payable and mortgages.

✔ **Net worth,** or **owner's equity,** constitutes worth in terms of money that would be divided among the owners if the institution were to go out of business.

alize an annual net gain of at least 5% (based on revenues over expenses) to replace assets as needed.

Many hospitals have historically derived a percentage of income from sources other than operations (e.g., fund-raising and interest or dividends on investments). However, utilizing such money as operating income is not a sound financial practice. The hospital budget should reflect expenses that can be covered by anticipated revenues from operations. It should not count on investment income to cover general expenses of daily operations. The situation is comparable to a family living beyond the earnings of its breadwinners and tapping savings accounts or investment accounts on a consistent basis. In such a case, annual family budgets are developed and include savings account income to cover expenses. After a short time, that source of income is depleted and the family has lost in two ways: (1) those emergency moneys or special-project moneys are gone, and (2) the family has built a lifestyle that the annual earnings of the breadwinners cannot support.

PUBLIC PERCEPTION OF HEALTH CARE INSTITUTIONS

During the past decade, national controversy has arisen in the health care community regarding the public perception of hospitals being managed as a business while claiming tax-exempt status. Recent tax rulings by the Internal Revenue Service have pitted revenue-starved communities against major hospitals and medical centers. At stake are large amounts of property tax revenues being waived because of the non-profit status of health care institutions. The tax-exempt status of such "profitable" institutions, which are perceived by the public as either limiting access or refusing health care to those community members without insurance or the financial resources to pay for their care, is under review.

The historic public view of hospitals as being charitable institutions providing care for all who come to their doors is being transformed into the view of a large, multi-faceted corporation or integrated network system whose primary mission is to produce a positive bottom line, as evidenced by intense competition for pay patients. In the future, more institutions will be challenged about their tax-exempt status as local governing agencies examine the financial activities of their community-based health care providers against their mission statement.

Recent headlines outlining the profitability of health maintenance organizations (HMOs) and, specifically, the actual earnings of select senior managers of those plans have aroused the anger and suspicion of many Americans. In many cases, people accurately perceive the amount and quality of health care services as having deteriorated or having the potential to deteriorate under managed care delivery systems. News stories have pointed to anecdotal evidence of the "disasters" of managed care: the newborn sent home with undiagnosed jaundice or the patient whose cancer was overlooked until it was too late. In an effort to counteract what is seen to be unsafe patient care practices dictated by profit concerns, several state legislatures have passed, or are contemplating passage of, legislation that will dictate the types and amounts of care patients will receive while in the care of state-licensed health care facilities.

The successful health care management team will plan with their governing body to effectively recognize and integrate the health care needs of their community into their strategic plan, while conserving resources and maintaining a positive bottom line.

FINANCIAL PERFORMANCE REPORTS

The formal reports that measure a health care entity's financial performance are the *financial statements,* which include the income and expense statements and the balance sheet.

Income and Expense Statement

The income and expense statement lists all the revenues, expenses, and net income or loss for a given period, usually on a monthly or annual basis. Any type of revenue can constitute income (e.g., dividends or interest on investments). In a business, the entity should operate on the income generated from the service it provides. See Figure 7-1 for a sample income and expense statement.

Balance Sheet

The balance sheet lists an institution's assets, liabilities, and net worth, as of a specific date. All an organization's assets must equal the total of the liabilities and net worth (fund balance) combined. To be in balance, the two totals must equal. Figure 7-2 is an example of a balance sheet.

Seaside Health System
Operating Income and Expense Statement
January 1—December 31, 199•
($000)

Gross revenues		$76,000
Deductions	$(25,000)	
Net revenue		$51,000
Operating expenses		
Salary costs	$25,000	
Other	15,000	
Bond expense	4,000	(44,000)
Net Income		$ 7,000

Fig. 7-1 An income and expense statement.

```
                        Seaside Health Systems
                            Balance Sheet
                         December 31, 199•
                             ($000)

ASSETS
Current assets:
    Cash                                                $ 2
    Accounts receivable*                                  6
    Inventories                                           2
        Total current assets                            $10
Land, plant, and equipment              $20
    Less: accum depreciation              8               12

Total Assets                                            $22

LIABILITIES AND NET WORTH
Current liabilities
    Accounts payable†                                   $ 4
    Notes payable                                         1
        Total current liabilities                       $ 5

    Bonds payable                                         3
        Total liabilities                               $ 8

Net worth
    Retained earnings                                   $14

Total Liabilities and Net Worth                         $22
```

*Accounts receivable is classified as assets because it is the amount of money owed to the hospital for the services already rendered (i.e., insurances billed, but money not yet received).

†Accounts payable is classified a liability because it is a cumulation of all the debts owed vendors for services already rendered to the hospital that will be paid for within the year.

Fig. 7-2 A balance sheet.

INSURANCE OVERVIEW

As stated earlier, health care providers are generally paid for their services by third-party payers, as opposed to individual payers or self-pay. The process of indirect payment from individuals for their care has been part of the national debate over the rising costs of health care. In the past, consumers never felt the pinch of high health care costs because their insurance companies paid the bill and their employers paid the cost of the insurance premium.

With the rising cost of employee health care negatively affecting the competitiveness of American products as compared to their foreign counterparts, employers across the country have banded together in business coalitions to demand lower costs, improved quality and customer service, and quantifiable outcomes from their providers of health care services. In addition to the business sector's revolt against the status quo of health care, both federal and state governments are demanding increased access for all people, with less reimbursement available for providers. Health care reform, managed care, and the integration of health care providers into vertical or horizontal networks have all evolved to meet the demands of the buyers of health care services. In this section health care reimbursement models that have been developed to attract and secure contracts to provide beneficiary services are briefly described.

Types of Insurance Plans

Indemnity. Indemnity insurance is an insurance plan that allows members to choose their own health care providers, who are paid on a fee-for-service basis and are not usually controlled through prior authorization or utilization controls. Beneficiaries may have a deductible to meet annually and a small co-pay with each encounter.

Fee-for-service benefit plan. Fee-for-service benefits are included in insurance plans that have generally paid for health care services on a full-charge basis. Historically, these plans have imposed few, if any, limitations on health care providers (hospitals, physicians), or alternate offsite providers. Reimbursement has been traditionally based on three factors, as follows:

1. Indemnity fee schedules/predetermined payments per procedure or service
2. Usual, customary, and reasonable fee schedule
3. Relative value units or the assignment of dollar values to a coded listing of services based on complexity of service

The two major categories of fee-for-service plans are as follows:

1. Basic hospitalization (with or without basic medical/surgical coverage)
2. Comprehensive hospitalization and medical/surgical coverage

Deductibles are usually associated with fee-for-service insurance arrangements; they are the amount of medical expenses that the individual must pay before a third-party payer will assume any liability for payment of benefits. The deductible can be either a fixed amount of money or the value of certain services over a given period (e.g., the deductible is equal to the charges for the first day of hospitalization).

As health care costs rose and insurance premiums followed, alternative delivery systems were developed to provide hospital and professional services on other than the charge, or fee-for-service, basis. Examples of alternative delivery systems include:

- Integrated Delivery Network
- Managed Care Organization
- Medicare Health Maintenance Organization
- Health Maintenance Organization (HMO)

- Preferred Provider Organization (PPO)
- Individual Provider Arrangement (IPA)

Integrated delivery network. An integrated delivery network is a provider of a continuum of either horizontal or vertical health care services, including one or more acute care hospitals, skilled and intermediate care facilities, outpatient and ambulatory surgery centers, home care agencies, and physicians who either are employees of the group or are managed by utilization protocols, established to competitively negotiate for contracts to provide care to a given beneficiary population.

Managed care organization (plan). A managed care organization provides its beneficiaries with a network of patient care services, (e.g., physician, inpatient and outpatient, ambulatory or home care services) for a set, agreed upon payment. This plan utilizes different types of control mechanisms to successfully manage the financial risk of providing health care services (e.g., case management, utilization control, other cost containment measures).

Medicare health maintenance organization (senior risk program). This is an alternative insurance product for Medicare beneficiaries that allows commercial insurers to contract with the Health Care Financing Administration (HCFA) to provide similar Medicare-covered services. Providers must have a contract with such insurers to provide beneficiary care. The advantages of such a program are that beneficiaries do not have to submit paperwork for payment, do not have a co-payment or deductible, and may have a richer benefit package. However, beneficiaries are limited in the number of providers they may go to and the number or types of services allowed. Beneficiaries are able to opt in, return to Medicare fee-for-service, and go back on a monthly basis.

Health Maintenance Organization. An HMO is a health care organization that provides comprehensive health service to its enrolled population for a fixed periodic payment.

Capitation is the term used to describe the fixed rate of payment (per member, per month) received by a health care provider on a periodic basis to cover a specified amount of health care services. All HMOs use a capitation rate when budgeting for their service area.

The ability to predict health plan premiums or costs based on the statistical analyses of financial, utilization, and demographic trends in a given area is found in actuarial services.

Preferred Provider Organization. A PPO is a health services organization of health care providers who have negotiated a special, usually reduced rate to attract insurance plan beneficiaries. Beneficiaries receive better cost coverage by using a contract provider; they can use a noncontracted provider, but will be responsible for a co-payment or additional fee-for-service payment.

Individual Provider Arrangement. An IPA is an organization that contracts with health care providers for the provision of medical services in their own offices for prepaid or managed care plans. One of the first alternative delivery plans was the prepaid plan. This is an insurance plan that offers its enrollees a defined set of benefits provided by a panel of providers within a specified geographic area. Kaiser Permanente was one of the first employers on the West Coast that provided such a plan, starting about 50 years ago.

Managed Care or Discounted Services

All of the above plans have a common denominator—the demand for discounted services. Discounts or deductions from revenue are the contracted amounts deducted from patient care revenues that health care providers must write off. Any or all of the plans may also negotiate a daily rate for the delivery of all health care services or only selected services, regardless of the actual services provided.

For example, a hospital or a home care organization may have a discount arrangement with a local HMO that reimburses 80% of charges for the guarantee of all local enrollees to utilize the contract services. The 20% difference would be deducted from the gross revenue, as well as the actual expense of providing the services. Across the nation, third-party payers are actively negotiating preferential rates with health care providers to try and control health care costs to their beneficiaries. In 1995, it had been noted that 21.1% of the insured in the United States were insured in a managed care plan, with individual state penetration as high as Massachusetts and California with 42.1% and 38.4%, respectively, to a low of Alaska and Wyoming with 0%.

It is very important for all managers and their staff to understand the concept of discounted services or managed care. Their health care facility may have a multitude of insurance providers demanding discounted services before allowing their enrollees to go to that facility. Each plan may have different preauthorization rules, lengths of stay, and types of service requirements that must be *observed, understood,* and *applied* appropriately to maintain financial viability.

Payer Mix

Payer mix is the distribution, usually expressed as a percentage, of all the sources of reimbursement for a health care provider. A typical example of a payer mix at a small urban hospital in the Northern California area is as follows:

- 40% Medicare
- 17% MediCal (Medicaid per diem or capitated)
- 5% Commercial (100% of total charges paid)
- 33% HMO/PPO (discounted contracts and Medicare Senior Risk)
- 5% Self-pay/No-pay

As you can see, approximately 95% of anticipated revenues have been or will be discounted—Medicare through the prospective payment system for DRGs; MediCal with a structured rate system per diem or capitated; HMO/PPO through discounted arrangements; and, most probably, write offs for the self-pay/no-pay (usually working individuals without insurance who do not qualify for Medicaid funds).

When charges are revised reflecting the increased cost of providing a service, the average discount is added back in to reflect true costs. In this scenario it is easy to comprehend why charges are rising so fast—to react to the demands for increased discounts from the payers. Staff members and managers need to understand the correlation between the gross charge and the net charge. In some cases, health care facilities may be averaging $.50 on each dollar of health care revenue because of discount arrangements.

CASE MANAGEMENT

Case management is a term that has developed a variety of meanings over the past few years, dependent on who was defining the term—the insurance carrier, the hospital, the home care organization—and from what perspective. There have been concerted efforts from both individual professionals and the national professional organization for case managers to agree upon a common definition of case management that would span all patient care sites.

Case management has been defined by the Case Management Society of America ". . . as the collaborative process which assesses, plans, implements, coordinates, monitors and evaluates options and services to meet an individual's health needs through communication and available resources to promote quality cost-effective outcomes."[6]

With the emergence of integrated health care delivery systems, the ideal case management model should shift from the narrowly-focused, institution-based one to a more wide-spectrum episode of illness-based, in order to more effectively coordinate patient care. Many health care facilities have enhanced and merged their discharge planning, utilization review, and in some cases social services departments into a more comprehensive case management staff. Those case managers are given the responsibility to plan for and monitor a patient's progress through the health care system, based on the patient's diagnoses, established treatment protocols and clinical paths, and utilization parameters. Working collaboratively with managed care plan representatives, physicians, and other health care professionals, case managers strive to provide the patient with the least disruptive care delivery system, with an efficient use of limited resources, while still striving to meet the assessed needs of the patient, both in the facility and back in the community.

Case management is important in the budget and resource management process within a health care setting. It allows for a reasonably accurate method to predict resource utilization of certain patients with given diagnoses, based on historic data, and it provides a foundation on which to gauge budget adherence when comparing actual expenses to budgeted expenses for certain patient categories.

THE BUDGET PROCESS

A budget is a document that outlines, for a specific period (usually 1 year), the plan an organization has developed for the consumption of resources. It involves the forecasting of revenue-generating activities and the resources used to achieve those goals. Nurse managers are usually involved in the development of three types of budgets:

1. Capital
2. Operating
3. Personnel

There are also different types of budgets, varying according to how they are generated and viewed during the budget cycle. A budget cycle is the period of time that the budget addresses—monthly, yearly, or multiple years. However, in most health care institutions, the budget cycle is on an annual basis following the fiscal year of the institution. Budgeting styles differ as well, as defined in Manager's Tip 7-2.

Capital Budget

A capital budget outlines the forecasted buying of large, fixed assets or types of equipment that depreciate (e.g., furniture, buildings, diagnostic imaging equipment). Usually the finance department will generate a payback analysis before approving the purchase of such budget items to ascertain whether the equipment can generate enough revenue to pay itself off over a given amount of time.

Depreciation is the amount/portion or cost of an asset that can be attributed to a certain operating period.

To meet Medicare regulations, capital budgets are forecasted over a 3-year period. However, they are reviewed and revised annually and as necessary as needs change. Figure 7-3 provides a sample capital acquisition summary.

Most payback analysis and net present value determinations can be generated with finance computer software. However, the nurse manager must supply the number of procedures and cost-related items that are estimated from the new piece of equipment, the amount of patient charge per procedure, and the total expense of operating the equipment. In that way, the finance department staff can determine whether the equipment can pay for itself within a stated period.

MANAGER'S TIP 7-2

BUDGETING STYLES

✔ A **fixed budget** is a budget amount that does not fluctuate with volume or staffing levels.
✔ A **flexible budget** is a budget that can be adjusted either up or down depending on the volume of service, which gives a manager a more accurate accounting of the costs incurred during a certain time frame.
✔ **Zero-based budgeting** refers to the process of planning and reviewing operations from the bottom up. It is not just an add-on of a certain percentage each year to account for volume increases or other indicators. The manager must review the expected service, what resources that service will require, and the cost of each of the resources for inclusion on the requested budget.

Seaside Health System
Budget Calendar Year 199•
Capital Acquisition Summary
($500.00 or more per item and 3 or more years of useful life)

Dept. priority	Proposed buy date	Item description	Replace/ upgrade	Number needed	Estimated cost of each item	Estimated total cost (including tax)

Attach as much supporting data as possible for each item, along with Capital Budget Form C-1. Return to senior manager for review and approval by September 1, 199•.

_____ Department

Manager Signature   Date

_____ Line

Administrator Approval   Date

Fig. 7-3 A capital acquisition summary.

Not all capital expenditures should be analyzed on payback analysis or net present value. If equipment is needed for regulatory or safety reasons, those reasons should be documented first and receive a priority rating of #1. However, the above method is a good way to determine the allocation of limited capital money.

Operating Budget

An operating budget describes the day-to-day operational expenses of a unit (excluding personnel costs). These types of costs include, but are not limited to, medical and nonmedical supplies, electricity, small equipment items (usually under $300 to $500 [i.e., stethoscope or sphygmomanometer]), and outside education expenses.

Ideally, all unit managers should create budgets using the zero-based method, which implies casting out all elements and components of all processes of care to be delivered (e.g., all alcohol swabs, betadine swabs, and IV tubing needed for budgeted patient care). However, that is not always possible for all budget categories. For this reason, it is important for the new nurse manager to review all the budget categories used for the past few years and determine appropriateness and continued applicability.

The categories that can be determined as direct costs and to which zero-based budgeting can be applied make the forecast more realistic and sustainable. An example of such a process includes the budgeting for an oncology unit with an estimated 100 admissions over the next 12 months. If the standard protocol called for IV lines for each patient and the lines were to be changed every 24 hours, and the length of stay was averaged at 3 days per patient, the manager could get an approximation of how many tubing lines to order.

$$100 \text{ patients} \times 3 \text{ lines per patient} = 300 \text{ tubing lines}$$
$$300 \text{ lines} \times \$25 \text{ each} = \$7500$$

Zero-based budgeting is very tedious, especially for a unit that uses a tremendous amount of supplies or other budgeted items. However, depending on the amount of time allotted to formulating budgets and the ability to control costs, it should be done at a minimum every few years to determine accuracy and serve as a monitoring system.

Understanding the mechanism of how costs have been applied to a budget and how the cost can be reduced from a budget provides the nurse manager with more fiscal control of the unit. It also makes reporting and understanding variances much easier to learn.

Personnel Budget

Finally, a personnel or full-time equivalent (FTE) budget is the document that forecasts the actual need for unit staff 24 hours per day, 365 days per year. Nursing personnel of FTE budgets differ from those of other hospital or health care setting departments in that, in addition to the estimated number of patient days being forecasted, the nurse manager must estimate the acuity level of the patients to more accurately determine the level, competency, number, and mix of nursing personnel needed to care for those patients.

The definition of an FTE is a personnel standard that allows for measuring and planning the staffing budgets. An FTE is equal to one person working 8 hours a day, 5 days a week, 52 weeks a year (2080 hours). It can be expressed in decimals as 1.0 (full-time) or .5 (half-time). An FTE does not necessarily mean one person; it can be two, three, or four workers providing enough hours to represent one person working a full-time shift. Figure 7-4 provides an example of a personnel budget form.

CLASSIFICATION OF COSTS

Costs incurred in the delivery of a service or the making of a product are called total costs and may be either direct or indirect, variable or fixed. A solid understanding of the types of costs and how they relate to your unit will allow you to make more appropriate decisions on how to cut costs, determine break-even points, and measure the effectiveness of any action.

Staff	(Productive and Nonproductive, exclude relief) POSITION SHIFTS								
Position Description	Position Class	AM	PM	NIGHT	199• Total FTE	Annual holiday days accrual	Holiday percent replace	Average sick day usage	Sick percent replace
Position Description	Position Class	Vacation FTE	Holiday FTE	Sick FTE	Non-productive FTE				

Fig. 7-4 A personnel budget form.

A **cost center** is any department or unit of the organization that has been designated as an area that accumulates costs. A nursing unit may have more than one cost center. More effective management can be accomplished by segregating costs and analyzing the benefits against the expenses in each center.

Fixed Costs

A fixed cost is a cost that does not change with the level of volume (e.g., the number of patients).Mortgage, loan, and bond payments are examples of fixed costs. Certain departments are considered fixed cost, or overhead, departments, such as medical records, admitting, the business office, and administration.

	Educ/ orientation days usage	Educ/ orientation percent replace	Non- productive total days					Holiday over- time hours	Annual stand- by hours	Annual call- back hours
	Relief FTE	Educ/ orientation FTE	Stand- by FTE	C/B FTE				Productive FTE	Total FTE	FTE Vari Productive STD

Fig. 7-4, cont'd A personnel budget form.

Variable Costs

A variable cost is a cost that is associated only with a specific activity (e.g., supply costs). Dressing supplies are considered a variable cost if a patient is being treated for a wound because the amount or type of supply utilized may vary. Variable costs may go either up or down with census shifts and are the first to be analyzed when operations are being reviewed.

Direct Costs

Direct costs can be allocated directly to the making or delivery of an item or service (e.g., nursing care hours in an intensive care unit or supply costs).

Indirect Costs

Those costs associated with the provision of services, but which cannot be directly linked to one specific area or service, are indirect costs. Generally, these costs are spread over the entire organization or areas of the organization based on some approved allocation method (e.g., number of FTEs or square footage of department pro-rated over total of classification). Some examples of these costs would be security, housekeeping, and utilities.

Budgets can be defined as both planning documents and control documents—two methods of ensuring financial viability in this dynamic marketplace. The margin for error is decreasing because reimbursement tightens while the cost of providing services increases daily as a result of new technologies and equipment, as well as higher salary demands by all health care personnel.

THE ROLE OF THE NURSE MANAGER IN THE BUDGET PROCESS

Historically, nurse managers have not been perceived as astute financial managers. Their expertise was in the clinical area, and the expectation was that the finance department administration and management would worry about reimbursing the cost of providing nursing service. But for nurse managers to successfully participate in negotiations between all health care departments vying for decreasing budget moneys, they must speak the same language and understand fiscal processes. Nurse managers must also be able to enter into the budget process without personalizing any budgetary actions. Staff cutbacks are sometimes inevitable solutions to the daily decreases in reimbursement for care. Special programs or increases of staff members must sometimes wait until the financial outlook improves or revenues are generated to pay for those services.

To plan more realistically and effectively, a nurse manager must be organized and consistent during the budget planning process, anticipating all changes that may occur within the budgeted time frame.

Budget Assumptions: Getting Ready to Start

Initially, all departmental objectives and goals must be analyzed to give the nurse manager direction in allocating given resources.

New projects and added or deleted services must be taken into account, along with the ongoing service of the unit. Historic data about estimated patient days or encounters, levels of acuity, or types of patients are also needed to make a more educated budget estimate. Knowledge of equipment needs, physician requests, and regulatory requirements is also essential for proper budgeting. Manager's Tip 7-3 lists questions for the manager to address when making primary budget decisions.

It is important to note that *budgets as planning and controlling documents are only as reliable as the data that were used in the development of the plan.* Changing requirements, service levels, or charge structures may be revised, and the budget document

MANAGER'S TIP 7-3

QUESTIONS TO ADDRESS WHEN MAKING BUDGET DECISIONS

✔ Do the benefits justify the costs?
✔ Is the budget consistent with the health system's strategic goals and objectives?
✔ Is the budget reasonable and realistic?
✔ Will the organization be able to support the budget?

may not be as relevant as it was when prepared. The nurse manager must be able to discern those changes that occur between development and implementation of the unit budget and reflect those changes once the budget period begins.

Recessionary cutbacks in tax revenues have forced certain state and local governments to reduce health care allocations immediately and across the board to all providers in their jurisdictions (e.g., the 1991 California MediCal cuts and state legislature's inability to pass a budget, thus resulting in the issuing of "warrants," or IOUs, for payment to health providers). Those health care entities with a large percentage of state Medicaid patients risk serious, if not fatal, financial duress if banking institutions refuse to accept the warrants as funds. Plans of action must be in place to meet such demands, including the issuance of loans or the reduction of services to stay financially viable.

The budget approval process is a dynamic function. Completed documents are submitted to higher management to be compiled and included in a larger document. For that reason, all department or service budgets are reviewed in relation to the prioritized needs of the organization.

Based on the organization's needs and financial abilities, a nurse manager may not receive all that has been requested during the budget process and thus must cut some costs from the budget. But the manager must be able to understand and distinguish the unit's core service and needs to more efficiently make the required cuts. Again, it is important that the new nurse manager not personalize any budget cuts because such behavior is counterproductive to successful management. Discussions should be ongoing between the unit managers and their senior management staff during the budget process to address the possibility of such problems.

BUDGETARY INDICATORS

Once settled in your new position as nurse manager with a basic understanding of the fiscal process, set up a financial report filing system that allows you the ability to monitor your unit's activities. Following is a list of financial reports that are used in various organizations:

Unit Reports

Payroll report	Employee earnings and hours worked by pay period classified by type of hour (e.g., education, productive, meeting time, vacation, sick, etc.)
Productivity report	Usually a percentage of total or productive hours worked for a given number of units of service (i.e., patient days as compared to budget)
Budget variance report	A listing of general ledger accounts, with monthly actual costs-to-budget amounts and cumulative year-to-date (CYTD) actual costs-to-budget amounts. Any deviance, whether positive or negative, is called a variance
Supply variance report	A listing by department of all supply costs and associated variances as compared with the budget amounts

All reports should be filed separately in chronologic order with the most recent on top. If your institution produces computerized ledger reports, there are expandable notebooks used to store these documents. These should be stored by fiscal year or fiscal period for easy retrieval and review.

Variances

Variances are the differences between the budgeted amounts and the actual amounts. Usually a negative ($-$) variance means a positive bottom line. In monitoring variances during periods of higher-than-budgeted volumes (e.g., numbers of patients), the manager must be aware of the forces of flexible versus fixed budgeting techniques. Variances may look askew, but when adjusted for volume, appear right on target.

Review all reports to ensure they are complete and correct; report discrepancies immediately to your supervisor or finance office (per organizational policy). Variances should be analyzed quickly and discussed with your supervisor. Abnormal or negative trends are insidious in nature, and you must closely oversee this aspect of your operations to analyze such occurrences and develop plans of action to correct identified negative trends.

Productivity and Variance Reporting

For an example of a productivity report showing a personnel usage variance, see Figure 7-5. Different job classifications, as well as their corresponding productivity standards, are noted in the first two columns. The actual versus budgeted units of service for that pay period are noted in the third through the sixth columns. A negative number in the variance column notes less-than-anticipated units of service. The productive and nonproductive FTE blocks show the actual versus the budgeted amounts of personnel. However, these are fixed-budget figures and do not reflect the FTEs used as compared with the actual units of service.

In the total FTE block is a flexible budget figure. That figure determines the number of FTEs available based on the actual units of service. In other words, if your unit had budgeted 4 FTEs for 16 hours of service and only 12 hours of service were given, only 12 hours should have been used. If, in the above scenario, you had used only 3 FTEs, the productivity rating would have been 100%. If you used the full 4 FTEs (as your budget states), your productivity would be only 75%.

The two blocks in Figure 7-5 for productive and total hours per unit of service actually address the productivity standard used for your department. In the case of the ICU, the productive standard for ICU days would be 16.109 hours per day; the total standard would be 17.688 hours per day.

The salary variance of $3,115 denotes a loss of $3,115 during that pay period resulting from overstaffing the ICU by approximately 13% to 15%. The $3,115 is an average amount of dollars for personnel costs across the board in the hospital. It is used as a guide to denote in dollar amounts the loss the hospital incurs from staffing overages. The positive amounts, such as are noted in the laboratory and pulmonary function columns, show the amount of moneys saved by increasing or decreasing staff.

Monitoring figures pay period by pay period allows the manager to review operations and identify negative trends. However, because of dramatic census shifts, labor contracts, and holiday and sick coverage, the manager must also look at the productivity rating over a longer period—either month to month or on a quarterly basis.

ASK QUESTIONS

Once you organize all the reports you have received to monitor the operations of your unit, set up a meeting with your fiscal representative. Ask questions and clarify statements or accounts at that time. Be clear as to the purpose of each report and what the data can tell you about the operations of your unit.

PRODUCTIVITY MEASUREMENT

Once approval has been given to the unit budget, the nurse manager must be able to abide by the financial constraints of that budget while still providing quality patient care services.

Before development of the cost-containment and tight-reimbursement health care arena that has dominated the industry during the past decade, cost-based reimbursement did not stress the need to be productive and use scarce resources in an efficient manner.

Productivity has been measured in many industries, and standards have been developed that enable a manager to quantify the effectiveness of any staff. For a long time, the production of only goods, not services, was felt to warrant productivity

Seaside Hospital
Productivity Report PPE: 6/20/9•

Unit of Service					Productive FTE				Nonproductive FTE			Total FTEs	
Dept	Desc	Act	Bud	Var	Var%	Act	Bud	Var	Staff Var	Act	Bud	Var	Act	Fixed Budget
ICU	ICU DAYS	54	63	(9)	-15%	11.3	12.8	1.4	11%	2.4	1.3	-1.2	13.7	14.0
M/S	M/S DAYS	267	282	(15)	-5%	25.7	28.0	2.2	8%	3.9	3.1	-0.8	29.6	31.1
E.R.	ER VISITS	807	716	91	13%	14.0	13.3	-0.6	-5%	2.4	1.1	-1.3	16.4	14.4
O.R.	OR MINS	13,310	11,363	1,947	17%	14.7	11.6	-3.1	-26%	2.5	1.4	-1.1	17.2	13.0
NSG ADM	ADJ PD	813	895	(81)	-9%	6.7	5.5	-1.2	-22%	0.4	0.9	0.5	7.1	6.4
Home Health	H.H. VISITS	444	577	(133)	-23%	14.2	15.7	1.6	10%	0.7	2.0	1.3	14.8	17.7
Lab	TESTS	8119	7898	221	3%	13.7	13.2	-0.5	-4%	1.6	1.9	0.3	15.3	15.0
Pulm Func.	CAP UNITS	9,023	9,750	(727)	-7%	1.0	1.4	0.4	29%	0.1	0.1	0.0	1.1	1.5
Medical Records	ADJUSTED PT DAYS	813	895	(81)	-9%	7.1	6.1	-0.9	-15%	0.4	0.8	0.4	7.5	6.9

Fig. 7-5 A productivity report.

measurements. The introduction of time-and-motion engineers into patient care units was not accepted well by staff members. The staff felt that nursing care could not be measured and that any constraint would be detrimental to the quality of the service delivered.

But economic survival forced productivity standards into the forefront of operational management techniques in health care settings. All activities of patient care were thoroughly examined and dissected to determine the amount or consumption of labor hours needed to provide those services. The averages of all those hours were compiled to develop a patient care standard.

Total FTEs		Productive Hours/Unit of Service				Total Hours/Unit of Service					
Flex Budget	Flex Var	Act	Bud	Var	Var%	Act	Bud	Var	Var %	Salary Var	Pro%
11.9	−1.8	16.755	16.109	−0.646	−4%	20.310	17.688	−2.622	−15%	($3115)	87%
29.5	−0.2	7.707	7.939	.0232	3%	8.877	8.831	−0.046	−1%	($221)	99%
16.3	−0.1	1.387	1.490	0.104	7%	1.621	1.613	−0.008	−1%	($116)	99%
15.3	−1.9	0.088	0.082	−0.006	−8%	0.103	0.092	−0.012	−13%	($4357)	89%
5.8	−1.3	0.661	0.493	−0.168	−34%	0.696	0.572	−0.124	−22%	($2527)	82%
13.6	−1.2	2.551	2.179	−0.372	−17%	2.675	2.454	−0.220	−9%	($1663)	92%
15.4	0.1	0.135	0.133	−0.002	−1%	0.151	0.152	0.001	1%	$199	101%
1.4	0.31	0.009	0.012	0.003	27%	0.010	0.013	0.003	23%	$445	130%
6.3	−1.2	0.695	0.549	−0.146	−27%	0.734	0.618	−0.116	−19%	($1323)	84%

Fig. 7-5, cont'd A productivity report.

PRODUCTIVITY RATINGS

Productivity rating is measured as a percentage:

$$\text{Standard} \div \text{actual} = \underline{\quad} \%$$

For example, if the standard for a home care nurse is 2 hours per visit, and the payroll records reflect that the average time spent per visit over a given time frame was 2.5 hours, the rating would be 80%. The usual variance is ±5%.

If the standard was 2 hours per visit and the nurse averaged 1.5 hours per visit, the rating would be 133%. That is a positive variance and reflects an overall savings to the home health agency.

FINANCIAL STANDARDS

There are many types of standards: national, industrial, local, and institutional. A standard is developed for use in a manager's facility, and the forecasting, budgeting, and actual review of operations must be consistent with the productivity standard that was designed to monitor the work of that individual department.

If a manager wants to develop a departmental standard, the following criteria need to be examined and then calculated into an amount of time per patient care service. First, a standard of quality must be agreed on for a given service, and then the average amount of time necessary to complete that service would constitute the production standard. Various methods can be used to gain that information: (1) an actual time-and-motion study, (2) an average formulated over a given period for the same type of services, (3) historic data, (4) benchmarking data from a similarly focused and sized facility, or (5) an educated guess if there are no data available.

BREAK-EVEN ANALYSIS

In learning how to be efficient in the management of your unit, you must develop the ability to determine a break-even analysis. Generally, all services or products offered by a business should be able to show a profit or should at least break even on costs.

However, breaking even is not possible in some health care situations, and the decision must be made whether to keep such services and balance their costs with other services. An example of such a costly service would be a trauma center or emergency service. Because of the specialized and expensive staff and equipment required to maintain the legal status of a trauma center on a 24-hour, 7-days-per-week basis, most facilities do not break even on this service. Most of the patients do not have sufficient insurance to cover all expenses, if they have insurance at all. However, it is a needed and vital service to the community.

Calculating Break-Even Points

The point at which the revenues equal the expenses is called the break-even point. A quick method to determine the break-even point is to divide the fixed cost of a service by the contribution margin per unit of service (see the definition below of contribution margin). Break-even analysis is very important in health care facilities because hospital buildings generally have very high fixed costs.

Budgetary Example in a Home Health Agency

For example, in a home health agency, the following information is given:

Monthly fixed costs: $10,000
Revenue per visit: $100
Direct cost per visit: $50
Contribution margin per visit $50

Contribution margin = (Revenue per visit − Direct cost per visit)

The break-even point (or the point at which the next unit of service's contribution margin is considered profit) would be:

$10,000 ÷ $50 = 200 visits

Contribution margin. The contribution margin is the amount of revenue left after the direct costs of providing the service are subtracted.

For example, the direct salary cost of a home health visit is $45 per visit, and the supply cost is $5, while the charge to the patient or payer is $100 per visit:

Direct cost: $45 + $5 = $50

The contribution margin would be the difference between the revenue and the direct cost, or:

$100 − $50 = $50

The contribution margin ($50) is then applied to the indirect, overhead, or administrative costs of doing business.

FUTURE TRENDS

As the health care industry continues its reforms and integrates CQI/TQM and fiscal responsibility into its case management structure, patient outcomes should improve and become more predictable.

Large employers, such as companies in the automobile industry, point out that they pay $300 to $500 of the revenue generated per new car for health care benefits for their employees. Just as consumers demand quality products off the automobile assembly line, health care consumers are demanding a standardized set of services that offers comparable outcomes.

This is a new concept to health providers—the argument has always been that health care is not quantifiable, as is the manufacturing sector of the economy. However, studies are showing that a wide divergence in standard practices for the same set of diagnoses or symptoms exists all across the country.

Large Business Groups on Health (LBGH, a lobbying group for business entities) is collecting and disseminating data on local hospitals and physician providers to the community denoting positive and adverse trends of service. LBGH is demanding that health care providers take a proactive stance for cost-effective, quality health care.

Once standards are clearly defined and routinely monitored, incentive systems can be put into place to reward those employees who use the best quality indicators, CQI/TQM, and patient satisfaction to turn their health care facility into a well-managed and effective organization.

Outcomes Management

Along with the demand for improved quality and decreased costs, health care buyers are demanding the quantification of what is being done to and for patients. They want to be able to compare patient care between similar settings to determine if the services are cost-effective. In the past, treatment varied with each practitioner and each setting in which it was delivered. However, with increased focus on patient satisfaction and the continual improvement of care processes, a need for the quantification of the results of such care arose.

Paul Ellwood, a leading futurist in outcomes management, described this emerging phenomenon as ". . . the technology of patient experiences designed to help patients, payers, and providers make more rational medical care–related choices based on better insight into the effect of these choices based on better insight into the effect of these choices on the patient's life."[7] Outcomes research has proceeded in earnest in all patient care settings, especially in acute care hospitals.

Outcomes measurement is the ability to measure the progression of a patient from one point in time to another. In the past the traditional definition of outcomes included cost, mortality, and morbidity—data collected by the Health Care Financing Administration (HCFA). Currently, there are many different methods to quantify outcomes; however, the most common areas to measure are:

- Clinical (traditional medical outcomes)
- Functional (both physical and social functioning)
- Well-being (mental/emotional health—pain, energy)
- Satisfaction with care
- Cost (what the patient and the system can/will bear)

Patients must be quantifiably assessed before the beginning of the movement across a care or protocol regimen in order to validate progress. In order for the data to be valid and reliable, it is imperative that commonalties in care or protocols are established and well-documented so that variances can be noted and reviewed and systems revised to provide a more positive care outcome. The aligning of patient processes, related outcomes, and cost of care will provide valid budgetary guidelines, both for a broad universal basis for health care and for specific, unit-based budget planning in a local health care setting.

Considerations for Home Care Managers

UNIQUE CHALLENGES IN FINANCIAL AND RESOURCE MANAGEMENT

Home health care is in the midst of an operational revolution as a result of its unprecedented growth over the past ten years, the emergence of managed care, and the impending shift in Medicare reimbursement (the largest payer of home care services). Home care managers have not always had to be as fiscally conservative as their acute care counterparts, primarily due to the mechanics of cost-based reimbursement. However, with the intertwining of capitation, Medicare managed care, and proposed prospective payment, those cost-based days are definitely in the past.

The home care manager is unique in many ways. The patient care delivery model already actively includes home care aides and attendants, as well as multidisciplinary team members, such as physical and occupational therapists, speech language pathologists, and medical social workers. Services are provided in the home setting, with management concern for staff safety both in driving to and from the home, as well as while in the patient's home—a major challenge. Successfully managing a staff who cannot be continually supervised from one delivery point is demanding. Financial and resource management is another complex challenge to the successful manager.

The majority of home care expense lies in direct and indirect personnel costs. Fixed costs are small, relative to an inpatient facility where patients are housed, fed, and cared for on a 24-hour basis. Hospital-based home care managers usually have had the additional challenge of trying to educate their hospital superiors on the intricacies and differences in home care budgeting and management, especially during times of downsizings and layoffs. Hiring freezes in patient care personnel encompassing the home health agency as well as other care facilities in an organization may harm the growth potential of the home care agency, since the visit volume is dependent on the number or qualified, oriented staff available to serve new and ongoing referrals. In many agencies closely aligned to an acute care setting that cares for the same population of patients, it has been noted that an inverse relationship exists between the census of the home care agency and the acute care facility, especially when the treatment of acute exacerbations of chronic diseases makes up the majority of both entities' patient loads.

BUDGETING

Home health care intermittent services, as differentiated from continuous case services, may be budgeted in a variety of ways. The primary method of home health care budgeting is visit cost (based on cost report accounting methods).

VISIT COST METHOD

Visit costs can be divided into two major areas:
- Direct (cost of clinical personnel time and transportation).
- Indirect (administrative staff, other variable and fixed costs).

The ratio of direct to indirect can be manipulated by management as determined by needs and other mandates; however, generally, a good "rule of thumb" should be as follows:

65%—Direct cost

35%—Indirect cost

Continued.

This method allows the manager to analyze cost-flexing based on contracted rates per visit, as opposed to a flex charge. It also allows the management team to decide what costs will make up the 35% when examining managerial, supervisory, and administrative personnel or needs of the organization. The costs can be broken down further within each category, such as:

Direct Costs:

- Personnel costs
  1. Patient care costs.
  2. Staff education.
  3. Administrative costs (meetings, team conferences, etc.).
  4. Documentation.
  5. Benefit costs (vacations, education and sick leave, etc.).
- Transportation costs
  1. Mileage.
  2. Toll or other costs.
  3. "Bonus" mileage (additional reimbursement for certain areas).

Indirect Costs

- Supplies
  1. Reimbursable medical supplies (attributed to individual patients).
  2. Nonreimbursable medical supplies.
  3. Office supplies.
- Administrative staff
  1. Managerial supervisory staff.
  2. Administrative/clerical/other staff.
- Other expenses
  1. Office space.
  2. Office telephone/cellular phone/utility expenses.
  3. Small equipment (noncapital).
  4. Subscriptions, books, etc.
  5. Management services (accounting, etc.).
  6. Other expenses.

PRODUCTIVITY STANDARDS

Productivity in home care has traditionally centered on number of visits per day per clinician to case loads per care manager. Standards should be used as a guiding management principle, with the caveat that there may be variances related to the geographic coverage of the agency and the clinician case load. Some agency staff may visit patients within a five-mile radius in large urban areas, whereas in rural areas it is not uncommon for staff to travel over 100 miles per day to care for their patients.

Generally, the following represents visit standards for the various disciplines (however, this should not be utilized without accounting for patient acuity and treatment regimens and level of services):

Skilled nursing: 5 to 7 visits per day (includes admission visits)
PT, OT, SLP: 6 visits per day
MSS: 4 to 5 visits per day
Home health aide: 5 to 6 visits per day

Agency management staff should assess the types and complexities of patients being seen and determine visit standards based on internal data, as well as external comparisons. Education, team and staff meetings, and continuous quality improvement efforts need to be analyzed and incorporated into visit standards, along with the organizations geographic coverage that has been described above.

Summary

Health care finance is a complex and demanding field, and nurse managers are an essential link in maintaining cost-effective, quality-oriented care. By understanding the role of cost accounting in the planning, delivery, and evaluation of care, the nurse manager can provide the best advocacy for patient care services in health care.

Financial managers are usually trained in the accounting or finance fields and usually do not have the education or expertise to make patient care decisions that involve cutbacks or reductions in services. Their focus is on improving the hospital's bottom line and providing sound financial decisions.

Nurses with business acumen and finance knowledge blend the best of both worlds and provide the most equitable perception of the budgeting process. Always be aware of the forces that are affecting the delivery of your patient care and be able to adapt to new and challenging situations.

References

1. Scholtes PR et al: *The team handbook,* Madison, WI, 1989, Jointer Associates.
2. Heidbreder J: Looking for the light—not the heat, *Healthcare Forum Journal* January/February 1993, pg. 26.
3. Marrelli TM, Hilliard LS: *Home care and clinical paths: effective care planning across the continuum,* St. Louis, 1995, Mosby.
4. Shillinglaw G, Meyer E: *Accounting: a management approach,* ed 7, Homewood, Ill, 1983, Richard D Irwin.
5. Anthony N, Reece J: *Accounting texts and cases,* ed 7, Homewood, Ill, 1983, Richard D Irwin.
6. Case Management Society of America: *Standards of Practice,* Little Rock, Ar, 1995, CMSA.
7. Ellwood PM: Outcomes management: a technology of experience, *New Engl J Med* 318(23):1549, 1988.

For Further Reading

Bruce C: Financial concepts in home health care, *JONA* 22(5):29, 1992.

Felteau A: Budget variance analysis and justification, *Nurs Manage* 23(2):40, 1992.

Hoss SF: Calculating capitation rates. *CARING Magazine* August 1995, 72-77.

Kerfoot K, Rohe D: Nursing management considerations: innovations for nurse managers to improve productivity, *Nurs Econ* 7(4):228, 1989.

Loevinsohn HT: A new perspective on scheduling: freedom and cost control, *Nurs Manage* 23(7):56, 1992.

Marrelli TM, Hilliard LS: *Home care and clinical paths: effective care planning across the continuum,* St. Louis, 1995, Mosby.

Maturen V, Zander K: Outcomes management in a prospective pay system *CARING,* June 1993.

Moss MT: Nursing tools: a global perspective *Nursing Management* June, 1994.

Murray JA: Benchmarking: a tool for excellence in palliative care *Journal of Palliative Care* 8(4):1992.

Porter-O'Grady T: *Nursing finance—budgeting strategies for a new age,* Rockville, Md, 1987, Aspen.

Schwartz WB, Mendelson DN: Hospital cost containment in the 1980s: hard lessons learned and prospects for the 1990s, *N Engl J Med* 324(15):1037, 1991.

Shikiar MS, Warner P: Selecting financial indices to measure critical path outcomes *Nursing Management* 25(9):58, 1994.

Tzirides E, Waterstraat V, Chamberlin W: Managing the budget with a fluctuating census, *Nurs Manage* 22(3):80B, 1991.

Wilburn D: Budget response to volume variability, *Nurs Manage* 23(2):42, 1992.

The following is a list of key financial terms that can be very helpful to you while learning your way as a new nurse manager.

Accounting The process of identifying and measuring an economic variable. Managerial accounting refers to the information that is prepared to assist managers in making decisions on how to use limited resources effectively and efficiently.

Acuity level A measured level that describes the severity of illness in patients by a weighted statistical method. Usually most acuity systems have four classifications of patients that describe the amount of time a nurse spends daily with each type of patient (i.e., ICU patients may have an acuity level of 4, denoting 1:1 RN:patient ratio). It was calculated using formulas that measured nursing functions in terms of actual time.

Adjusted average per capita cost (AAPCC) An estimate of the total payment for services a managed care payer would make for a unique category of services divided by the number of beneficiaries eligible for the services. This estimate is usually used in negotiating capitated agreements.

Aligned To be in accord with another similar management project or endeavor; working towards the same goal.

Arbitration A process of dispute resolution, principally employed by labor unions as a tactic to resolve a member's dispute with management, or a process to resolve perceived employee-related discrimination or termination.

Autocratic A style of management that does not allow others to make decisions and utilizes a rigid, structured style of leadership that does not include the input of others—a negative leadership style.

Bargaining unit A union group that is represented as a unified entity, usually made up of individuals who have related job titles or technical occupations within an organization.

Burnout The point where an individual, usually a manager, becomes overstressed and ineffective in her/his job; can also describe work group or organization.

Buy-out Financial takeover of a health care organization or unit within an organization by a larger or financially more prosperous entity; also the termination of an established employment contract.

Capitated risk The financial risk involved in not being able to accurately estimate the cost of and appropriately contract for care or services to a capitated population.

Capitation A set dollar amount established to cover the cost of health care services delivered to an individual. The amount is based on the number of members in the plan, not the amount of services used.

Capitation management The process of gathering as much information on the population to be capitated and understanding the key characteristics of that population in order to manage the financial risk involved in providing care or services.

Card-signing Activity in which a union asks nonunion health care employees to sign cards requesting an organization-wide election that might vote a union into existence.

Certificate of Need (CON) Document provided by a state governing body to a health care institution at the institution's request that allows the institution to build additional physical facilities or provide services to handle more customers.

Chain of command Term that reflects the lines of report and power structure within the health care organization, thus clarifying who reports to whom.

Chief Executive Officer (CEO) The main administrator of a hospital or health care organization; usually indicates that the administrator is also a member of the governing body.

Chief Financial Officer (CFO) A second-tier executive with comprehensive control of the financial systems; has responsibility for financial stability and compliance efforts.

Chief Medical Officer (CMO) A senior physician manager, usually reporting to the CEO of a health care organization with responsibilities over the medical functions and medical staff of the organization.

Chief Nursing Officer (CNO) A senior nurse executive (NE) who reports to the CEO with overall responsibility for the nursing services provided in the health care organization.

Chief Operations Officer (COO) Individual responsible for all critical operational facets of a health care organization; reports to the CEO.

Cost-based reimbursement Reimbursement to health care providers based on the aggregation of allowable costs, up to a certain limit (e.g., cost caps). This system of reimbursement was originally established for Medicare program providers and is quickly disappearing with the advent of capitation and managed care.

Cost control Management approach that encourages the insightful utilization of financial resources in the interest of getting maximum benefit from each dollar spent and effectively maintaining fiscal responsibility and budgetary integrity.

Cost shifting The act of increasing rates to one segment of the patient population to offset losses incurred by another segment, such as Medicaid or indigent patients.

Depreciation Erosion, over time, of the quality and effectiveness of certain resources within a health care institution, and the resultant financial practice of incorporating this erosion into fiscal and tax considerations.

Gross revenue/income The total amount charged for a service.

Hours per patient day (HPPD) The number of nursing care hours provided per patient per 24-hour day.

Liabilities The financial obligations of the hospital or other health care organization (i.e., accounts payable or loan amounts).

Medicaid program A state health insurance program for those individuals meeting certain financial guidelines that is supported by the federal government in association with funds from a given state. Not all states have Medicaid programs, and the programs and their coverage vary from state to state.

Medicare program The federally funded health insurance program for those individuals over the age of 65 or disabled. It was started in 1965 and totally revolutionized the delivery of health care in the United States. It reimbursed hospitals and other health care providers on a cost-based system. The health care system then experienced rapid growth because there were no incentives built into the program to conserve or properly use resources.

Currently, the Medicare program is undergoing extensive scrutiny and revision to meet the growing needs of the burgeoning older population. Hospitals have been taken out of the cost-based system, and the prospective pay, or DRG, system has taken its place.

Medicare-certified home health agencies are still currently cost-based. Studies are being conducted to determine the best method to establish a prospective payment system for the rapidly growing home care industry in the near future.

Net income The difference between the gross revenue and what remains after all expenses have been deducted.

Nonproductive hours Paid hours that are not associated with the provision of care or service (i.e., vacation, sick, and education leave).

Outliers Cases in which a patient's length of stay exceeds the national average by 20 days or a 1.94% standard deviation, or in which the cost of treatment exceeds the national average diagnostic-related group rate by $12,000 or 150%, whichever is greater.

Patient classification system A system to classify patients using different criteria sets. The goal of the patient classification system is to allocate nursing personnel to specific units (i.e., staffing matrix).

Productive hours Paid hours that are associated with provision of care or service, including regular time, overtime, and holiday time.

Prospective payment system The third party payment system that establishes certain payment rates for services regardless of the actual cost of care provided. The Medicare diagnostic-related group system for inpatient acute care services is the most widely known example of this type of payment. The prospective payment system was established in 1981 under the Tax Equity and Fiscal Responsibility Act (TEFRA).

Relative value units A numerical value that has been coded to reflect the relative complexity of a given service, such as time, skill, and overhead costs for a certain procedure. Many third-party payers attach a dollar value to these units in calculating reimbursement rates. An example of a service measured in RVUs is rehabilitation services (physical therapy).

Risk pool An incentive pool of moneys, over and above the direct payment made to a service provider, that is distributed to a determined number of providers if certain predetermined financial outcomes are met.

Staffing mix The type and ratio of professional personnel (RNs) to other patient care personnel. This mix varies from hospital to hospital and is gaining in popularity as the need to decrease personnel costs becomes more evident.

Nurse extenders or licensed vocational/practical nurses in tandem with an RN are two examples of using a varied staffing mix. This is a move away from the all-RN staffs demanded by the nursing industry in the 1970s and 1980s.

Sub-capitation A subset of capitated moneys set aside for a particular group of services (e.g., home care services under a hospital-controlled plan or home medical equipment as a subcapitator to a home care organization).

CHAPTER 8

LEGAL ISSUES AND RISK MANAGEMENT

ELIZABETH HOGUE

This chapter focuses on significant legal issues. Discussion of legal issues in nursing management could fill *several* books, and it is often difficult for the new nurse manager to know where to focus attention in terms of legal issues. In addition, the new manager's difficulty in discerning significant legal issues may be further complicated by the staff's initial tendency to raise numerous questions or concerns about legal issues. In the absence of effective management, staff members may seek structure and stability in their work environment through the law. Once effective nursing leadership is in place, the tendency to see everything as a legal issue will disappear. Understanding the legal aspects of supervision can help the nurse manager provide such leadership and allay staff members' concerns.

LEGAL ASPECTS OF SUPERVISION

Nurses are generally responsible for the acts and omissions of all of the practitioners whom they supervise. Their liability is based on legal theory called *respondeat superior,* which literally means "let the master say." The theory is that since supervisors control what practitioners do, they are therefore legally responsible for their errors.

The only exception to this rule occurs when, despite appropriate supervision, practitioners take it upon themselves to do something that is entirely outside the scope of their job functions. A classic example of this conduct involves nurses who voluntarily provide care to patients in their homes after they have been discharged from the hospital, facility, or home health agency. As long as management is able to demonstrate that a policy was established that prohibited this conduct, liability for injuries to patients during such "detours" may rest solely with the practitioners.

Questions of appropriate delegation of allowable functions to certain types of practitioners is controlled almost exclusively by state laws. That is, state licensure statutes govern which functions related to patient care may be delegated to certain types of practitioners. Nurse managers must thoroughly understand these statutes in the states in which their organization provides services in order to ensure that functions

187

are properly delegated. Any questions or areas of uncertainty should be referred to the appropriate state licensure boards for written clarification.

Many nurse managers are understandably concerned about the scope of their responsibilities for everyone who falls within their chain of command. They certainly cannot provide direct supervision to each practitioner whom they supervise on a daily basis. This valid concern serves to reinforce the importance of hiring and retaining practitioners who provide care to patients in an appropriate manner. It also underscores the need to take prompt disciplinary action with regard to practitioners who do not meet established standards.

Even though every practitioner's actions cannot be supervised directly, significant legal issues exist that always merit the attention of competent nurse managers. New managers should immediately focus their attention on these issues and continuously monitor developments in the following areas:

- Negligence
- Consent to treatment, including the patient's right to refuse treatment
- Employment issues

NEGLIGENCE

Health care providers often equate negligence with something going wrong. In fact, there are risks associated with treatment. Just because something goes wrong does not mean that any legal liability exists. Rather, there are four components that every patient must be able to prove were involved to show that nurses were negligent:

1. Duty
2. Breach
3. Causation
4. Injury

All four of these components must be involved to prove negligence. If patients fail to prove even one of these elements, they lose their cases. Thus these elements can serve as a checklist for the new nurse manager to use to manage risks and evaluate the likelihood of legal liability. If she/he can defeat even one of the components, no legal liability exists.

A determination that there is no legal liability is certainly not all that should concern the nurse manager. Managers may have significant ethical, quality assurance, employment, and licensure concerns that should be pursued even when no legal liability exists. However, it is helpful to eliminate concerns about legal liability even when other serious considerations require resolution.

It is also important to remember that involvement of these elements constitutes the definition of negligence that is actually used by the courts. That is, when courts attempt to determine whether providers are negligent, they consider these elements in relation to each case to determine liability. This is true regardless of the state in which nurses provide care. The definition of negligence in New York is the same as in California. The legal definitions of duty, breach, causation, and injury are discussed below.

Duty

Duty is the obligation owed by providers to their patients. Thus the existence of a provider-patient relationship is a prerequisite to liability.

The duty owed by nurses to their patients is a duty of reasonable care. Of course, the key question then becomes: What is reasonable? The law says that what is reasonable is what other reasonably prudent nurses do under the same or similar circumstances. Nurses know what other nurses do by examining standards of care. Standards of care define nurses' duties to their patients. Sources of such standards of care are listed in Box 8-1.

The Importance of Policies and Procedures

Policies and procedures constitute perhaps the most important source for standards of care. Developing appropriate standards of care through policies and procedures is certainly a double-edged sword for nurse managers. Although it provides an opportunity to establish standards that are appropriate for institutions and staff members, the law requires strict adherence to these standards once they have been developed.

In addition, developing policies and procedures is an exceptionally tedious task for several reasons. First, some nurses believe that policies and procedures should cover every possible contingency associated with the policy subject. Nurses who share this belief want such policies so that they feel they have clear guidance. Other nurses, however, believe that policies and procedures should provide only broad guidance, within which nurses should exercise appropriate professional judgment. Obviously, finding a balance between these two competing goals is necessary. Policies that are too detailed often prove useless because staff members do not have the time or inclination to read through volumes to understand procedure. Conversely, promoting clarity of expectations of staff members is one of the basic tenets of effective nursing management.

---

box 8-1
SOURCES OF STANDARDS OF CARE

- The employer's internal policies and procedures
- Court decisions
- Standards of professional nursing organizations such as the American Nurses Association (ANA) and the National League for Nursing (NLN)
- State licensure statutes
- Requirements of third-party payers
- Standards of accreditation organizations such as the Joint Commission for the Accreditation of Healthcare Organizations (JCAHO)

Developing standards of care though policies and procedures is further complicated by the sheer number of individuals and committees that typically review a new or revised policy or procedure. Often, what goes into the process bears little resemblance to the final result.

Despite these obstacles, nurse managers must persist in developing and maintaining appropriate policies and procedures. A key to success is to avoid thinking that this process is ever complete. Nursing policies and procedures should be under almost constant review and scrutiny; they are not static. Rather, they change often because of experience, judgment, and new clinical developments. Manager's Tip 8-1 presents five key steps for developing policies and procedures as a means of risk management. If nurse managers follow these steps, they will have greater assurance that they appropriately manage risk by careful definition of duty in terms of policies and procedures.

Breach

Nurses may breach their duty to patients by doing something they should not do, which is commonly referred to as an *act*. They may also fail to do something that they should do, which is often referred to as an *omission*. In many malpractice cases, patients are able to prove that providers committed more than one act or omission. Yet, they *need* prove only *one* act or omission to prove a breach.

For example, in one recent court case, a man was brought to the emergency room with a chest wound. He was evaluated to see if he needed a thoracic surgeon. It was determined that he did not have such a need. He was reevaluated an hour later, and it was determined that he, indeed, needed a thoracic surgeon. The surgeon was called but did not arrive for over an hour. On the surgeon's arrival, the patient was rushed into the operating room, where he died. The family sued, claiming that if the surgeon had arrived earlier, the patient would not have died. During the course of discovery, the attorney for the patient's family found an emergency room policy that stated that if the thoracic surgeon was called and did not arrive within 30 minutes, the patient

MANAGER'S TIP 8-1

KEY STEPS TO MANAGING RISK
THROUGH POLICIES AND PROCEDURES

- ✔ Review policies and procedures at least annually.
- ✔ Involve different staff members in reviewing policies and procedures so that various points of view are obtained and the staff has an opportunity to review standards of care.
- ✔ Make needed changes promptly.
- ✔ Ensure that all staff members are informed of changes in policies and procedures.
- ✔ Ensure that all new staff members read and understand the policies and procedures.

must be transferred to another hospital. The family won this case because the nursing staff breached its duty as established in emergency room policies and procedures.

Causation

A patient must show that the act or omission of the nurse caused injury or damage. The best way to define causation is in terms of "but for." That is, but for the action or inaction of the provider, the patient would not have been injured. Another way to consider causation is in terms of what courts call "foreseeability." That is if providers should have foreseen that their act(s) or omission(s) would cause injury or damage to a patient, the injury was foreseeable and therefore caused by providers. Conversely, if providers could not have foreseen that their act(s) or omission(s) would cause injury or damage to a patient, the injury was not foreseeable and therefore was not caused by providers.

Time is certainly a consideration with this requirement. For example, when a patient who is released from a mental health institution causes injury or damage to an individual after release, it is tempting to find a causal connection between the patient's release and the injuries sustained. Nurses recognize, however, that an individual's mental status may change very rapidly. Therefore no causal connection may exist whatsoever between release and the injuries.

Nurses sometimes ask how long of a period must elapse before causation is no longer a concern. This period varies depending on the circumstances of individual cases. Providing specific rules is thus impossible. A good general rule is that the longer the period between the providers' action or inaction and the occurrence of the injury, the less likely that providers will be held liable.

Injury

To be held liable, nurses must injure or damage their patients. Most of the time the courts insist on a physical injury to establish liability. Courts require proof of physical injury for several reasons. First, if the alleged injury is not physical, patients may be faking their injuries. Courts have evidentiary requirements that must be met to prove injury. If the claimed injury is mental or emotional in nature, it is almost impossible to prove. Second, the courts recognize that a certain amount of irritation and inconvenience simply accompany being alive. It is not the job of the courts to address all of these inconsequential irritations and inconveniences. Rather, individuals are generally required to accept life's daily aggravations that are relatively insignificant. Unless patients can show a physical injury, their complaints may fall into the category of mere irritation and inconveniences, not legal liability. Finally, judges are increasingly distressed about their overcrowded dockets. In many jurisdictions there are so many cases pending that it takes several years for a civil, noncriminal case to come to trial. Courts recognize that caseloads will increase many times over if they start considering cases involving claims for emotional injuries only. They therefore normally insist the claimant have a physical injury before they will find providers liable.

Extreme and outrageous behavior. The one exception to this general rule occurs when the behavior of providers is what the courts call "extreme and outrageous." Extreme and outrageous behavior is outside of the acceptable bounds of civilized behavior. Extreme and outrageous conduct is illustrated by the case in which a woman was in the delivery room about to deliver a baby. Her husband was with her at her head. She died precipitously. The father rushed around to his deceased wife's side and put his hand on her abdomen. He could feel the infant still moving. He turned to the delivery room staff and asked them to perform an emergency caesarean section to save the life of the infant. The staff refused. He stood in the delivery room, begging and pleading with the staff, until the infant died.

In this case, there may have been liability for the death of the mother. Certainly there was liability for the death of the infant. But the court also acknowledged liability directly related to the father, even though his injuries were emotional only. The court did not require a physical injury because it was clear that the father was not faking emotional injury in view of the circumstances. The court was also certain that the father's injuries amounted to more than mere irritation and inconvenience. Finally, even though court dockets are crowded, the courts are extremely interested in hearing this type of case because of the egregious conduct of the providers.

Thus unless physical injury exists or extreme and outrageous conduct on the part of providers occurs, there is no legal liability. The focus of appropriate risk management is therefore on avoiding injuring patients. Good risk management truly amounts to damage control.

Nurse managers continually struggle to avoid certain common types of liability for negligence. They must work hard to control risk related to the types of negligence outlined in Manager's Tip 8-2.

Negligent Premature Discharge

Negligent premature discharge, a relatively new area of potential liability for negligence, merits special attention. Concerns about negligent premature discharge are di-

MANAGER'S TIP 8-2

FIVE COMMON TYPES OF NEGLIGENCE

- ✔ Failure to properly monitor and observe patients.
- ✔ Improper diagnosis, particularly meningitis in pediatric patients and myocardial infarctions.
- ✔ Falls.
- ✔ Foreign objects left in patients during surgery.
- ✔ Negligent premature discharge.

rectly related to changes in the activities of third-party payers. Third-party payers now command the authority of providers with their assumed decision-making authority regarding patient care. Whereas providers previously made decisions regarding patient care, payers are now the gatekeepers to the health care delivery system. In view of this change, providers have begun to question why they may be held liable for the results of payment decisions of payers.

In response, payers argue that they do not write orders, including discharge orders. Providers are free to render as much care as they determine patients need. Payers are saying only that they will not pay for such care. Further, payers argue that, in many instances, they are simply enforcing a contract of insurance. Once benefits required by the contract have been provided, they are under no obligation to pay for additional care, regardless of the clinical condition of patients.

Providers, however, recognize the reality of the health care delivery system today, which is that payment decisions are, in essence, treatment decisions. Courts are considering the question raised by this reality to determine if payers should be held responsible for the injuries or damages that result from payers' adverse payment decisions. To date, three court decisions have addressed this issue.

Wickline versus The State of California. In the 1987 case of *Wickline versus The State of California,*[1] Mrs. Wickline had vascular disease. She had surgery, followed by a complicated recovery. Her physician wanted to keep her in the hospital to observe her for further complications. The Medicaid program, however, determined that no further payments would be made for acute care.

Mrs. Wickline's physician asked the Medicaid program for an additional extension of payment for acute care. Specifically, he asked the Medicaid program to pay for 8 additional days of care. Medicaid agreed to pay for 4 additional days.

At the end of the 4 days, the physician took no further action, and Mrs. Wickline went home. She developed further complications that ultimately resulted in the amputation of one of her legs. She then sued the Medicaid program. She claimed that the program had a duty to her to make payment for needed care that was breached when payment was refused for additional acute care. Medicaid's adverse payment decision, claimed Mrs. Wickline, caused injury to her in the form of the amputation of her leg.

It is important to note that there were alternatives that could have been used to limit risk in this case. For example, home care might have been an appropriate way to continue to monitor Mrs. Wickline for additional complications outside of the acute care setting. Even if nurse managers cannot ensure payment for the type or length of care that they regard as most desirable, it is important to arrange for other available care that may help to limit risk.

The court considered Mrs. Wickline's claim against the Medicaid program. It first recognized a so-called "changed reality" in the health care delivery system. That is, the court acknowledged that payers now make treatment decisions. Therefore, said the court, payers should be liable for adverse payment decisions that harm patients.

The one condition placed on this shift of liability from providers to payers was that providers must satisfy what the court called "duty to protest." In other words, the court said that providers would not be liable for results of adverse payment decisions so long as they protest payment decisions that they think will injure patients.

Because the physician in Mrs. Wickline's case did not protest the decision to terminate payment after the additional 4 days, the court did not find the Medicaid program liable in this case. The physician was not liable either because he was not a defendant in the case. The court made it clear, however, that from then on it would hold payers liable if they persisted in adverse payment decisions in view of protests by providers.

Valro versus Blue Cross and Blue Shield of Michigan. In the case of *Valro versus Blue Cross and Blue Shield of Michigan,*[2] workers at General Motors (GM) Company decided that they wanted more mental health and substance abuse benefits. GM agreed to provide the additional benefits but wanted to self-insure for them because these benefits can be expensive to offer.

GM went to Blue Cross and Blue Shield of Michigan and asked Blue Cross to run a pilot program to assist in developing these benefits. Blue Cross agreed. Both parties signed an agreement that, among other factors, made it clear that the pilot program would include a rigorous utilization review (UR). It would include preauthorization, precertification, concurrent review, and prospective and retrospective review.

Blue Cross then signed agreements with individual mental health providers to treat patients in the pilot program. All of the participants were satisfied until the UR program became so rigorous that it interfered with the providers' ability to deliver patient care or receive payments for providing care. They thought that the activities of Blue Cross amounted to the practice of medicine and sued them.

The court considered the providers' claims. In the court's view, the providers were simply attempting to ensure payment for fulfilling their ethical and legal duty to provide care to patients. The court came very close to calling them greedy wimps and termed the basis of the providers' lawsuit "strange stuff" on which to base a claim.

Thus the decision in the *Valro* case is inconsistent with that in the *Wickline* case. Specifically, *Wickline* says that providers are not required to treat patients if payment is denied, and, when patients are injured as a result, payers, not providers, are liable if payment is denied despite the providers' protests. *Valro,* however, says that providers have a legal and ethical obligation to provide care whether or not they receive payment.

Wilson versus Blue Cross and Blue Shield of Southern California, et al. In the case of *Wilson versus Blue Cross and Blue Shield of Southern California, et al,*[3] decided in 1990, Mr. Wilson was hospitalized in Los Angeles for depression and anorexia. His physician, Dr. Taft, recommended inpatient care for 3 to 4 weeks. This recommendation was conveyed to Blue Cross.

Blue Cross contracted with a utilization review organization, Western Medical Review, to consider whether payment for claims such as Mr. Wilson's should be authorized. Dr. Wasserman at Western Medical Review considered Mr. Wilson's claim. He determined that he would authorize payment for the few days of inpatient care that Mr. Wilson had already received, but would not authorize payment for any additional inpatient care.

This decision was relayed to Dr. Taft and Mr. Wilson. Mr. Wilson had no other way to pay for his care and was discharged from the hospital.

Within the period during which Mr. Wilson probably would have been hospitalized, if his request for inpatient care had been authorized, he committed suicide. His parents then sued Blue Cross, Western Medical Review, and Dr. Wasserman, claiming that Mr. Wilson was negligently prematurely discharged as a result of the adverse payment decision.

The case was dismissed at the trial level based partly on Dr. Taft's failure to protest the adverse payment decision. On appeal, the court said that the previous ruling in the *Wickline* case was wrong. That is, payers are liable for the adverse payment decisions made that injure patients, whether or not providers protest these adverse payment decisions. This determination may serve as a useful precedent, permitting courts in other jurisdictions to reach a similar conclusion that payers are now liable for injuries that occur because of failure to pay for needed care.

In view of these court decisions, which are clearly inconsistent in some respects, nurse managers may well ask how to take appropriate action. The best advice at this time is to fulfill the duty to protest adverse payment decisions. This recommendation is based on the conclusion that such protests are good risk management. It is also based on the importance of the nurse's role as a patient advocate. If nurses do not speak for patients in the face of adverse payment decisions, it is unlikely that anyone will do so. Most patients do not understand the complex health care delivery system well enough to be their own advocates.

Nurse managers must be prepared to monitor developments in the area of liability for premature discharge. The last word has by no means been spoken on this important issue by courts and legislatures.

INFORMED CONSENT

Informed consent is not required for routine or emergency treatment. Routine care often includes physical examinations and drawing blood. Emergency treatment usually occurs when danger to life or permanent injury to patients' limbs is threatened.

Informed consent is required for treatment that is neither routine nor provided in response to an emergency. Generally, the need for valid informed consent increases in direct proportion to the risk of the treatment.

Prerequisites

The following two prerequisites must be met to obtain valid informed consent:
1. The patient must have the capacity to give consent in terms of chronologic age and the ability to understand information.
2. The patient's consent must be voluntary.

Generally, patients must be of legal age before they can consent to treatment. The age at which an individual is legally considered to be an adult varies from state to state but is usually at either age 18 or age 21. Exceptions to this requirement include:

- Minors who are emancipated because they are married, have borne a child, or are economically independent—the laws on this category vary from state to state.
- Minors who seek treatment for certain types of conditions such as sexually transmitted diseases, mental illness, or substance abuse—laws regarding these exceptions also vary from state to state.

Patients must also be able to understand information to give valid consent. Generally, this requirement means that they must be able to understand the consequences of their choices regarding treatment. Patients who have been found to be incompetent by the courts clearly lack capacity to understand information. Patients who have not been declared incompetent may, nonetheless, lack the necessary level of mental capacity. The best method for evaluating capacity is to use a mental status examination and to document the results in patients' records just before obtaining informed consent.

You should note that the law recognizes that capacity (the ability to understand information) may vary from moment to moment. Confused patients may suddenly seem much more lucid. It is appropriate to seek informed consent during such moments. Consent under such conditions is valid even after the patient becomes incapacitated once again.

A patient's consent must be voluntary (i.e., there can be no fraud or duress). Providers cannot tell patients that they are going to perform one treatment and actually perform an entirely different treatment. Providers walk a fine line between informing patients of the consequences of their refusal of treatment and threatening them. Manager's Tip 8-3 lists the information required for informed consent.

MANAGER'S TIP 8-3

INFORMATION NEEDED FOR
INFORMED CONSENT

Patients who satisfy the prerequisites for informed consent must receive the following information:
- ✔ Description of the proposed treatment.
- ✔ Possible benefits of the proposed treatment.
- ✔ Significant risks associated with the treatment.
- ✔ Description of alternative treatments.
- ✔ A clear acknowledgment of their right to refuse treatment.

When obtaining informed consent, the provider must give a description of the proposed treatment because consent is valid only when a patient understands the treatment to be received. A patient cannot provide valid consent to a treatment that she/he does not understand.

Benefits of proposed treatment must never be described in absolute terms or as guarantees of results. If benefits are presented to patients as guarantees, a contract may be created that is breached by providers if they fail to deliver the promised result. Providers must speak of *possible* benefits from proposed treatment.

A provider is not required to share *all* risks with patients. Rather, a provider is required to share those risks that are either statistically significant or are especially important to patients in the provider's opinion. For example, if proposed surgery involves even a slight possibility of injury to a violinist's hands, this risk must be disclosed.

Alternative treatments must also be described. These may include medications, physical therapy, surgery, diet and exercise, or whatever could be of benefit to the patient.

Finally, the unqualified right of patients to refuse any treatment must be acknowledged as part of the process of obtaining informed consent. Providers should make a clear statement to this effect, which should be specifically acknowledged by patients.

Patients who consent to treatment after the prerequisites have been met and the above information has been given have given valid informed consent. Verbal consent is acceptable.

It is important, however, to document the patient's consent. Providers use several methods to accomplish this goal. The most popular vehicle is undoubtedly a consent form, which is useful only when it documents the specific information given to the patient. Other providers use progress notes summarizing the consent process. Audio and video recordings are also acceptable means of documenting informed consent.

Nurse managers should understand that it is the physician's job to obtain valid informed consent. Nurses may ask patients to sign forms documenting that they have given informed consent. Their signature on such forms as witnesses means that they saw the patient sign the form; their signature does not verify that patients received appropriate information. But nurse managers must also realize that the nursing staff has a vested interest in making sure informed consent is obtained because health care is almost always provided as a team. When one member of the team fails to perform or to adequately protect the team, the whole team is at risk, not just one member.

Suppose, however, that patients cannot meet the prerequisites of informed consent because of their chronologic age or lack of ability to understand information. Who may give substitute consent on behalf of such patients? Manager's Tip 8-4 on p. 198 lists sources of substitute consent and presents additional information that nurse managers may find helpful.

MANAGER'S TIP 8-4

THOSE WHO CAN GIVE SUBSTITUTE CONSENT ON BEHALF OF PATIENTS

✔ **Parents on behalf of minors.** In the case of separation or divorce, either the custodial or the noncustodial parent may consent unless she/he is prohibited from doing so in a separation agreement or a divorce decree. Nurse managers should educate staff to obtain copies of relevant documents and to place copies of these documents on patients' charts to certify that appropriate individuals gave consent on behalf of minors.

✔ **Courts.**

✔ **Guardians of the person.** Courts appoint two types of guardians or conservators: guardians of the property and guardians of the person. Only guardians of the person may consent to health care. Staff must obtain a copy of any decree of guardianship and place it on the patient's chart to document valid informed consent.

✔ **Attorneys-in-fact.** Attorneys-in-fact are appointed to act on behalf of patients in powers of attorney. Powers of attorney are very flexible instruments. Nurses must therefore obtain a copy of any power of attorney under which an individual claims authority to evaluate the scope of their powers. Powers of attorney may be executed only by patients who have mental capacity. When patients become permanently mentally incapacitated, it is too late to sign a power of attorney. Durable powers of attorney survive the incapacity of patients. The laws governing powers of attorney vary from state to state.

✔ **State statutes.** Some states have passed laws that permit individuals to make decisions regarding health care in the absence of a guardian or attorney-in-fact. There is significant variation among the state statutes.

WITHHOLDING AND WITHDRAWING TREATMENT
No Code Orders

"No code" or "Do not resuscitate" orders are a form of withholding treatment. It is important for nurse managers to understand, however, that these orders permit providers to withhold *only* treatment related to resuscitation if patients need such measures. Such orders do not apply to withholding nourishment, hydration, or IV fluids.

No code orders may be entered by physicians at their discretion for terminally ill patients after consultation with competent patients or family members. Physicians are required to provide these orders.

No code orders may not be transferred between institutions. Patients who had no code orders in long-term care facilities must have a new order entered when admitted to a hospital.

Some institutions permit partial no code orders. Partial no code orders are undesirable from an administrative point of view. It is extremely difficult for staff members to remember what each patient's no code order permits.

Verbal no code orders. There is a clear difference of opinion regarding verbal no code orders. The best practice appears to permit them only under the following circumstances.

- They are given in the presence of two witnesses.
- They are valid for a very limited period before a written order is required, preferably 24 to 48 hours.

Withholding Other Forms of Treatment

Withholding or withdrawing other forms of treatment is always acceptable if the decision is made by competent adult patients. Difficulties arise, however, when family members or next of kin want to make decisions regarding withholding or withdrawing treatment. The question is: Under what circumstances may treatment be withheld from patients who lack capacity?

First, the providers must make a determination that the patient is either terminally ill or in a persistent vegetative state. This determination should be documented in the chart.

The question then becomes who can make decisions on behalf of the patient. The most important court decision that addressed this issue was *Cruzan versus Director, Missouri Department of Health*,[4] a 1990 decision of the U.S. Supreme Court. In this case a young woman, Nancy Cruzan, was in an automobile accident. When rescue personnel reached the scene, Ms. Cruzan had no pulse or respiration. These two essential functions were restored at the scene of the accident, and she was transported to a local hospital. The initial diagnosis was cerebral contusions compounded by significant lack of oxygen. Neurologists determined that Ms. Cruzan had probably been deprived of oxygen for approximately 12 to 14 minutes.

She remained in a coma for several weeks and then progressed to a semiconscious state. She was able to take some nourishment. To ensure proper nourishment and hydration, however, physicians asked her husband for permission to insert a gastrostomy tube. Her husband gave consent and the tube was implanted.

Despite valiant efforts, Ms. Cruzan remained in a vegetative state. That is, her body functioned almost entirely by its internal controls. It was able to maintain temperature, heartbeat, pulmonary ventilation, digestive activity, and reflex activity of muscles and nerves, which permits low-level conditional responses. But she exhibited no behavioral evidence of self-awareness or awareness of her surroundings.

She remained in this state for several years. When it appeared unlikely that Ms. Cruzan would regain her mental capacity, her parents asked the hospital to remove the gastrostomy tube and to stop nourishment. Hospital personnel refused the request. Her parents filed suit and the case was eventually heard by the U.S. Supreme Court.

The Court said that each state has the right to safeguard the process for making decisions regarding withholding or withdrawing treatment. Each state is free to require whatever evidence it desires to accomplish this goal.

The Court recognized that family members do not always act in the best interest of patients. Therefore each state may decide to refuse to permit family members to make decisions on behalf of incompetent patients unless substantial proof shows that the decision made is one that the patient would also make. Substantial proof of patients' wishes may be expressed in durable powers of attorney or living wills.

Thus it is important for nurse managers to recognize that the requirements of the state in which they practice are paramount. At the extreme, states can refuse to permit withholding or withdrawing of treatment unless there is a clear statement from patients themselves about their wishes in the event of terminal illness or a persistent vegetative state.

To encourage clarity regarding patients' wishes, Congress passed the Patient Self-Determination Act, which became effective on December 1, 1991. This act requires providers to obtain information from patients about their wishes regarding future health care. Such information is commonly called an *advance directive*. Specifically, providers must:

- Develop written policies and procedures to implement patients' rights to make decisions concerning future health care through the use of durable powers of attorney or living wills (advance directives) as permitted by state laws.
- Provide all adult patients with written information about their rights under the laws of the state in which care is provided, including the right to consent to or refuse treatment, the right to sign advance directives, and a statement of the provider's policies governing implementation of patients' wishes.
- Document in patients' files whether they have executed advance directives.
- Provide education for all nursing staff members regarding advance directives.

Compliance with this statute will undoubtedly assist nurse managers in clarifying issues of withholding and withdrawing treatment.

EMPLOYMENT

Regardless of practice setting, health care is a labor-intensive business. New nurse managers may feel lost in a maze of employment-related laws and court decisions, particularly those relating to discrimination and termination of the employment relationship. Two key questions are as follows:

1. How can the new nurse manager avoid discrimination against workers?
2. Under what circumstances may workers be terminated?

Discrimination

As most nurse managers already know, both federal and state laws prohibit discrimination on the basis of race, sex, handicapping condition, and religion. The practical steps outlined in Manager's Tip 8-5 will help nurse managers ensure they do not vi-

MANAGER'S TIP 8-5

STEPS TO AVOID DISCRIMINATION

✔ Identify the essential job functions of all positions for which individuals are responsible. "Essential job functions" is a technical term. New nurse managers may need assistance from their HR departments to identify essential job functions and put them in writing in the form of job descriptions.

✔ Accept that reasonable accommodations are required so that individuals can perform essential job functions if the need for modifications is in any way related to a handicapping condition.

✔ Carefully follow the written essential job functions in carrying out all personnel activities, including hiring, evaluations, promotions, transfers, disciplinary actions, and terminations.

✔ Document all personnel actions in terms of the essential job functions.

MANAGER'S TIP 8-6

FIVE GUIDELINES TO HELP IN AVOIDING LIABILITY FOR UNLAWFUL TERMINATION OF EMPLOYEES

✔ Employee handbooks and policies and procedures must contain clear, unequivocal statements that they do not create a contract of employment.

✔ Managers must strictly adhere to their own policies and procedures, including definitions of circumstances that warrant immediate termination of employment.

✔ Except when immediate termination is warranted, managers must discipline workers progressively. They must first counsel workers, including development of specific corrective action, before taking more serious action.

✔ Managers must thoroughly document all disciplinary action, especially counseling and corrective action.

✔ Consistency in following procedures and applying rules to all employees is essential.

olate these laws. New nurse managers who follow these guidelines will be successful at managing issues of employment discrimination.

Unlawful Termination

Similar steps may be taken to avoid liability for unlawful termination of workers who are not governed by a union contract (see Manager's Tip 8-6). Generally, in the absence of any kind of contract, nurses can be hired and fired at will. Nurses are generally so-called "at-will" employees. Employees' attorneys have tested the absolute nature of this doctrine in recent years. Nurse managers may unwittingly fall into the trap of taking action that amounts to the creation of a contract without realizing that they have done so, thereby destroying their ability to terminate employees. Although it is often difficult to find the time and energy to follow these steps, they are vital to avoiding personnel problems.

Considerations for Home Care Managers

LEGAL ISSUES FOR HOME CARE MANAGERS

Nurse managers who are responsible for home care services should take special note of the following issues:

■ Exercise care with regard to hiring and retaining staff members. Remember, supervision in home care is less intense than in institutional settings, so only practitioners who can operate effectively with a relatively great degree of independence should work in home care.

■ All patients admitted or readmitted to the agency should be appropriate for home care services. Staff must perform a global assessment of appropriateness that includes evaluation of care needed, whether the patient can care for self or a reliable primary caregiver is available to assist patients, and whether the environment of patients' homes will support home care services.

■ Staff must accomplish appropriate follow-up on their communications with physicians. That is, staff must report all changes in signs and symptoms to physicians. They must then obtain a response from physicians' offices regarding the changes that they have reported. When physicians order changes in plans of care, those changes must be implemented promptly.

■ Staff must refuse to implement inappropriate orders from physicians. An area of particular concern in this regard is wound care. Physicians may not be familiar with relatively recent changes in standards of care and may continue to order care that has become obsolete. Nurses are responsible for making certain that they do not act on physicians' orders that result in inappropriate care.

LEGAL CONSIDERATIONS: DELEGATING NURSING TASKS*

Delegation of nursing tasks to unlicensed individuals carries serious patient care and legal implications. Nurses practicing in a home care setting must be concerned especially about the nursing tasks they delegate to the unlicensed individuals who provide care in the home under the nurse's supervision. If care is improperly provided and harm results to the patient, the nurse will be held responsible. More and more frequently in malpractice lawsuits, licensed nurses are held liable for improper delegation or inadequate supervision of delegated tasks. Also actions taken by State Boards of Nursing against a nurse's license based on delegation issues have been increasing.

To avoid liability for the delegated acts of others, the following considerations are recommended:

*From Guarino KS: Legal considerations: delegating nursing tasks, *Home Care Nurse News* 2(7):5, 1995.

Continued.

Considerations for Home Care Managers

- Recognize when you are delegating a nursing task. Any action which falls within your state's definition of nursing practice may only be performed by an unlicensed individual under delegation by a licensed nurse.
- Check your state's nurse practice act and regulations on which nursing acts may be delegated to a non-licensed individual, and which nursing acts may not be delegated.
- Check your home health agency's policies and procedures on delegation of nursing tasks and on requirements for supervision of unlicensed individuals.
- Delegate only those nursing tasks which are within the area of your responsibility as a licensed nurse.
- Evaluate whether, in your opinion, the delegated task can safely be performed by an unlicensed individual.
- Prior to delegating a task, assess the client's nursing care needs to assure that the delegated task can be appropriately performed by an unlicensed individual for that particular client.
- Prior to delegating a nursing task, verify the competence of the unlicensed individual to whom you are delegating.
- If you are in a situation where you determine that delegation may not appropriately or safely take place, do not delegate the task, but rather perform it yourself.
- Instruct the unlicensed person in performance of the task and verify that the unlicensed person is competent to perform the task. Return demonstrations are recommended.
- Direct or supervise the performance of the nursing task by regularly evaluating the nursing tasks performed by the unlicensed personnel.
- Assess the client to assure the nursing tasks performed by the unlicensed individual are effective in the care of the client.
- Assure accurate documentation of all tasks performed in the patient care setting.
- Correct any situation where an individual under your supervision is performing nursing acts incompetently. Once you know, or should have known that an unlicensed individual is unsafe, you are under a duty to assure that the individual is removed from the patient care setting.

Even if you are not sued as a result of delegated nursing tasks, your license may be at risk for acts improperly delegated or improperly supervised. To defend either a legal claim or an action against your license by the Board of Nursing, you must be able to show that you took all of the steps itemized above and that you established effective mechanisms for monitoring the unlicensed individuals under your supervision. It is essential that you create a process whereby the unlicensed individuals are provided with well-defined expectations and reporting requirements, and that you have a consistent means of assuring they were meeting those expectations. Be able to show that you trained the unlicensed individuals well (or assure that they have been well-trained), that you were available to them, and that you were consistently aware of how they performed the nursing tasks you delegated to them.

Remember that the licensed nurse is ultimately responsible for making the decision whether to delegate and under what circumstances the delegation is appropriate. Agencies cannot delegate nursing tasks. Even if your employer has protocols that require unlicensed individuals to perform nursing tasks, an individual with a nursing license will be held responsible if the unlicensed individual performs the task improperly.

SUMMARY

The information in this chapter is by no means exhaustive. There is much more for the new nurse manager to learn in the area of legal issues, and readers are encouraged to seek further information when issues with legal implications arise. A glossary of legal terms is included in the appendix of this chapter for the reader's information.

But new managers who arrive at their offices on the first day in their new positions with no more than the information provided in this chapter are well on their way to success in managing the various risks associated with managing nursing personnel. This can be accomplished by remembering to:

1. Continuously monitor the quality of patient care to limit legal liability.
2. Assist patients in giving valid informed consent and making decisions regarding withholding and withdrawal of treatment.
3. Identify essential job functions and apply them in relation to all personnel functions, discipline employees progressively, and avoid creating contractual obligations unless you intend to do so.

References

1. *Wickline v State of California,* 192 Cal App 3d 1630, 239 California Reporter 810, 1986.
2. *Valro v Blue Cross and Blue Shield,* 708 F Sup 826, ED Michigan, 1989.
3. *Wilson v Blue Cross of Southern California,* Cal App 2d, 271 California, Reporter 876, 1990.
4. *Cruzan v Harmon,* 760 S W 2d 408, Missouri 1988, en banc, *aff'd sub nom Cruzan v Director, Missouri Department of Health,* 110 S Ct 2841, 1990.

APPENDIX 8-1

GLOSSARY OF LEGAL TERMS

The author relied heavily on *Black's Law Dictionary,* ed 5, St. Paul, Minn, 1979, West Publishing, to prepare this glossary. Readers should make further use of this excellent resource when necessary.

Actual damages Compensation for actual injuries or losses such as medical expenses or lost wages.

Affidavit A written statement of facts given voluntarily under oath.

Allegation The written statements by a party to a suit concerning what the party expects to prove.

Amended complaint A corrected or revised version of the document filed in court by the plaintiff to being a suit.

Amicus curiae Literally, "friend of the court." Persons or organizations with a strong interest in or views on a suit may ask the court in which the suit is filed for permission to file a brief to suggest a resolution of the case consistent with their views. *Amicus curiae* briefs are often filed in appeals of cases involving a broad public interest such as civil rights cases.

Appellant The party who appeals the decision of one court to another court.

Appellate brief Written arguments by attorneys required to be filed with an appellate court stating the reasons why the trial court acted correctly (appellee's brief) or incorrectly (appellant's brief). The contents and form of appellate briefs are often prescribed by the rules of various court systems. Appellate briefs usually contain a statement of issues presented for review by the appellate court, a statement of the case, argument, and a conclusion stating the precise action sought by the party submitting the brief.

Appellate review Examination of a previous proceeding.

Appellee The party in a case against whom an appeal is brought. Sometimes also called the "respondent."

Assault Any conduct that creates a reasonable apprehension of being touched in an injurious manner. No actual touching is required to prove assault.

Assumption of the risk A defense to plaintiffs' claims based on the theory that plaintiffs may not recover for injuries to which they consent. To prove that the plaintiff assumed the risk, the defendant must show that: (1) the plaintiff had knowledge of a dangerous condition, (2) the plaintiff appreciated the nature or extent of the danger, and (3) the plaintiff voluntarily exposed herself/himself to the danger.

Attorney-in-fact Any person authorized by another to act in her/his place either for a particular purpose or for the transaction of business affairs in general. This authority is conferred by a document called a power of attorney.

Battery An unconsented, actual touching that causes injury.

Borrowed servant rule A theory of liability or negligence that is used to extend liability beyond the person who actually committed negligent acts to include those who had the right of control over the negligent actions.

Brief A written statement prepared by an attorney arguing a case in court. A brief contains a summary of the facts of the case, the pertinent laws, and an argument of how the law applies to the facts supporting an attorney's position.

Burden of proof The requirement of proving facts in dispute on an issue raised between the parties in a case.

Captain of the ship doctrine This doctrine imposes liability on surgeons in charge of operations for negligence of assistants during period when those assistants are under the surgeons' control, even though the assistants are also employees of a hospital. This doctrine extends the borrowed servant rule to the operating rooms of hospitals.

Cause of action The fact or facts that give a person the right to begin a suit.

Common law As opposed to laws created by legislatures, the common law consists of legal principles based solely on usages and customs from time immemorial, particularly the ancient, unwritten laws of England.

Complaint The first document filed in court by the plaintiff to begin a suit.

Conservator Any individual appointed by a court to manage the affairs of an incompetent person.

Continuance Adjournment or postponement of a session, hearing, trial, or other proceedings to a subsequent day or time.

Contributory negligence A defense to a claim of negligence. Any act or omission on the part of the complaining party amounting to a breach of the duty the law imposes on everyone to protect themselves from injury that contributes to the injury complained of by the plaintiff.

Counterclaim Claim presented by a defendant in opposition to the claim of the plaintiff. If the defendant establishes her/his claim, it will defeat or diminish the plaintiff's claim.

Cross-complaint A defendant or cross-defendant (plaintiff) may file a cross-complaint based on (1) any claim against any of the parties who filed the complaint against her/him *or* (2) any claim against a person alleged to be liable whether or not the person is already a party to the suit. The claims in a cross-complaint must (1) arise out of the same transaction or occurrence as the original suit *and* (2) make a claim or assert a right or interest in the property or the controversy that is the basis for the claim already made.

Cross-defendants Plaintiffs who, subsequent to suing defendants, are then countersued by the defendants. Defendants in a suit brought by defendants.

Cross-examination The questioning of a witness by an adverse party to test the truth of her/his testimony or to further develop it.

Declaratory judgment Provided for in state and federal statutes. A person may seek a declaratory judgment from a court if there is an actual controversy among the parties, and the party asking for the declaratory judgment has some question or doubt about her/his legal rights. The judgment is binding on the parties both presently and in the future.

Defendant The person defending or denying; the party against whom a civil lawsuit is brought or the accused in a criminal case.

Defense A response to the claims of the other party stating the reasons why the claims should not be recognized.

Demurrer An argument in which the defendant admits the facts in the plaintiff's complaint, but claims that the facts are insufficient to require a response.

Deposition Advice by which one party asks oral questions of the other party or of a witness for the other party before the trial begins. The person who answers questions is called a deponent. The deposition is conducted under oath outside of the courtroom, usually in one of the lawyer's offices. A transcript, or word-for-word account, is made of the deposition.

Directed verdict When the party with the burden of proof fails to prove all necessary elements of the case, the trial judge may direct a verdict in favor of the other party because there can only be one result anyway.

Docket A list or calendar of cases to be tried during a particular period prepared by employees of the court for use by the court and attorneys.

Due process clause Two clauses in the U.S. Constitution, one in the Fifth Amendment applicable to the U.S. Government, the other in the Fourteenth Amendment that protects persons from actions by the states. There are two aspects: (1) procedural, in which a person is guaranteed fair procedures, and (2) substantive, which protects a person's property from unfair governmental interference. Similarly, clauses are in most state constitutions.

Due process of law An orderly proceeding in which a person receives notice of the proceeding and the subject matter of the proceeding and is given an opportunity to be heard and to enforce and protect her/his rights before a court or person(s) with power to hear and determine the case.

Equal protection clause A provision in the Fourteenth Amendment to the U.S. Constitution that requires every state to treat individuals in similar circumstances the same in terms of rights and redress of improper actions against them.

Ex parte On one side only; by or for one party; done for, on behalf of, or on the application of one party only. A judicial proceeding, order, or injunction is *ex parte* when it is granted at the request of and for the benefit of one party only without notice to any person adversely interested.

False imprisonment A tort that consists of intentionally confining a person without her/his consent.

Felony A crime of a more serious nature. Under federal law and many state statutes, a felony is any offense punishable by imprisonment for a term exceeding 1 year or by death.

Guardian Any person responsible for managing the property of and protecting the rights of another person who, because of youth or lack of understanding, is incapable of managing her/his own affairs.

Guardian ad litem A special guardian appointed by a court to prosecute or defend, on behalf of a minor or incompetent person, a suit to which the minor or incompetent person is a party.

Harmless error Any trivial error or an error that is merely academic because it did not affect important rights of any party to a case and did not affect the final result of the case. Harmless error will not serve as a basis for changing a decision of the court.

Implied consent Signs, actions or facts, or inaction or silence that indicates that consent is given.

In loco parentis In the place of a parent; instead of a parent; charged with a parent's rights, duties, and responsibilities.

Infliction of emotional distress Conduct going beyond that usually tolerated by society that is calculated to cause mental distress *and* that actually causes severe mental distress.

Informed consent A person's agreement to allow something to happen that is based on a full disclosure of facts needed to make the decision intelligently.

Intent Design, resolve, or determination that serves as the basis for a person's actions. Intent can rarely be proven directly but may be inferred from the circumstances.

Interrogatories A tool to elicit information important to a case before trial. Interrogatories are written questions about the case submitted by one party to another party or witness. The answers to interrogatories are usually given under oath (i.e., the person answering the questions signs a sworn statement that the answers are true).

Judge a quo Literally, "from which." A judge of a court from which a case was taken before a decision is made.

Judgment of nonsuit A decision by a court against plaintiffs when they are unable to prove their cases or refuse or neglect to proceed to trial. A court decision that leaves the issues undetermined.

Judgment notwithstanding the verdict (inov) A judgment entered by order to the court for a party, even though the jury decided in favor of the other party. A motion for directed verdict must usually be made before a judgment, notwithstanding the verdict.

Jurisdiction The right and power of a court to decide a particular case.

Jury instructions Statements made by the judge to the jury regarding the law applicable to the case the jury is considering that the jury is required to accept and apply. Attorneys for both sides usually furnish the judge with suggested instructions.

Justiciable controversy Courts will decide only justiciable controversies That is, courts will decide only cases in which there is a real, substantial difference of opinion between the parties as opposed to a hypothetical difference or dispute or one that is academic or moot.

Leave to amend Permission or authorization given by a judge to any party to a suit to correct or reverse any document filed by the party with the court.

Locality rule To show negligence according to the locality rule, a plaintiff must prove that the defendant practitioner failed to render care considered reasonable in the same or in a similar geographic location.

Misdemeanor Criminal offense less serious than a felony and usually punished by a fine or imprisonment in other than a penitentiary. Any criminal offense other than a felony.

Motion for a new trial Request to a judge to set aside a decision already made in a case and to order a new trial on the basis that the first decision was improper or unfair.

Motion for summary judgment An application made to a court or judge to obtain a ruling or order that all or part of the other party's claim or defense should be eliminated from further consideration. This motion is made when a party believes there is no significant disagreement concerning important facts among the parties *and* the law supports the position of the party making the motion. A motion for summary judgment may be directed towards all or part of a claim or defense. It may be made on the basis of the pleadings or other portions of the record in the case, or it may be supported by affidavits and a variety of outside material.

Motion to dismiss An application made to a court or judge to order that the plaintiff's suit be eliminated from further consideration by the court or judge. This motion is usually made before a trial is held and may be based on a variety of reasons: for example, insufficiency of the plaintiff's claims or improper service of process of the plaintiff's suit on the defendant.

Motion to intervene/Plea in intervention A written request to a court to become a party to a case filed in the court based on an interest in the results of the case.

Negligence The failure to do something a reasonable person would do or doing something a reasonable person would not do.

Nominal damages A very small amount of money awarded to plaintiffs in cases in which there is no substantial injury. Nominal damages are awarded to recognize technical invasions of rights or breaches of duty or in cases where the injury is more substantial but the plaintiff fails to prove the amount.

Parens patriae Literally, "parent of the country." Refers to the role of each state as sovereign and guardian of persons under legal disability. This concept is the basis for activity by states to protect interests such as the health, comfort, and welfare of the people.

Per quod Literally, "whereby." A phrase used to designate facts concerning the consequences of defendant's actions on the plaintiff that serve as the basis for an award of special damages to the plaintiff.

Petition A formal, written request to a court asking the court to take certain action regarding a particular matter.

Physician-patient privilege The right of patients not to reveal or have revealed by their physicians the communications made between patients and physicians. The privilege is established in most states and therefore varies from state to state. The privilege belongs only to the patient and may be waived by the patient.

Plaintiff A person who sues in a civil case.

Pleading The formal, written statements by the parties to a suit of their respective claims and defenses.

Power of attorney A document authorizing another person to act on one's behalf. The other person is called the attorney-in-fact. The power of the attorney-in-fact is revoked on the death of the person who signed the power of attorney. The powers given to the attorney-in-fact may be general or for special purposes.

Prejudicial error Any error that substantially affects the legal rights and obligations of a party. A prejudicial error may result in a new trial and the reversal of a decision by the court.

Pretrial conference A meeting between opposing attorneys and the judge in a particular case. The purpose of the meeting is to define the key issues of the case, to secure stipulations, and to take all other steps necessary to aid in the disposition of the case. Such conferences are called at the discretion of the court. The decisions made at the conference are included in a written order that controls the future course of the case.

Pretrial discovery Any device used by parties before trial to obtain evidence for use at trial such as interrogatories, depositions, or requests for admission of facts.

Prima facie case Sufficient evidence presented by the plaintiff on which a decision that the plaintiff's claims are valid can reasonably be made.

Proximate cause The dominant cause or the cause producing injury. Any action producing injury, unbroken by any efficient intervening cause, and without which the injury would not have occurred.

Punitive damages Money awarded to the plaintiff over and above compensation for actual losses. Punitive damages are awarded in cases where the wrongdoing was aggravated by violence, oppression, malice, fraud, or wickedness. They are intended to compensate for mental anguish, shame, or degradation or to punish or make an example of the defendant.

Remand To send back. The sending back of a case by an appellate court to the court in which it was previously considered to have some further action taken on it.

Request for admissions Written statements of fact concerning a case that are submitted by the attorney for a party to a suit to the attorney for another party to the suit. The attorney who receives the request is required to either admit or deny each of the statements of fact submitted. Those statements that are admitted will be treated by the court as established and need not be proved at trial.

Res ipsa loquitur Literally, "the thing speaks for itself." Although the plaintiffs cannot testify to the exact cause of injury, they can prove (1) that the instrument causing injury was in defendants' exclusive control and (2) that the injury they sustained does not normally occur in the absence of negligence. Plaintiffs who prove both of these things can recover damages for negligence even though the exact circumstances of injury are known.

Res judicata A legal principle that says that once a *final* decision is made on a matter, the same question may not be raised at a later date.

Respondeat superior Literally, "let the master say." A basis for extending liability to include the employer for the wrongful acts of an employee. The doctrine is inapplicable where injury occurs when the employee is acting outside the legitimate scope of employment.

Retrial A new trial of a case that has already been tried at least once.

Stare decisis Literally, "to abide by or adhere to decided cases." The policy of courts in the United States to apply previously established principles of law to all future cases where the facts are substantially the same, even though the parties to the suit are not the same.

State action Activity of a state necessary to trigger the protection of the Fourteenth Amendment of the U.S. Constitution for private citizens.

Statute of limitations Legislative enactments establishing limits on the right to sue. Statutes of limitations declare that no one may sue unless the suit is filed within a specified period after the occurrence or injury that is the basis for the suit.

Stay A stopping by order of a court. A suspension of the case or some designated proceedings in it. A stay is a type of injunction with which a court freezes its proceedings at a particular point. It can be used to stop the case altogether or hold up only some phase of it.

Stipulation A voluntary agreement between opposing attorneys concerning disposition of a point that alleviates the need for proof of this point or for consideration, signed by the attorneys for all of the parties and placed on file as part of the court record.

Third-party defendant A party brought into a suit by the defendant who was not a party to the transaction on which the suit is based, but whose rights and liabilities may be affected by the suit.

Tort A private or civil wrong or injury for which a court may award damages. Any civil suit except a suit for breach of contract. Three elements of every tort claim are

(1) existence of a legal duty by the defendant to the plaintiff, (2) breach of this duty, *and* (3) resulting damage to the plaintiff.

Transcript A word-for-word written record of a trial, hearing, or other proceeding.

Trial An examination and determination of issues between the parties to a case by a court.

Trial by court Judicial examination and determination of issues between the parties in a case.

Trial by court or judge A trial before a judge only, in contrast to a trial before a judge *and* jury.

Vicarious liability Indirect legal responsibility.

Voir dire Literally, "to speak the truth." Refers to the preliminary questioning that the court or attorneys conduct to determine the qualifications of a person to serve as a juror in a particular case.

Writ of certiorari An order of an appellate court used when the court exercises discretion about whether or not to hear an appeal. If the writ is denied, the court refuses to hear the appeal, and the decision of the court that previously heard the case remains in effect. If the writ is granted, the appellate court will reconsider the case and perhaps change the decision of the lower court.

Writ of error A writ issued from an appeals court to a trial court requiring the trial court to send the record of a case to the appeals court for reconsideration. The writ is based on errors of law apparent from the record. It is the beginning of a new suit to reverse a decision of a lower court and is not a continuation of any suit in a lower court.

Writ of habeas corpus Literally, "you have the body." The primary function of this writ is to force the release of a person from unlawful imprisonment.

CHAPTER 9

TAKING CARE OF YOURSELF AND YOUR STAFF

PATRICIA M. FEENEY

MAINTAINING BALANCE UNDER STRESS

Nicholson, a registered nurse and certified Stress Management Program Director through the American Institute of Preventive Medicine, proposed a definition of stress as it applies to the nursing profession. After reviewing the work of Hans Selye and many others, Nicholson suggested that stress in nursing is

> . . . a phenomenon that is characterized by a response to a certain occurrence. This response may be interpreted as positive or negative by the individual and can affect biologic processes, which may result eventually in wear or tear on one's physical, psychologic, behavioral, and/or emotional well-being.[1]

Stress in the Nursing Profession

Careers in nursing and nursing management bring with them careers in managing stress. It is important to your personal and professional long-term success as a nurse and nurse manager to integrate effective stress management skills into your life.

A critical element in managing stress in the nursing profession is accepting that stress does and always will exist. Some of these stresses are unique to our profession. Foxall and others[2] compared the frequency and sources of nursing job stress perceived by intensive care, hospice, and medical-surgical nurses. Although the groups assigned different degrees of stress to various aspects of their work, the overall frequency of job stress was similar among the three groups.

Numerous studies detail the sources of stress experienced by nurses. Although many of these stresses may be identified in non-health care settings, many stresses found in the nursing profession are products of the environment. Examples include dying patients, cardiac arrests, communicable disease, and upset families.

Stresses in the nursing workplace that also are identified in non-health care settings, such as increased workload and conflicts with staff members, can be intensified in the health care setting. These common or universal job stresses affect nurses more because they directly affect patients and their care.

Nurse Managers: A Twofold Responsibility

As a nurse manager, you accept a twofold responsibility in stress management: (1) guiding and supporting your staff as they experience stress and (2) coping with stress as it affects you. Although these responsibilities seem self-evident, many managers are not successful in supporting their staff, themselves, or both. Sadly, a failure to support one or the other generally results in a failure to support both.

For example, if your concern rests primarily with your own stress and coping mechanisms, your staff will recognize this fact. Eventually, they will resent your lack of support and may begin to experience excessive stress themselves. Over time, these feelings may result in high staff turnover, decreased staff performance, and unhappy patients and physicians. These factors in turn lead to excessive stress for you.

Conversely, if your concern is exclusively for your staff, eventually you will become emotionally drained, resentful, and overly stressed. As these feelings take their toll on your well-being, your ability to manage and support your staff will diminish. This diminishing performance in turn will lead to excessive stress for your staff.

It is imperative that you understand the importance of attending to the needs of your staff, as well as to your own needs—consistently and simultaneously.

Stress Evaluation Exercises: Introduction

This chapter contains stress evaluation exercises. These exercises are designed to help you identify and evaluate stress in your work environment. The exercises include stress self-knowledge, stress coping mechanisms, and signs of unmanaged stress. You may use these exercises alone or in brainstorming sessions with your peers. The exercises may also be used in staff support groups that are conducted by a professional facilitator.

The stress evaluation exercises are tools to help you identify stress and its accompanying problems. In most cases, you and your staff will be able to respond to stress effectively. However, you may find that you, an individual on your staff, or your staff as a group is experiencing stress beyond normal levels or is developing a serious problem in response to stress. If so, seek professional support for yourself or the employees experiencing the problem. Please refer to the section, "When You Identify A Serious Staff Problem," of this chapter for further discussion.

SOURCES OF STRESS IN THE PATIENT CARE ENVIRONMENT

Once you are committed to monitoring and managing stress in the workplace, a clear understanding of the sources of stress is critical. Undoubtedly, you have a good sense of the types of events or situations that create stress for you. Most nurse managers have spent a considerable part of their career in staff level positions and are well acquainted with the rigors and challenges of the profession.

It is important to note that the areas of stress that affect you may not be the same as those that most affect the members of your staff. For example, off-shift scheduling affects people differently and may affect them differently at various points in their lives. Working the night shift profoundly affects some people's sense of emotional equilibrium and their sleep patterns. Yet, some nurses enjoy an occasional rotation to nights and some happily choose to work nights full-time.

Caring for dying patients is stressful. Yet for some nurses, caring for a dying patient is not experienced as a negative stress. These nurses may exercise hidden strengths and qualities and be deeply satisfied by the experience. For other nurses, caring for a dying patient may be deeply depressing.

It is helpful to review an inventory of the sources of stress in the patient care workplace so that you can be sensitive to the differences among your staff members and guard against generalizing your experiences to them.

Lees and Ellis investigated a variety of common stresses in their study[3] of nursing staff, nursing students, and students who left nurse training. The stresses they identified are listed in Box 9-1, with the stresses most frequently cited appearing at the top of the list.

Simms and others investigated some of these same stresses in their study[4] of nursing burnout. Box 9-2 on p. 218 lists the exhausting activities cited by nurses in their study. The activities at the top of the list are those most frequently cited.

Staff may experience additional stresses when they care for patients with specialized needs or with an illness such as AIDS or hepatitis, which can be threatening to one's own health. Although caring for a patient with a communicable disease may cause anxiety for nurses, there are several other, less visible, special-care situations that may concern nurses.

Some of these situations are those that pose a real or imagined threat to the health of the nurse or the nurse's family. For example, nursing personnel in neonatal inten-

---

box 9-1

COMMONLY OCCURRING STRESSES

- Understaffing.
- Dealing with death and dying.
- Conflict with nurses.
- Overwork.
- Conflict with doctors.
- Hours.
- Cardiac arrests.
- Responsibility/accountability.
- Training junior staff.
- Dealing with relatives.
- Lack of resources (beds/equipment).
- Aggressive patients.
- Study/examinations.

- Carrying out certain nursing procedures.
- Feeling inadequate to carry out procedures.
- Seeing patients in distress.
- Staff rough with patients.
- Conflict with others (administrators, dieticians).
- Child abuse.
- Dealing with overdose patients.
- Living in nurses' home.
- Open visiting.
- Working off-shifts.
- Disorganization of workloads.
- Being in a new situation for the first time.
- Heat in the hospital.

Lees S, Ellis N: The design of a stress-management programme for nursing personnel, *J Adv Nurs* 15:946, 1990.

---

box 9-2

EXHAUSTING ACTIVITIES

- Decreased staffing.
- Negativism on part of staff.
- Demanding families.
- No time for breaks or lunches.
- Increased patient load.
- Too many patients.
- Dealing with difficult people.
- Being on feet all day.
- Routine patient care.
- Transferring patients in beds.
- Mandatory overtime.
- Running errands.
- Problems with other departments.
- Dealing with staff conflict.
- Patients and families unwilling to accept diagnosis.
- Patients who are self-abusing.
- Paperwork.
- Cardiac arrests.
- Caring for debilitated patients.
- Meetings in other buildings.
- Not being busy.
- Being on call.
- Orienting new staff.
- Repetitive teaching.
- Scheduling and staffing.
- Responding to alarms.
- Trying to alleviate patient's pain.

Adapted from Simms L, et al: Breaking the burnout barrier: resurrecting work excitement in nursing, *Nurs Economics* 8(3):185, 1990.

---

sive care units are frequently called on to hold or otherwise manage infants during x-ray procedures. If the infant is in isolation, does the nurse contaminate a lead apron (creating the need for time-consuming decontamination), put on and cover the apron, or simply hold the infant without protecting herself/himself from the radiation? This kind of decision, invariably made in a split second, may create stress for the nurse making the decision.

Nurses on oncology units regularly manage chemotherapy agents and waste products of patients receiving these agents. The threat of possible exposure to mutagenic chemicals may bring considerable stress to the nurses managing these patients. Nurses who plan to have children, particularly those who are pregnant or actively trying to become pregnant or father a child, may experience additional stress in care settings where they may be exposed to mutagenic chemotherapy agents, communicable diseases, radiation, and other threats to their ability to bear or father a healthy child.

In addition to the stresses intrinsic to the workplace, nurses, like all people, may experience personal problems that magnify the stress at work.

STRESS EVALUATION EXERCISE: STRESS SELF-KNOWLEDGE

Develop a list of all possible sources of stress in your workplace. Recognize that there are no "rights" or "wrongs" in your evaluation and that not every stress identified will apply directly to you or to every nurse on your staff. The purpose of your evaluation is simply to identify sources of stress, not to assign blame for the stress or to provide solutions.

By limiting the first task at hand to a simple process of identification, the pressure to solve—or deny—problems is eliminated.

STRESSES FOR NURSE MANAGERS

The nurse manager is vulnerable to stresses that are inherent to the twofold role of nurse and manager (see Box 9-3).

One source of stress is a result of the nurse manager's position in the organization. New managers typically are first-line supervisors and must report to a supervisor above them. In fact, there may be several layers of personnel between the nurse

---

box 9-3

OTHER SOURCES OF STRESS FOR THE NURSE MANAGER

- Feeling "sandwiched" between your staff and your supervisor.
- Being responsible for patient care/client services delivered by each member of your staff.
- Accepting fiscal responsibility for your area of supervision.
- Being responsible for staff turnover in your area of supervision.
- Serving as liaison in physician-nurse relationships.
- Serving as liaison in staff-upper management relationships.
- Having responsibility for staff education and training.
- Handling conflicts with role expectations from your staff and your supervisor.
- Handling internal role conflicts concerning your responsibilities as a nurse and as a manager.
- Scheduling staffing for your area of supervision.
- Making unpopular decisions.
- Facilitating communications between your staff and upper management, especially when faced with implementing unpopular decisions.
- Evaluating staff.
- Setting reasonable, objective goals for your staff and monitoring performance.
- Taking disciplinary action against a staff member.
- Terminating a staff member.
- Hiring a staff member.
- Responding constructively to unmanaged stress among your staff.
- Recognizing the signs of unmanaged stress among your staff.
- Working with staff who refuse to be accountable for self and professional behavior.
- Recognizing signs and symptoms of unmanaged stress within yourself.
- Facilitating open communication among your staff with each other and with you.
- Conducting staff meetings.
- Accepting criticism from your supervisor and from your staff.
- Taking a vacation from your job.
- Learning to delegate appropriately.
- Being seen as the "bad guy" by your staff.
- Being regarded as "omnipotent" by your staff.
- Having little orientation for your management role.
- Dealing with employees who merely want a "job," and are not committed to their profession or career.
- Keeping a balance at work when your personal problems seem to be following you to work.
- Managing an employee who brings her/his personal problems to work.
- Other stresses you have identified.

manager and top management. This "layering" of management can be a significant source of stress.

For example, when you receive top management's communications through your supervisor, she/he may alter the positioning or emphasis of the communication to motivate you to act positively. This is not necessarily a problem. In fact, you will find yourself doing the same in your communications with your staff. As you become an effective manager who is more acquainted with the staff, you will learn how to report information so that the staff members understand the content and are motivated to take positive action.

However, this filtering of information can become a problem for you when your supervisor, committed to her/his own agenda, misinterprets information and communicates misinterpretations to you. You then receive communication that is inconsistent with top management's message and possibly inconsistent with the organization's objectives. You, in turn, communicate this misinformation to your staff, who ultimately may experience their own stress related to this situation.

Managing an employee with a personal problem warrants a brief discussion. Employees' personal problems are just that—*their* personal problems. Nonetheless, if one of your employees is experiencing difficulty in her/his personal life, be it financial, marital, child-related, or so forth, it is not uncommon for the employee to bring the problem to work. Sometimes an employee may be so stressed and distracted by personal concerns that her/his job performance is affected. Although you must address the employee's performance deficits, it is especially important in these circumstances to do so with compassion.

If an employee confides a personal problem to you, it will be important to keep a balance between showing concern and caring and trying to correct the problem. Keep in mind that you are not a therapist and are not equipped to psychologically counsel your staff. You cannot remedy your staff's personal problems. Sometimes the greatest support you can offer is to suggest that the employee seek guidance from an Employee Assistance Program (EAP), community resource, or trained professional. Examples of resources are discussed in the section, "When You Identify a Serious Staff Problem."

You have probably become acquainted with many of the sources of stress on the nurse manager's stress list. It may also be helpful to brainstorm sources of stress with your peer group. Discussing sources of stress with other first-line managers can help validate your perceptions. This process also can strengthen your peer relationships.

THE MANAGER-STAFF RELATIONSHIP

To understand the stress you experience as a nurse manager, it is helpful to examine the nature of your relationships with your staff and with your supervisor.

A guiding principle behind successfully managing your staff is a clear understanding of the psychology at work. As simplistic as this sounds, this psychology often is neglected when a nurse manager is caught up in day-to-day operational management responsibilities.

How the Staff View the Manager

Regardless of your age, experience, and education, generally your staff will view you as an authority figure. This authority is vested in you because you have a supervisory job title.

Your staff will expect you to respond to their needs, alleviate the stress of their job, and guide them through troubled times. Over time, the authority your staff vests in you must be proven, or the staff will lose the respect for you that is important to successful manager-staff relationships. Nonetheless, knowing that you arrive on the job with a certain measure of authority can boost your confidence as you face the challenges ahead.

But what does this authority mean? At first glance, it seems great. People will listen when you speak. People will work harder and do their best if they believe you are aware of their performance. You have at your disposal several ways to motivate your staff: pats on the back, performance reviews, certificates of merit, continuing education days, and other perks you can provide.

However, your position of authority brings with it some other, less desirable, effects. People will listen when you speak, but they may criticize you for what you say, regardless of whether the blame is accurately assigned. For example, if you have to report staff cutbacks that have been formulated by upper management, *you* may be blamed for the cutbacks. If you correct someone's nursing technique, you may be considered "too hard," "unrealistic," or "out of touch with the real world."

Staff cutbacks and correcting a nurse's technique may be necessary, but they will still create stress for you and your staff. As the manager, you must be aware of this inherent stress so that you communicate with your staff in a positive way, without placing undue stress on them or on yourself.

Open Communication

Effective communication as a nurse manager is not measured by how much your staff likes you. Rather, it is measured by how well you relate verbally and nonverbally in a clear, respectful manner, listening to your staff, encouraging comments and constructive criticism, and creating an environment in which each individual's opinions are respected. As the manager, you ultimately must make decisions on matters related to personnel and operations in your area of responsibility. These decisions—although not always popular—must be respected.

A manager who has created an environment of open communication may experience what appears to be a lack of support in the face of an unpopular decision. Staff members who feel comfortable expressing disagreement and concerns will be more apt to criticize—and sometimes do so unfairly. It will be important to remember that the staff are simply expressing openly what they would think covertly in a less communicative environment. Even if you are unable or unwilling to alter your decision, listening attentively to your staff's dissatisfaction will provide a degree of relief from the stress brought on by your decision.

Do not underestimate your staff and expect that unpopular decisions will necessarily make you unpopular. Sometimes a manager finds unexpected support in the face of a tough decision. This support may not be apparent until the staff has had the opportunity to assimilate the decision. In most cases, your staff will recognize a fair or necessary decision for what it is and respect you for making it.

Regardless of your staff's response to an unpopular decision, you must bear in mind your first priority: to live up to your job responsibilities to the best of your abilities. This generally means doing what is best for the patients/clients first, and then for your staff.

Balancing Your Emotional Needs and Your Job Responsibilities

Because your job can be draining, take care to see that your emotional needs are met in constructive ways. Avoid using your staff as the key source of your emotional support. This does not mean you must tense up if one of your staff extends a helping hand or offers a kind or caring remark. (This would be wonderful!) However, keep in perspective how much you can expect of your staff. Although you may come to enjoy being with and care about many of your staff members, relying on them to support you emotionally is not fair. If you become dependent on one or more of your staff members for support, your judgment will be clouded and it will be difficult for you to do your job.

Although most nurse managers want their staffs to like and care about them, focusing on this desire can create serious problems. Most experienced nurse managers know that it is difficult to do a good job *and* be liked all of the time. Some nurse managers—just like some of the population at large—have a strong emotional need to be liked. If this is true of you, it is important that you continually assess your performance to be sure you are doing your job, not running for office. In fact, even experienced managers may be vulnerable to the desire to "run for office' when things seem particularly tough in running their department, clinic, or home health agency.

Conversely, some managers, in an attempt to establish their authority, tend to go overboard and create an environment akin to a police state. This pitfall, as well as "running for office," seems particularly common with first-time managers and is an understandable mistake. It's difficult to gauge how to present oneself, or how strong to come on with the staff, when the nurse manager has had no previous management experience.

Inventory of Your Management Practices

You may want to take a mental inventory of your management practices. The quiz in Box 9-4 presents questions designed as triggers to help you evaluate your behavior and to build a healthy work environment—an environment in which your staff feels able to communicate with you and contribute to decision-making, but is

box 9-4

MANAGEMENT PRACTICE QUIZ — QUESTIONS TO ASK YOURSELF

	YES	NO
1. Before I report a management decision to my staff, do I worry about what the staff will think and say about me (more than what they will think and say about the decision)?	___	___
2. When I report an unpopular decision, do I usually say, "I didn't have anything to do with this," "It's not my fault," or another "Don't get mad at me" statement?	___	___
3. Do I back down from enforcing policies because I do not want to deal with the resentment of the staff?	___	___
4. When I make the work schedule, am I guided first by my interest in serving the needs of my staff (rather than my commitment to serving our patients/clients)?	___	___
5. Do I subtly try to align my staff with me against my supervisor?	___	___
6. Do I speak negatively about my supervisor to my staff?	___	___
7. Do I find myself trying to do my staff's work to gain their acceptance/approval?	___	___
8. Are my efforts to help my staff with their work impeding my ability to meet the requirements of *my* job?	___	___
9. Do I avoid terminating an employee when it is necessary?	___	___
10. Do I show favoritism to any member of my staff?	___	___
11. Do I give good performance evaluations to all my staff regardless of performance?	___	___
12. Is it clear to my staff how they can earn "perks," such as extra education days, bonuses, or other privileges?	___	___
13. Do I strike a balance between lending hands-on assistance to my staff and managing my department so that my staff does not routinely need this assistance?	___	___
14. Do I provide ample opportunity for my staff to express their concerns and needs?	___	___
15. Whenever possible, do I request input from my staff in making decisions that affect our department?	___	___
16. Do I ask for input from my staff on things they would like to see change in our department?	___	___
17. Do I clearly explain how much change I can and cannot effect?	___	___
18. Whenever possible, do I request input from my staff in determining how to execute management decisions?	___	___
19. Do I set clear verbal and written expectations and goals for my staff?	___	___
20. When an employee does not meet expectations, do I provide clear verbal and written guidelines and expectations for improvement?	___	___
21. Do I understand and follow human resource guidelines in taking disciplinary action with members of my staff?	___	___
22. If I take disciplinary action against an employee, is it the same action I would take against *any* employee with the same record?	___	___

respectful of your responsibilities as a manager. The questions also will help you measure your management "comfort level" (i.e., how well you are accepting the nurse manager's responsibilities). Following the questions are guidelines to evaluate your responses.

The first 11 questions address fundamentals of your responsibility as a nurse manager and your ability to execute these basics effectively. If you responded "yes" to any of these questions, you may be resisting the psychologic jump from staff nurse to nurse manager or you may need additional guidance or training in effective management. Take a serious look at your thinking and your management practices. You probably need to adjust both. If you answered "no" to these questions, you have a good start in defining your role as a nurse manager.

The rest of the questions address your ability to (1) facilitate open communication with your staff and (2) create a fair, supportive work environment. A "yes" response to these questions indicates a commitment to these goals. If you answered "no" to any of these questions, consider the consequences of your management practice in question. For example, if you fail to set clear guidelines for performance improvement, it will be difficult for an employee to meet your expectations. You will create a stressful work environment—one in which an employee may never really understand what you expect. Or, if you fail to follow human resource guidelines for disciplinary action, you will create an unpredictable and stressful work environment. In addition, your disciplinary actions may be overturned in grievance procedures, greatly weakening your credibility. As you examine the consequences of your management practices, you will probably realize that the energy you invest to create a predictable, positive workplace will pay great dividends.

How the Manager Views the Staff

The way the manager views the staff is generally given less attention than the way the staff views the manager. Just as a certain authority is vested in the manager, the manager enters this role with beliefs about employees. These beliefs vary, depending on the manager.

For example, some managers may view their employees as children to be cajoled, scolded, rescued, and praised. Some managers may view their employees as a group of potential friends and supporters who will meet their emotional needs for love and acceptance.

Ideally, a manager will view employees as valuable members of the team—a group of people who can cooperate in creating a successful work environment. Although the manager must provide guidance, leadership, and support, her/his self-respect and respect for the employees will not falter.

How a manager views her/his staff generally depends more on the psychologic make-up of the manager and less on the actual history or potential of the staff. Because of this, it is important to assess your beliefs before you get too far into your job. The more you understand about how you view your staff, the easier it will be for you to avoid intensifying stress and creating problems with your staff. Also, this under-standing will help you identify problems for what they really are, not for what you may believe them to be.

For example, if you are the type of manager who tends to view your staff as chil-dren, you may unknowingly create stress and resentment among the ranks. Few adults want to be treated like a child.

If you feel threatened by your staff, not only will this be evident to the staff, your management judgment will be impaired. It's difficult to make fair decisions and carry out your responsibilities if you are preoccupied with protecting your own interests.

If you view your staff as potential friends, you may create an adolescent environ-ment with an "in crowd" and an "out crowd." This is not effective in the adult world of providing services to patients, carrying out responsibilities, and building careers.

Although these examples of manager beliefs may be ineffective and sometimes even destructive, most managers enter their roles with a little of each of these, as well as other points of view. What is important is that you understand how you ac-tually *do* see your staff—before you determine how you think you *should* see your staff.

As you determine how you actually see your employees, you are in a better posi-tion to change your point of view, if necessary, and to develop effective management practices.

Ideally, you come to your manager role with a healthy respect for your staff and yourself—a respect that all human beings deserve, whether they are one of the best nurses in town or one of those who needs help developing. On this premise you can build a realistic and effective view of your staff—one in which stress is manageable and all are able to thrive.

Inventory of Your Beliefs About Your Staff

Box 9-5 on p. 226 presents a quiz to help you clarify your management practices re-garding your beliefs about or preconceived notions of your staff. The questions are designed as triggers to help you think about and develop or change your beliefs.

Following the inventory are guidelines for you to evaluate your responses to the first eight questions. The rest of the questions will help you reflect on how comfort-able and confident you are in your role and in "what makes you tick" as a nurse manager.

"Yes" responses to the first five questions generally indicate a positive, respectful attitude towards your staff.

If you respond "yes" to any of the next three questions, you may be experiencing problems with your management role (i.e., recognizing the boundaries between you and your staff, as well as recognizing your responsibility to be objective and fair). For example, if you find you are generally irritated when your staff is dissatisfied, you may be personalizing their reactions. Your irritation may stem from your own dif-ficulties in recognizing boundaries.

box 9-5

BELIEFS ABOUT YOUR STAFF—QUESTIONS TO ASK YOURSELF

	YES	NO
1. Do I invite feedback from my staff?	___	___
2. Do I invite constructive criticism of management policies or practices, including my own?	___	___
3. Do I communicate my staff's concerns to my supervisor?	___	___
4. Do I discuss star performers with my supervisor? Do I discuss problem employees with my supervisor?	___	___
5. Do I communicate openly with my staff about the overall operations and goals of the institution or business? Whenever possible, do I inform them of any information handed down to me?	___	___
6. Am I easily irritated when my staff expresses dissatisfaction with a policy or management practice? Why?	___	___
7. Do I discuss staff members' personal or work-related problems with other staff members? Why?	___	___
8. Are there staff members to whom I give preferential treatment? Why?	___	___
9. Do I think someone on my staff wants my job? Why do I think this? Would this person or someone else on my staff be able to do my job? What have I done to explore her/his professional growth objectives? What have I done to encourage capable staff members to consider a management job in this institution or elsewhere?	___	___
10. What do I think of my previous managers? Was anyone exceptionally good? Exceptionally poor? Why?	___	___
11. How did my previous managers view their staffs? Do I share any of these views? How did their opinions of their staffs affect the staffs? Were the managers' opinions of their staffs justified? Why do I think this? Did their opinions of their staffs become self-fulfilling prophesies? Why do I think this?	___	___
12. What are the positive lessons I have learned from my previous managers? How can I incorporate these lessons into my management style?	___	___
13. What aspects of my previous managers' styles do I want to avoid? Why? How can I avoid repeating management practices that could be mistakes?	___	___
14. How do I think my present supervisor views me? Is this justified? Why? Is this effective and productive? Why?	___	___
15. Do I want to pass on this view of subordinates to my staff? Why? How can I do or not do this?	___	___

COPING MECHANISMS

Although many sources of stress are in the nursing workplace, individual nurses cope differently with these stresses.

In their study of critical care nurses, Robinson and Lewis[5] reviewed various coping mechanisms, including adaptive and maladaptive mechanisms (see Box 9-6). Adap-

---

box 9-6

COPING MECHANISMS

- Take vacation.
- Watch television or read.
- Problem-solving.
- Hobbies.
- Discuss problems with family.
- Caffeine (coffee, tea, or soft drinks).
- Exercise.
- Consider changing jobs.
- Work harder and enjoy less.
- Overeating.

- Progressive relaxation techniques.
- Deny problems.
- Alcohol.
- Absenteeism.
- Imagery.
- Meditation.
- Smoking.
- Self-hypnosis.
- Drugs to relax.
- Discuss problems with coworkers.

Robinson JA, Lewis DJ: Coping with ICU work-related stressors: a study, *Crit Care Nurs* 10(5):86, 1990.

tive coping mechanisms are positive responses to stress and require no intervention. Maladaptive coping mechanisms indicate a negative response to stress and call for stress management intervention.

As you can see, this list includes adaptive and maladaptive coping mechanisms. Although the study characterized various mechanisms as either adaptive or maladaptive, some of these coping mechanisms could fall into either category. For example, discussing problems with one's family may prove to be adaptive for one individual but maladaptive for another.

The way a nurse copes with stress in the workplace is highly individualized. Coping mechanisms that work for one may not work for another. In addition, a coping mechanism that works for a nurse under low-level stress may not work for that same nurse under higher levels of stress.

For the purposes of this discussion, those coping mechanisms that cause additional, albeit different, physical or emotional stress in a nurse are maladaptive coping mechanisms. Generally, behaviors such as overeating, overworking, drinking alcohol, smoking, and so forth eventually cause additional stress in the nurse.

Stress Evaluation Exercise: Coping Mechanisms

Earlier in this chapter, you were asked to list as many sources of stress in your work environment as you could identify. As a follow-up to this exercise, now list all coping mechanisms you can imagine. Do not exclude those coping mechanisms you consider to be maladaptive. After generating your coping mechanisms list, consider those coping mechanisms that may be helpful and those that may not be helpful. Identify reasons some coping mechanisms may be adaptive and some maladaptive. You may further define coping mechanisms in terms of their usefulness for various levels of stress (e.g., taking a vacation may be appropriate as temporary relief from long-term stress, and reading or watching television may be effective as relief from short-term stress brought on by a rough day).

If you are doing this exercise with some of your peers, take ample time for discussion. Resist the temptation to push your personal agenda. Rather, learn from each other and broaden your understanding of how people cope with stress.

UNMANAGED STRESS IN THE PATIENT CARE WORKPLACE

Recognizing the signs of unmanaged stress in the workplace is critical to the nurse manager's ability to respond constructively to her/his own and the staff's needs.

Understanding the sources of stress in the patient care workplace and the accompanying coping mechanisms is a prerequisite to understanding what you and your staff are experiencing. When a stressful situation continues for an extended period, or when coping mechanisms are maladaptive or are failing, stress may become unmanageable.

Unfortunately, early signs—and even later signs—of unmanaged stress often go unnoticed. In fact, some managers first recognize that stress is spiraling out of control when staff members resign in legion numbers. Staff members themselves may not even recognize the early signs.

For various reasons, nurse managers often fail to recognize early stress signals. Most managers have risen through the nursing ranks. They have often been conditioned by their supervisors to ignore stress until it reaches mountainous proportions. Thus "It's always been like this" becomes a way to minimize the seriousness of stressful situations. Some nurse managers bring to their jobs a history of ignoring their own signs and symptoms of unmanaged stress, as well as inexperience in recognizing others' signs of unmanaged stress. In addition, the new nurse manager has not had the experience of viewing stress from the vantage point of a manager and claiming responsibility for helping the staff to manage it.

Breakwell,[6] in analyzing the stresses experienced by those in the health care profession, discusses the effects of stress as being both psychologic and behavioral (see Box 9-7). The psychologic effects are seen in changes in one's thinking, as well as in one's emotions.

Stress Evaluation Exercise: Signs of Unmanaged Stress

Nurse managers would do well to monitor themselves and their staffs for the changes brought on by unmanaged stress. Because many of these changes are subjective symptoms, astute nurse managers must learn to observe staff members for the objective signs that usually accompany these subjective symptoms. Box 9-8 on p. 230 presents a stress inventory checklist.

FAILING TO MANAGE STRESS: A COMMON PITFALL

Once a nurse manager learns to identify signs of stress in the workplace, the next step is problem-solving and responding to this stress. Failing to respond constructively to stress in the workplace is a common pitfall for nurse managers.

---

box 9-7

EFFECTS OF UNMANAGED STRESS

SOME CHANGES IN THINKING AS DESCRIBED BY BREAKWELL[6]
- Deteriorating memory.
- Declining concentration and attention span.
- Dissipating powers of organization and long-term planning.

SOME EMOTIONAL CHANGES
- Depression.
- Hostility.
- Defensiveness.
- Feelings of powerlessness and worthlessness.
- Cynicism.
- Mood swings.
- Hypochondria.
- Personality changes (e.g., a shy person becomes gregarious or vice-versa).

SOME BEHAVIORAL EFFECTS OF STRESS
- Decreased energy level.
- Disrupted sleep.
- Increased drinking and/or smoking.
- Absenteeism from work.
- Diminished sex drive.
- Lack of enthusiasm
- Lack of interest in activities and hobbies that once were satisfying.

SOME CHANGES BROUGHT ON BY CHRONIC, UNRELIEVED STRESS (MAY BE SUBTLE)[7]
- Feeling overwhelmed.
- Fatigue, angry outbursts, depression.
- Forgetfulness and disorganization.
- Guilt and self-sacrifice.
- Feeling disillusioned.
- Passivity.
- Distancing yourself from your patients.
- Letting yourself go.
- Substance abuse.
- Physical illness.

Often managers minimize the toll stress can take on themselves and their staffs, ignoring even late warning signs of stress's wear and tear. There are many reasons for this failing. For example, a nurse manager may ignore the effects of stress because of a fear of impotence (e.g., "There's nothing I can do about it, so I'll ignore it.") Unfortunately, this attitude of impotence—no matter how toughly exhibited—is communicated to the staff. When one experiences impotence in the face of stress, the stress is magnified, creating an even more strained environment. On the contrary,

----------------- box 9-8 -----------------

STAFF STRESS INVENTORY CHECKLIST

As a manager, you can take stock of what you are seeing in your staff's behavior by asking yourself questions that address Wilson's[7] list of symptoms. You may ask yourself the questions in reference to an individual on the staff or in regard to the staff as a whole. For the purposes of this discussion, assume that you are considering one individual.

FEELING OVERWHELMED

Is she slow to start at the beginning of the workday? _____
Does she "jump right in," before having had the chance to organize the workday? _____
Does she dart from task to task without a clear sense of purpose or control? _____
Does she seem to respond mostly to the "squeaky wheel" (or patient), rather than acting on priorities? _____
Does she express a fatalistic attitude about the workload (e.g., "Oh well, it's not going to get done anyway.")? _____
Does she consistently have to work overtime to complete assignments? _____
Has she failed to complete assignments? _____

FATIGUE, ANGRY OUTBURSTS, AND DEPRESSION

Does he lose his temper at the slightest provocation? _____
Does he respond rudely or abruptly to patients? _____
Is he rough with patients? _____
Has he become quiet or unusually reserved? _____
Has he lost his sense of humor? _____
Does he get tearful with little provocation? _____
Does he remark that the job is "getting to him"? _____
Has he been absent from work more often than is considered average absenteeism? _____
Does he say he is depressed? _____
Has he shown personality changes? _____
Has he become disinterested or apathetic about work? _____
Has he become disinterested or apathetic about other aspects of his life? _____

FORGETFULNESS AND DISORGANIZATION

Is she making more than the normal amount of mistakes? _____
Are you seeing an increase in her incident reports? _____
Does she forget aspects of patient care? _____
Does she forget to report patient problems appropriately? _____
Is she failing to recognize patient problems or to make logical deductions about patient problems? _____
Are her usual thinking abilities impaired? _____
Does she seem distracted? _____
When you address her, does she sometimes seem not to hear you? _____

Adapted from Wilson LK: High-gear nursing: how it can run you down and what you can do about it, *Nursing '89*, 19(12):81, 1989.

Continued.

······················· box 9-8, cont'd ·······················

GUILT AND SELF-SACRIFICE

Is he coming to work when he is ill? _____

Is he consistently skipping lunch or work breaks to catch up on work? _____

Is he consistently working overtime? _____

Does he consistently volunteer for distasteful tasks, overtime assignments, and holiday shifts? _____

FEELING DISILLUSIONED

Does she express resentment about the nursing profession? _____

Does she express envy of people in other professions or regret that she became a nurse? _____

Does she remark that the actual practice of nursing is much different from what she learned in school? _____

Does she express regret that she can never deliver the type of care she would like to deliver? _____

Does she express feelings of hopelessness about nursing (e.g., "It will never change.")? _____

PASSIVITY

Does he take abuse from coworkers or physicians? _____

Does he remark that "it's not worth" disagreeing with difficult individuals? _____

Does he seem indifferent about problem-solving? _____

Is he among the first people you consider when you must assign a distasteful task (because you know there will be no resistance)? _____

Is he described as a wimp by coworkers? _____

DISTANCING ONESELF FROM PATIENTS

Does she refer to patients as disease entities, rather than as people (e.g., "the hepatitis in 22")? _____

Does she respond irritably to patients who "interrupt" tasks with questions or requests? _____

Does she limit conversation with patients by speaking only when absolutely necessary? _____

Does she ask patients to make their requests all at once so she can limit interactions with them? _____

Does she focus almost exclusively on the physical aspects of caring for patients, rather than also considering the psychologic aspects? _____

Does she make remarks about family members who "interfere" with patient care by asking questions or making requests? _____

Is she "cold" or "cool" to patients? _____

LETTING ONESELF GO

Has he gained or lost weight recently? _____

Is his appearance sloppy or haphazard? _____

Continued.

---

box 9-8, cont'd

SUBSTANCE ABUSE

Is she drinking more coffee or smoking more cigarettes? _____
Has she said she is taking something to sleep? _____
Has she been late to work? _____
Has she been absent from work more often than is considered average absenteeism?

_____

Has she joked or commented about excessive "partying"? _____
Is she showing any of the physical or psychologic signs of chemical dependency? _____
   (Refer to later section, "When You Identify A Serious Staff Problem.")

PHYSICAL ILLNESS

Has he had excessive absenteeism because of illness? _____
Does he seem to have an inordinate number of colds, headaches, or gastrointestinal problems? _____

---

the sense that one can effect change, regardless of degree, provides a feeling of hope and empowerment.

A second reason nurse managers may fail to respond constructively to stress is a false sense of their own invulnerability. This sense of invulnerability—"That doesn't bother me," "I've been in nursing 10 years (or 3 or 5 years); I'm used to that,"—often is no more than a way of building up to the burnout so many nurses experience. A nurse who appears immune to the emotional roller coaster of nursing may in fact be closer to burnout than suspected.

For example, distancing oneself from and depersonalizing patients (e.g., "the colon cancer in 13-A" or "the three 'total-cares' I had today") help a nurse avoid feelings of frustration, fear, or grief but are poor substitutes for accepting and sharing these feelings with others.

In the long run, trying to be invulnerable leaves one vulnerable to frustration, depression, and burnout. And a nurse manager who, by example, fosters such invulnerability in her/his staff also fosters burnout in her/his staff.

A third reason nurse managers may fail to respond constructively to stress is a misguided belief that managers are expected to "roll with"—rather than respond to—stressful situations. Often managers are concerned that acknowledgment of the stress level in their area may indicate a deficiency in their management skills. This concern is heightened when a manager's own supervisor appears unaware of or invulnerable to stress.

You may be able to identify other reasons nurses and nurse managers fail to respond constructively to stress. Regardless of the explanation, the result is the same: failure to respond constructively to stress leads to increased stress. When you are able to recognize unmanaged stress, you are better able to respond to stress in the workplace with effective coping mechanisms. You will also be better equipped to respond to the needs of your staff and help them in enhancing their adaptive coping mechanisms.

WHEN YOU IDENTIFY A SERIOUS STAFF PROBLEM

Occasionally you will identify an employee who has a serious problem. This problem may be caused by job stress, personal difficulties, or a combination of factors.

If you are concerned that an employee's performance may be impaired because of chemical dependence, or that she/he may be experiencing serious emotional problems or depression, you need to request guidance. You can speak with your EAP counselor, the staff social worker or psychologist, the psychiatric nurse specialist, or a professional outside your organization.

It generally is best to use your organization's resources first. People within your organization may know the employee, or your organization may have resources or policies to respond to these types of problems.

If you do seek assistance from an outside professional to guide you in your dealings with an employee, resources are usually available. Most cities have emergency or crisis hotlines for referrals to appropriate organizations, many of which will discuss your concerns about your employee free of charge. Hospital emergency rooms frequently keep hotline and other organization listings.

Discuss your concerns with your supervisor and determine a course of action. If your supervisor is not responsive, these cases—because of their serious nature and possible consequences—obligate you to take your concerns up your organization's chain of command or to HR, the EAP counselor, or other professional until you get assistance.

The Chemically Dependent Employee

It is important for nurse managers to be aware of the problems of alcohol and other chemical dependencies in the health professions. Bissell,[8] a nationally recognized expert on addicted health care professionals, and Jones[8] conducted research indicating the severity of chemical dependency in the nursing profession. Their research suggests that approximately 5% of the 1.5 million registered nurses in the United States are dependent on alcohol or drugs.

Selbach[9] cites job strain—including factors such as the nursing shortage, work overload, and dealing with illness and death—as a traditional source of the frustration and stress contributing to a nurse becoming chemically dependent. She cites rotating shifts, night duty, chronic stress, tension, fatigue, and anxiety as factors that can lead to insomnia and the initial use of chemicals to unwind, relax, and sleep. In addition, most nurses are women, and many actually have two full-time jobs, nurse and mother, and try to be "superwoman" at both.

A word of caution: the chemically dependent nurse, like many others dependent on drugs or alcohol, often does not embody the stereotype of the debilitated addict.

In fact, some chemically dependent nurses are excellent workers who show no sign of their dependency until late in the disease. The chemically dependent nurse may be a high achiever, an individual who has done well in school and in past jobs and may have been the model employee/spouse/friend/parent before the dependency. She/he often is a compulsive individual, which is a trait that can lend itself to good patient care but which can also cause the nurse to create unrealistic expectations of herself/himself at work and in other areas of life. These expectations can produce the stress overload the nurse believes is alleviated by using drugs or alcohol. Box 9-9 lists signs of the chemically dependent nurse.

Many health care facilities have policies concerning the chemically dependent employee, including policies to assist the employee in seeking treatment. Although terminating a chemically dependent employee may appear to be a quick fix, the terminated employee probably will not seek treatment. In fact, she/he will probably

---

box 9-9

SIGNS OF THE CHEMICALLY DEPENDENT NURSE

Numbers 1 through 7 are signs identified by Patton, an occupational health nurse and EAP coordinator. Other common signs follow.

1. Too many medication errors.
2. Frequent absences from the nursing unit.
3. Too many controlled substances wasted and/or spilled.
4. Consistently incorrect narcotics count.
5. Signs out more controlled substances than do others.
6. Rapid, extreme, and inappropriate mood changes.
7. Patient complaints of the ineffectiveness of pain medication when administered by individual. (This could be a sign that the nurse is substituting saline or sterile water, emptying capsules, or substituting nonnarcotic tablets.)
8. Excessive absenteeism.
9. Tardiness.
10. Getting by at work, but not performing beyond the bare minimum needed.
11. Failure to complete assignments.
12. Leaving responsibilities to other staff.
13. Sloppy, illogical, nonexistent, or meaningless charting (often by rote and could apply to any patient).
14. Excessive incident reports and/or failure to file incident reports.
15. Excessive mistakes.
16. Abnormal physiologic reactions resulting from drug or alcohol use, such as headaches, diarrhea, lack of sleep, and withdrawal symptoms.
17. Inappropriate behavior or quick flashes of temper.
18. Personality changes.
19. Obvious physical signs of drug use, such as slurring speech, rapid speech, smell of alcohol, confusion, or weight loss.
20. Accusations that people are "out to get" or are against her/him.
21. Blaming others and refusal to take responsibility for actions.

From Patton J: Addicted nurses, *J Pract Nurs* 37(4):40, 1987.

move onto another job—the "geographic cure"—taking the chemical dependency into another workplace.

As a nurse manager facing the possibility of a chemically dependent employee, your responsibilities are twofold: (1) to see that your patients are receiving proper care from responsible employees and (2) to address the needs of the chemically dependent employee, including the right to privacy and the opportunity to seek help.

If you believe you have a chemically dependent employee on your staff, discuss the matter with your supervisor to determine a course of action (i.e., what policies your organization has in place, what professional person will guide you). If your supervisor is not responsive, continue to seek guidance.

The Employee with Emotional Difficulties

If you are concerned that an employee is severely depressed, disturbed, or suicidal, seek guidance immediately to determine how to handle the situation. If you have fears or concerns that an employee is "not right," these feelings are probably well founded. In these cases, you must provide for the safety of your patients and determine, with the help of your supervisor and a trained professional, how to support your employee. Again, if your supervisor is not responsive to your concern, seek guidance from others.

Other Serious Problems

Aside from chemical dependency and emotional difficulties, other serious problems that warrant attention may manifest themselves in your department as a whole or in a member or members of your staff. For instance, sometimes a staff member copes with stress by blaming you, another individual on the staff, or a small group of individuals for the stress. This scapegoating can become a way of life in the department and can devastate the person or persons being scapegoated. In addition, it never alleviates the stress in the department because it does not solve the problem.

Other problems that may arise in your department could affect almost everyone on your staff. The situation may be the result of long-term problems within your organization or department, such as excessive turnover, or it may be a problem that is clearly time-limited—whether it be 1 month or 1 year in duration. Examples of these situations include major management changes (e.g., a new CEO who effects many changes), a large construction or renovation project that disrupts daily activities, a flu epidemic that depletes the staff, or the introduction of computerized scheduling, which requires a period of adjustment while the "bugs" are worked out.

In some instances, you may recognize that many of your staff are experiencing a great deal of stress, but you cannot identify the source. If you think your staff as a group is feeling the strain of unmanaged stress, regardless of the source, it may be helpful to invite a professional to facilitate an ongoing staff support group. It is not recommended that a nurse manager try to lead these group meetings. The support group should allow for the sharing of feelings and personal interpretations, which only a trained professional should direct. In addition, if there are communication gaps between you and any of your staff members, a professional can help in closing these gaps. Discuss your options with your supervisor.

UNMANAGEABLE ENVIRONMENTS

Although most problems can be solved with time and the proper guidance and intervention, you may find yourself in a work environment in which the problems are so many or so deeply rooted that you are unable to be an effective manager. In this instance, it is generally best for you to leave the position.

There are many understandable reasons why you may leave a job. Some examples include a poor job match for you, a disagreement with the values or policies of a supervisor or organization, a realization that you prefer not to be a manager, or a realization that you are not ready to be a manager. Another understandable reason for leaving a job is the recognition that you are attempting to manage an unmanageable environment.

Generally, an unmanageable environment is characterized by two components: (1) a serious problem exists in the department or organization, and (2) you have little or ineffective management support in solving it. If your immediate supervisor shows little support or if the support is ineffective, you may be able to find help from someone else within your organization. Some problems, because of their serious nature, require you to seek this help when your immediate supervisor is not responsive. Some of these situations were discussed earlier in this chapter, under "When You Identify a Serious Staff Problem."

You may identify other serious problems that call for immediate attention. For instance, staffing that is so lean that patient care is threatened would require you to seek help beyond a nonresponsive supervisor.

A word of caution: when you secure problem-solving assistance or intervention from someone in your organization other than your supervisor, the immediate problem may be resolved, but you have not changed your environment. Although your first responsibility must be to solve the immediate problem, you must then evaluate your options and the viability of continuing as a manager with an ineffective supervisor.

Ineffective Management Support

A supervisor may demonstrate ineffective management support or a lack of management support to the nurse manager in many ways. For example, the nurse manager may be restricted from taking corrective action against employees who defy the policies of the organization or department. The manager may be prevented from taking disciplinary action against an employee who is rough with a patient. The supervisor may listen sympathetically to the nurse manager's concerns about the department, but offer no advice or direction. The nurse manager may be consistently scapegoated by the staff, and the supervisor may offer no guidance for dealing with this situation.

These are a few examples of how a supervisor may fail to support a nurse manager. In each case, the manager's inability to take action, to correct a problem, or to establish leadership authority will affect the morale of the staff, the quality of patient care, and the manager's ability to manage the department.

Sometimes a new nurse manager enters a job without knowledge of the department's history and resulting problems. Perhaps the staff members believe the previous manager was unfairly dismissed from the position. Or they may have experienced a long period without leadership and resent the arrival of the new manager. These factors alone do not necessarily create an unmanageable environment. However, if the new nurse manager receives little support and guidance from her/his supervisor, effective management could be difficult.

Box 9-10 presents a list of conditions that, when combined with ineffective support or a lack of support from management above you, could signal an unmanage-

---

box 9-10

SIGNS OF AN UNMANAGEABLE ENVIRONMENT

- An individual or group (or clique) of nurses holding the unspoken power in the division.
- Understaffing, with no plan or hope for improvement.
- Poor patient care.
- Staff scapegoating of you or a member of your staff.
- A chemically dependent employee.
- An employee stealing drugs, narcotics, or supplies.
- Widespread absenteeism.
- An employee coming in late to work, leaving early, or disappearing during the work day.
- An employee who physically or emotionally abuses patients.
- An employee who defies the policies of the organization.
- An employee who shows you no respect (e.g., walking away from you when you talk, shouting at you, ignoring you).
- A staff that is divided along lines of race, gender, professional status, levels of competence, tenure, or other factors.
- A supervisor who makes management decisions based on any of the factors cited in the preceding point.
- A supervisor who maintains friendships with one or more staff members who do not support you or who undermine your authority.
- A supervisor who misrepresents you to upper management (e.g., lying about you, taking credit for your work).
- A supervisor who listens to the complaints of the staff (about you, your management, or other matters related to your department) without encouraging the staff to talk to you or without informing you of the conversations.
- An apathetic staff.
- An employee who defies your instructions, policies, and so forth.
- An employee who seems seriously depressed, disturbed, or suicidal.
- Other conditions you have identified.

able environment. You may be able to add items to this list. Included in the list are some additional destructive behaviors your supervisor could exhibit—behaviors that go beyond not showing support and are more actively destructive.

If you determine that you are in an unmanageable environment, it is important that you give yourself permission to resign your position. Sometimes nurse managers are reluctant to give up on a job, believing if they only try harder, conditions will improve. In an unmanageable environment, unfortunately, this often is not the case. By definition, this type of environment cannot be improved without radical changes in the leadership above.

If you resign a position because you believe the work environment to be unmanageable, you may want to request an exit interview with an objective nurse recruiter, personnel director, or other individual in an influential position who may be receptive to listening. Each organization is different, and you will have to determine your best course. Because patient care may be at stake, it is important to share your perceptions of the environment in the hope that the situation will be addressed. As you relate your perceptions, take care to provide only the facts, not your subjective feelings or intuitions about the situation. For example, relate problematic events in your department and how you attempted to get help to solve them.

Sometimes it is best to schedule an exit interview for a time after you have recovered from the immediate stress of your resignation. If you choose to pursue an exit interview, it will be important for you to conduct the interview calmly, presenting your information in a rational manner.

TAKING ACTION TO SUPPORT YOUR STAFF

Fortunately, most nurse managers do not find themselves in unmanageable environments. And in most cases, there are many steps a nurse manager can take to alleviate routine stress in the department. Everyone agrees that a nurse manager's support is critical to the staff's successful management of stress. Albrecht and Halsey[10] suggest that we consider "social support as verbal and nonverbal communication between recipients and providers, which reduces uncertainty about the situation, the self, and others . . . to enhance personal control."

Albrecht and Halsey Study on Support to Staff Nurses

Albrecht and Halsey[10] discuss the types of messages that are most helpful to a distressed nurse (see Manager's Tip 9-1).

Their study of staff nurses' stress and how their managers support them was very revealing. The nurses' perceptions of a manager's supportive behaviors were measured separately in four hypothetical stress situations. The combined results show that the manager's listening, offering reassurance, and giving advice were supportive behaviors that were valued by many of the nurses. Although the manager's taking action to solve the problem also was viewed as supportive, the results showed that this

MANAGER'S TIP 9-1

HELPFUL MESSAGES FOR THE DISTRESSED NURSE

✔ Reduce uncertainty by offering a new perspective on the problem (e.g., "Why don't you think about this?).

✔ Help increase feelings of control over the problem by allowing education days or teaching new skills.

✔ Help enhance a sense of control over the problem by providing tangible assistance (in a friendly, noncondescending manner).

✔ Offer acceptance and reassurance.

Modified from Albrecht TL, Halsey J: Supporting the staff nurse under stress, *Nurs Manage* 22(7):60, 1991.

behavior was not valued by as many nurses as were the manager's communication and advising behaviors.

However, one stress situation in which many of the nurses viewed the manager's action as supportive was when the staff nurses were working in an understaffed situation. Here, the manager's helping with the work was particularly valued. This makes sense because understaffing threatens the nurses' ability to provide good patient care, the driving desire of most nurses. However, even in this situation, many nurses also valued the manager's listening skills.

As a nurse manager, you must weigh each stressful situation and determine the steps you can take to support your staff. In some instances, active, as well as communicative, support is imperative, lest you become known for "all talk and no action." In the case of understaffing, it may be important to help in the immediate situation, then take action to see that understaffing does not become a chronic problem.

The lesson to be learned from Albrecht and Halsey's study[10] is not to underestimate the value of each of a manager's methods of offering support to the staff: listening, offering reassurance, giving advice, taking action, validating your staff's feelings, and helping your staff understand the perspective of other employees and of physicians.

In some cases, good communication skills or concrete suggestions will greatly alleviate staff nurses' stress. In others, you will need to combine this support with action.

To address some forms of stress, you may need to make changes in how your department operates. Be mindful of ways you can alter your work environment to alleviate stress. Include your staff in discussions of ways to modify operations for a smoother, less stressful work day. Enlist the guidance and support of your supervisor. Work with your supervisor to determine what changes you can and cannot effect and why. For example, if you have been unable to fill some vacant positions, what alternatives do you have to tide the staff over until the positions are filled? Is there a way to get more secretarial support? Can you employ temporary nurses? Can you draw more help from the float pool? Are there some nonpatient care activities that can be suspended until your positions are filled?

Drawing on the Work and Experience of Other Nurse Managers

Many nurse managers fall into the trap of thinking they are alone in dealing with staff stress. In addition to your supervisor and a myriad of other resource people within and outside your organization, consider the experience of your peers. Ask them how they support their staffs and consider if these techniques would work for your staff. Be sensitive to the differences in departments, personnel, and your personality versus the personalities of your peers. What works for them may not work for you. Also, you may find that you simply do not agree with the approaches of some of your peers. Nonetheless, your peer group may offer new ways of looking at conditions and new ideas for supporting your staff.

Another resource to consider is the nursing literature. Much has been written about stress in nursing and the allied health care professions. A trip to a nursing or medical library can result in a lot of new information. If you have specific concerns, such as the impaired nurse or the stress of dealing with death and dying, you can easily find articles on these topics. If there is no nursing or medical library in your facility or where you live, contact your local library to see if they carry any appropriate journals. Also, if your organization has an education or training department, consult with the director.

Subscribing to one or more of the nursing professional journals is a good idea, both for the clinical and management information. You may want to share subscriptions with some of your peers to cut costs and increase your access to various publications.

Communicating with Upper Management

An important way to support your staff is to communicate their concerns to your supervisor. By working with your supervisor, you may be able to generate additional ways to demonstrate support to your staff. Manager's Tip 9-2 provides further suggestions.

If your department is experiencing a particularly stressful situation, be certain to let them know that you and your supervisor are concerned. Tell the staff what you and your supervisor are able to do to support them. Often, your staff's knowing that you recognize their stress is the first step in alleviating it. Also, their knowing that you consider their feelings important enough to discuss with your supervisor lets them know that you care.

Humor

Humor can break the tension in even the most stressful situation. If you are attuned to the sensitivities of your staff and have a good sense of timing, you can use humor very effectively to make a tough day a little less stressful.

MANAGER'S TIP 9-2

LENDING SUPPORT TO YOUR STAFF

✔ Encourage camaraderie among your staff. Provide the opportunity for them to know each other as people, not just as nurses. Whenever possible, schedule breaks and meals for at least two nurses at a time.

✔ Sponsor a staff party away from the workplace a few times a year. A pot-luck dinner is an inexpensive way to get together and will encourage staff participation.

✔ Take time to know your staff. Ask about their families, friends, and school experiences. Take some of your breaks and meals with them.

✔ Let your staff know you. Do not discourage casual conversation. Let them know it is okay to ask you about yourself by volunteering information about your life and interests away from the job. However, do not overdo it by talking about yourself in a one-sided conversation.

✔ Allow time at regular staff meetings for your employees to ask questions and voice concerns. You can invite this communication broadly (e.g., "Is there anything anyone would like to discuss?") and specifically (e.g., "Does anyone have any questions or concerns about our new admissions policy?"). A combination of both techniques is most effective.

✔ Recognize unmanaged stress (e.g., "It seems this is a difficult time," "Are you okay?" "It would make sense that you would be stressed out today.").

✔ Listen. Listen. And listen again.

✔ If you are concerned that someone may be experiencing stress, talk to the person and offer reassurance and support with constructive problem-solving. In cases of severe stress, look to your supervisor and a trained professional for guidance.

✔ Provide time in the workday for your staff to think and reflect on the best way to organize and deliver their patient care.

✔ Provide regular staff in-services and updating of skills.

✔ Allow for education days for your staff to encourage them to develop professionally.

✔ Use your supervisor for assistance in supporting your staff.

✔ Help your staff learn to manage their time.

✔ Arrange staff coverage so that your employees are able to take vacation breaks on a regular basis.

✔ Offer words of support, recognizing your staff's good work and giving positive feedback frequently and freely.

As wonderful as humor can be, there are some basic guidelines concerning its use. For example, never make a joke at the expense of another person—present or absent—or at the expense of a group of people based on their gender, race, sexual orientation, and so on, regardless of whether a member of the group is on your staff. Hostile, bigoted, or demeaning humor may lead to feelings of insecurity among your staff (e.g., "When will she/he come after me or someone like me?").

In addition, it is important not to use humor at an inappropriate time, such as in a serious patient-care situation that requires concentration. Laughter at this time could have serious consequences for the patient. Also, do not use any form of humor that would show disrespect for a patient or the patient's family.

Particularly effective is lighthearted humor poking fun at yourself (however, not at your gender, race, sexual orientation, and so forth). If you are comfortable with self-deprecating humor, you can give your staff the chance to relax a little, as well as to see you in a more personal light, thus strengthening the bonds between you. According to Smith,[11] "Team spirit and improved staff morale are benefits reaped by the nurse manager who knows how to take her job seriously while taking herself lightly."

Smith[11] notes that it is difficult for most people to tell a scripted joke and get the desired effect, particularly to a group or to people with whom relationships are not well developed. For spontaneous situations, Lee[12] suggests that a comical remark about a personal event or predicament generally works best.

SUPPORTING YOURSELF

As was discussed at the beginning of this chapter, it is critical that you support yourself as you simultaneously support your staff from the effects of stress. Listed later are various ways to help you manage long-term and short-term job stress. However, there are individuals for whom these and other methods may not work. The following discussion addresses these individuals.

If you believe your environment is basically manageable, but you are having difficulty coping with the stress of your job, give yourself permission to get professional help, either from your EAP counselor, another in-house professional, or a professional counselor or therapist outside your organization. Remember, you are new to your job and to the stresses of being a manager. Even when you are an experienced nurse manager, there may come a time when you feel your coping mechanisms are failing you. Do not consider yourself inadequate if you are having problems dealing with the stress of your job. Discussing your situation with an impartial professional can help you to problem-solve, strengthen your coping mechanisms, or develop new ones.

If There Is No Hope in Sight

You may reach a point where you cannot handle the stresses of your job, despite the fact that the environment may be manageable (when viewed objectively), despite your best efforts to problem-solve and seek help, and despite your belief that you should be able to handle the stress. Or you simply may know it is best for you to leave your position because you are not able or do not want to invest the energy necessary to cope with the stress. If you have no reason to believe your situation will improve, give yourself permission to leave your job. Many nurses are drawn to their profession because of their gifts and inner needs to care for others. Although these qualities are admirable and serve others well, they do not always serve the caretaker well. Resigning a position does not mean you are a failure. It could be a way to take control of your life and afford yourself the type of care and attention you are so good at giving to others.

In most instances, your work environment will be manageable and you will be able to support yourself and your staff. Below are recommendations for supporting yourself.

Wilson[7] recommends the strategies in Manager's Tip 9-3 for nurses dealing with the stress of their profession. These tips apply to staff nurses as well as to nurse managers.

MANAGER'S TIP 9-3

SUPPORTING YOURSELF

✔ Develop a "can do" attitude. Consider the problems you *can* solve and focus on these, rather than all the problems you *can not* solve. These successes will help you feel capable, stronger, and more able to take on the next problem.

✔ Become more assertive. Feeling powerless in your relationships is a great source of job stress. Learn constructive ways to solve problems and communicate effectively with others—not aggressively, but calmly, directly, and with respect for yourself and others. Take a class or workshop in communications or assertiveness.

✔ Make overwhelming tasks manageable. Break down big tasks into their component parts. Then concentrate on completing each part. At the beginning of the day, instead of feeling powerless in the face of the next 8 to 10 hours of work, prioritize and write down your tasks for the next 30 minutes, 2 hours, 4 hours, and so on. Then take them a step at a time.

✔ Manage your time better. Combine tasks when you can. If you have to make a call, before you pick up the phone, consider if you have other matters to discuss with the same person or department. If you take a patient admission history, write it directly onto the form. Do not write it on scratch paper and copy it later onto the form. Learn to delegate when appropriate. Do not think you have to do *everything*. Learn what you must do to take care of yourself and what can be expected of others.

✔ Accept your failures, and do not take yourself so seriously. When you fail, look at what went wrong and why, and consider whether you could have done something differently. Learn from your mistakes and resolve to put this learning to use. Accept that you are human and that you will make mistakes. Learn to laugh at yourself sometimes and appreciate the good things around you.

✔ Nurture each other. Use your caretaking skills with one another. Cultivate friendships with people you trust.

✔ Nurture yourself. Learn to relax, listen to your body's needs for caretaking, exercise, and do something fun for yourself at least once a week.

Adapted from Wilson LK: High-gear nursing: how it can run you down and what you can do about it, *Nursing '89* 19(12):81, 1989.

More Tips for Taking Care of Yourself

Manager's Tips 9-4 and 9-5 offer other ways to support yourself and alleviate the effects of routine stress on a short-term and long-term basis. Work to stop a molehill of stress from building to a mountain. Many of these suggestions also could be helpful for your staff. We saved the best lists for last.

MANAGER'S TIP 9-4

SHORT-TERM STRESS: TIPS IF YOU ARE FEELING TENSE AT WORK

✔ Ask a coworker to relieve you for a few moments so you can adjust your thinking and put things in perspective.
✔ Take a few minutes to sit down, take some deep breaths, and relax.
✔ Step away from the work environment and stretch your arms and legs, touch your toes, and open and close your fists to release tension.
✔ Take a moment to think of an enjoyable time you had with a friend or family member. Let yourself smile.
✔ Take a moment to visualize yourself as a relaxed, capable individual who *can* solve problems.
✔ Take a few minutes to consult with a peer, ventilate, and perhaps get a different perspective.
✔ Make up your mind that the stressful situation at hand will not get the better of you.

MANAGER'S TIP 9-5

LONG-TERM STRESS: TIPS FOR THE REST OF YOUR LIFE

✔ Take time to "smell the roses" every day. Do something just for you, no matter how small. Watch a favorite television program, talk to a friend on the phone, take a walk, give yourself a pedicure, or curl up in bed an hour early and catch up on your reading.
✔ Get a manicure, facial, or a new haircut.
✔ Get regular physical exercise, such as walking, jogging, swimming, or gardening.
✔ Eat healthful foods. Limit caffeine and alcoholic beverages.
✔ Ventilate tension from work by talking for 5 or 10 minutes to a sympathetic listener—a spouse, friend, or coworker. Talk in general terms—"Two people died today," or "We had to work short today." Avoid detailed discussions or blow-by-blow accounts of your

Continued.

day, which only serve to make you relive the stress a second time, instead of relieving it. The object is simply to feel the support of someone who cares about you.

✓ Learn to meditate. Meditation is a good way to focus yourself and to relax. Fifteen to thirty minutes of meditation in the morning or evening will go a long way towards helping you keep perspective for the rest of your day.

✓ Build your relationships with your peer group. Sharing concerns, considering solutions to routine problems, and enjoying one another's company all are good ways to give and receive support.

✓ Schedule regular vacations, usually at 3-month or 4-month intervals. In the interim, a 3-day weekend can provide a great deal of relaxation.

✓ Leave work at work. Plan so that you are not taking home work on a regular basis.

✓ Cultivate outside interests that are unrelated to your work. Include individuals who are not in the health care field in your circle of friends.

✓ Ask your supervisor to set up time with you to brainstorm solutions to particularly stressful situations.

✓ Stay tuned to the stress level of your staff. The more quickly you address their stress, the less likely serious problems will develop.

✓ Participate in professional development, quality control, or other committees in your work setting. This involvement will help you become more familiar with your institution, help you to network, provide different perspectives on situations and problems in your job, and give you exposure for recognition for your good ideas and work.

✓ Be active in your professional organizations. Through this participation, you will learn nursing and management skills, as well as increase networking and strengthen peer relationships. As a result, you will feel stronger, smarter, and less stressed.

✓ Be realistic about the problems on your job. Not every problem is your responsibility, and you cannot solve the world's problems. Take responsibility for only those problems that are yours.

✓ Have realistic expectations of others. Eliminate the stress of being frustrated by inconsequential shortcomings of others.

✓ Keep a positive attitude. Bad attitudes are contagious and breed additional stress.

✓ Address and correct mistakes. Then forgive yourself and others for making mistakes.

Considerations for Home Care Managers

STRESS SYMPTOMS IN HOME CARE STAFF

The concepts and suggestions discussed in Chapter 9 apply to all nurse managers across the continuum as they struggle to care for themselves and their staff during this tumultuous period of health care. Stress can be demonstrated in various ways in home care and the manager needs to be aware of the symptoms in order to assist staff before they act in patient homes, or while driving to visits throughout the day. Examples could include staff being involved in automobile accidents while making visits as a result of lack of concentration or focus.

SUMMARY

This chapter reviewed stress in the nursing workplace and how it can manifest itself, stress-coping mechanisms, and signs of unmanaged stress. Examples of serious staff problems and recommended actions were discussed. Also, the unmanageable environment was explored, as were points on how to recognize this "no-win" situation.

Many suggestions were made about supporting yourself and your staff. Undoubtedly you can think of additional ways—ways that apply specifically to you or to your staff.

No single reference, person, or resource contains all the answers to a given situation or problem. Talk to your supervisor and your peers. Read professional journals. Continue your efforts to seek information and develop your own solutions to take care of yourself and your staff. The return on your investment will be great.

References

1. Nicholson L: Stress management in nursing, *Nurs Manage* 21(4):53, 1990.
2. Foxall MJ, et al: A comparison of frequency and sources of nursing job stress perceived by intensive care, hospice and medical-surgical nurses, *J Adv Nurs* 15(5):577, 1990.
3. Lees S, Ellis N: The design of a stress-management programme for nursing personnel, *J Adv Nurs* 15:946, 1990.
4. Simms L, et al: Breaking the burnout barrier: resurrecting work excitement in nursing," *Nurs Economics* 8(3):185, 1990.
5. Robinson JA, Lewis DJ: Coping with ICU work-related stressors: a study, *Crit Care Nurse* 10(5):86, 1990.
6. Breakwell GM: Are you stressed out?, *Am J Nurs*, 90(8):31, 1990. Article abstracted from Breakwell GM: *Facing physical vio-lence*, first published in London, 1990, The British Psychological Society in association with Routledge Ltd, and 1990, New York, Chapman & Hall.
7. Wilson LK: High-gear nursing: how it can run you down and what you can do about it, *Nursing '89* 19(12):81, 1989.
8. Bissell L, Jones D: The alcoholic nurse, *Nurs Outlook* 29:96, 1981.
9. Selbach KH: Chemical dependency in nursing, *AORN J* 52(3):531, 1990.
10. Albrecht TL, Halsey J: Supporting the staff nurse under stress, *Nurs Manage* 22(7):60, 1991.
11. Smith LB: Humor relations for nurse managers, *Nurs Manage* 21(5):86, 1990.
12. Lee BS: Humor relations for nurse managers, *Nurs Manage* 21(5):86, 88, 90, 1990.

For Further Reading

Albrecht TL, Halsey J: Supporting the staff nurse under stress, *Nurs Manage* 22(7):60-61, 64, 1991.

Bennett S, Robertson R, Moss P: Education: learning the pitfalls of codependency, *Nurs Manage* 23(2):80B, 1992.

Casey JL: Counseling nurse managers, *Nurs Manage* 20(9):52, 1989.

Cauthorne-Lindstrom C, Hrabe D: Codependent behaviors in managers: a script for failure, *Nurs Manage* 21(2):34, 1990.

Fortman R: Staff support groups: what works, what doesn't, *Hospice* 1(1):23, 1990.

Guntzelman J: Making frustration work for you, *Nurs 90,* 20(12):85, 1990.

Kaplan SM: The nurse as change agent, *Pediatr Nurs* 16(6):603, 1990.

Nicholson L: Stress management in nursing, *Nurs Manage* 21(4):53, 1990.

Patton J: Addicted nurses, *J Pract Nurs* 37(4):38, 1987.

Selbach KH: Chemical dependency in nursing, *AORN J* 52(3):531, 1990.

CHAPTER 10

WHEN BAD THINGS HAPPEN
TO GOOD MANAGERS

T.M. MARRELLI

Certain problems commonly faced in management are unpleasant or difficult for many managers. Hopefully you will not experience many of them. However, they do occur and should be addressed. These problems can be as simple as feeling vulnerable during the transition from nurse to manager and wanting to stay in the former role. You must put these problems into perspective. Although they alone are not usually good reasons for leaving a position that you otherwise would enjoy, they can make you feel like resigning. Some of the most common problems faced by new managers are discussed in this chapter.

SPECIAL PROBLEMS
When You Are Promoted and Your Friend Is Not

When you are chosen for a management position, a friend or close colleague who also applied for the position may feel hurt, disappointed, or resentful. Your friend's reaction may, in turn, make you feel sad, disappointed, or even guilty. These feelings can be incredibly uncomfortable and usually do not go away overnight. You must remember that you are now the manager and were chosen over your friend for a reason, although you probably should not verbalize this to your friend. In addition, no matter how happy your friend may appear for you, hurt feelings will probably arise. You cannot pretend that the relationship has not changed; it has by the nature of the hierarchy in the workplace. The change can be particularly difficult if you have been long-term peers and have experienced parallel careers and a close friendship. Although your goal may be to stay close friends, this may be difficult. It depends on you and your friend. The new manager must realize that favorites or perceived favorites cannot exist on a cohesive team. Therefore follow the suggestions in Manager's Tip 10-1 on p. 250 to ease the transition.

MANAGER'S TIP 10-1

DEALING WITH A CLOSE FRIEND AFTER YOUR PROMOTION

✔ Do not apologize even if you feel somewhat guilty about receiving the promotion.

✔ Do not give your friend favorable treatment. Your guilt may cause you to want to "protect" your friend, which will cause problems with other staff members.

✔ Try to ignore the situation if your friend teases you verbally about the position (e.g., referring to you as the big honcho). However, you will have to set limits on this behavior if it continues.

✔ You can try to maintain your social relationship, but you must accept that it will change. Obviously, your social relationship must be kept outside the work setting. Sometimes the relationship will deteriorate, and you may have to accept this loss.

✔ Work on achieving mutual respect. Bringing professional behaviors and effective interpersonal skills to these uncomfortable situations can help. The effort expended to maintain the friendship can be draining, and the transition period can be disheartening for new managers.

✔ Give this process time. Your friend may need space initially while getting used to the change. Eventually you and your friend may be able to resume the friendship.

✔ Discuss with other nurse managers how they have addressed and solved this problem. Such support can be beneficial to you in this uncomfortable situation.

Discomfort in an Unfamiliar Environment

As health care settings must now be more financially conservative in order to survive, some changes are being felt in the patient care environment. The new nurse manager can be easily overwhelmed by the red tape, politics, and sabotage that sometimes occur if she/he is not prepared to deal with them. The suggestions in Manager's Tip 10-2 can help you adjust.

Firing or Letting Go a Staff Member

Probably no management process is as difficult to be involved in as firing a staff member. This process can be especially challenging for new managers. When there are serious and ongoing problems with a staff member, discuss the situation with both your immediate supervisor and the HR manager. You should not attempt to handle this process without adequate support, particularly if the staff member's problems precede your tenure. For a more in-depth discussion of firing, please refer to Chapter 3, "Human Resource Management."

Times of High Stress or Anxiety

Maclaren said, "What does anxiety do? It does not empty tomorrow of its sorrow; rather it empties today of its strength" (Jan Maclaren, 1920). As nurses, we all know

---

MANAGER'S TIP 10-2

TIPS ON ADJUSTING TO A NEW ENVIRONMENT

✔ Talk to trusted peer nurse managers on an ongoing basis.
✔ Introduce yourself to everyone you can. Ask people to lunch or to tell you about their role in the organization. People love to talk about themselves and their accomplishments, and these meetings can give you the needed insight into the corporate culture that you would not find on the organizational chart or in the recruitment brochure.
✔ Watch how people communicate with each other (formal, informal, memos) and observe nuances that are unique to your work setting.
✔ Rely on both the grapevine and feedback. Unfortunately, in some environments, there is poor communication from the top levels to the ranks below. If you are in this type of environment, the grapevine may often provide more information than do formal communications.
✔ Try to remain objective. If your current setting operates differently from the last setting you worked in, give your new organization time to demonstrate how it works before judging and trying to implement major changes.

---

the symptoms of anxiety and stress. Probably few, if any, management positions exist in which stress is not a hallmark of daily life. You must remember that some stress is good and that the way you view your relationship to stress can help you master it. You must take steps to control stress or channel it into productive activities.

You can use the uncomfortable feelings stress creates as catalysts for needed change and to learn new or more effective behaviors. Yet, when you are stressed, you may not feel like doing anything that affects or solves the problem. At these times, you may want to meet with peers or other appropriate staff members such as the social worker or the psychiatric liaison nurse. Some facilities provide nurse managers with counseling to assist them through change and crisis and also to help them support their own staff. J.L. Casey, a nurse, said the following about this positive process:

> Through the counseling sessions, the clinician helped me to understand group dynamics and to learn how to support the staff effectively in times of stress or change. Also, she enabled me to gain an awareness of my own personal management style and of how others react to me. Indeed, the clinician's support has alleviated much of the stress of my new job. She has given me the courage to meet new challenges and to continue to grow and develop both professionally and personally.[1]

Please refer to Chapter 9, "Taking Care of Yourself and Your Staff," for an in-depth discussion on stress and stress management.

Unfulfilled Promises by Management

It can be disheartening when your supervisor makes promises that are not kept. This is why many employment counselors suggest obtaining a written job offer with all details specified before accepting a position. Unfulfilled promises can also occur with bonuses, promotions, or other aspects of your employment. Broken promises erode trust and can be damaging to morale and productivity. It is best to avoid making promises, either actual or implied, to your staff unless you are certain that you can fulfill the promises.

REORGANIZATION

As mentioned throughout this book, health care is in a tumultuous state. Downsizing, reorganizing, facility closings, merging, and disengaging are just a few of the many things occurring to organizations across the country. What can a patient care manager do to survive the stress of such times?

First of all, the downsizing of health care facilities is due to an increase in empty beds, as the paradigm of health care completes its massive shift from inpatient to outpatient settings. Patient care units are being merged with other units and staff are being relocated to other more flourishing departments, such as outpatient or ambulatory care services and community health care (home care) programs. As mergers and acquisitions occur, one facility and its staff may take precedence over the facility being bought out or merged with. Besides trying to increase market share and revenue opportunities, such mergers usually are aimed at increasing cost-effectiveness through the combination of support functions and other commonalities. Job loss is a threat to management staff as well as clinicians.

Because of forced resignations or layoffs, there may be major management shifts in a facility that has not been achieving projected revenue or expense projections. It is not uncommon for middle management to witness the complete change in senior management staff over a short period of time when a new CEO/administrator is brought in since she/he may recruit her/his own management team. Especially hard for new nurse managers is the possible loss of the person who recruited them for their management position and/or who has been their personal mentor. She/he may be perceived as a member of the "old order" and will be watched for signs of counterproductive behavior or attitude. Focus your attention on assisting your new supervisors, peers, and subordinate staff in the transition.

Since the philosophy of the organization and the corporate culture may change with the new management team, the nurse manager must step back, observe, and evaluate the new changes before taking any drastic steps. Give the new management team your support during this time, since it will probably be fraught with disorganization, conflict, and high tension. Encourage, motivate, and support staff during this time, protecting them from the bureaucratic and nonproductive tensions that might arise. However, keep them informed of the pertinent factual items that are necessary to accomplish the goals of the department. In their best-selling handbook, *Business as unUsual,* Price Pritchett and Ron Pound, of Dallas-based Pritchett & Associ-

MANAGER'S TIP 10-3

MANAGING AND SURVIVING ORGANIZATIONAL CHANGES

✔ Be a change agent.
✔ Keep a positive attitude.
✔ Give your troops clear-cut marching orders.
✔ Nail down each person's job.
✔ Promise change . . . and sell it (carefully).
✔ Don't give away your power.
✔ Focus on short-range objectives.
✔ Establish clear priorities.
✔ Raise the (performance) bar.
✔ Motivate to the hilt.
✔ Get resistance to change out in the open.
✔ Don't try to cover all the bases yourself.
✔ Create a supportive work environment.
✔ Provide additional job know-how.
✔ "Beef up" communication efforts.
✔ Protect quality and customer service.
✔ Take care of the "me" issues in a hurry.
✔ Reduce the level of job stress.
✔ Encourage risk-taking and initiative.
✔ Rebuild morale.
✔ "Ride close herd" on transition and change.
✔ Pass out more "psychologic paychecks."
✔ Go looking for bad news.
✔ Re-recruit your good people.
✔ Play the role of managerial therapist.
✔ Be supportive of higher management.
✔ Be more than a manager or supervisor . . . be a LEADER.[2]

From Pritchett P, Pound R: Business as unUsual, Dallas, 1988, Pritchett Publishing.

ates, Inc., delineate 27 tactics for managing and surviving organizational change (see Manager's Tip 10-3).

Corporate management tactics in an unstable economic environment may cause great stress and turmoil, testing the personal mettle of managers and staff alike. No matter what is occurring in your institution, do not allow yourself to get caught up in the negative side of power politics, such as backstabbing, backbiting, whining, and sabotage. Instead, be professional and humanistic at all times, focusing on your true objectives—enhancing the quality of service to the patients/clients entrusted to your care and developing your staff.

YOUR POSITION IS ELIMINATED

In the unlikely event your position is eliminated as a result of unit mergers or downsizing, hopefully you will have nurtured a positive relationship with senior management or with a network of health care professionals. Senior managers are continually searching for good managers to run patient care departments. By carefully using the skills outlined in this text, your chances of quickly being recruited for the new merged position, or a new, more exciting position borne out of the paradigm shift, is likely. Positive attitudes, "can-do" spirits, and the ability to successfully manage people are traits always in demand. Manager's Tip 10-4 provides suggestions for helping yourself and your staff through the change.

Unreasonable or Bad Managers

"In a recent study of 73 managers conducted by the University of Southern California, nearly 75% of the participants reported having had difficulty with a superior. Moreover, bad-boss behavior appears to be on the rise."[3] It is hoped that you never work for someone who expects more every day when you have no hope of getting the staff or other resources needed to do the tasks. The continual feeling that you can

MANAGER'S TIP 10-4

TAKING CARE OF YOURSELF

Once it has been determined that your managerial options at this health care setting are nonexistent, plan for your departure, both personally and for the staff you may leave behind:

✔ Ascertain what severance options you might have with your employer:
  • Management severance pay options vary between employers; however, a good rule of thumb is to provide one week of pay for each year of employment, with a minimum base of 4 weeks for middle management.
  • Health insurance coverage for the length of severance period if not longer (COBRA benefits are available per legislation).
  • Outplacement Services:
    ▪ Assistance with resume preparation (you should always keep up to date).
    ▪ Assistance with learning interview and job search techniques.
    ▪ Assistance with career counseling (if new career direction desired).
    ▪ Put in contact with professional recruiters.
  • Assistance with job search—networking within organization or health care community.
✔ Do not speak negatively about the organization or management staff (the health care world is ever shrinking and you might "burn your bridges").
✔ Prepare staff and unit for changes (as much as possible with time allotted).
✔ Write letters of recommendation for staff and request letters of recommendation for yourself from senior management.

never do enough can lead to burnout. The successful nurse manager must set limits and know what can be accomplished effectively and realistically in what time frames and with what resources. Network with your peers to validate your perceptions. You may find that you are not alone and that they may have developed coping skills to assist them in remaining fairly content in their positions. Their advice and insight may help you to cope with your situation.

Little or No Management Training

Perhaps your "management training" consisted of the regular staff nurse orientation accompanied by a videotape on assertive behavior and a 2-hour session on HR management! Then you were left to sink or swim. This is a problem. To successfully make the transition to management and function as an effective manager, the new nurse manager should receive structured training related to management issues, concepts, skills, and techniques. If you do not feel that you received the orientation you need, talk to your supervisor about your specific needs. Do not be embarrassed—you are entitled to an orientation commensurate with your responsibilities. To supplement formal educational offerings, you can also offer to lead a peer nurse manager workshop and have the new group define the topics on which orientation is needed. Responsibility for running these meetings can be rotated among the members. It might be helpful to invite and involve your facility's staff development coordinator. Reading the numerous books and journals available can also help you develop your management expertise. Educational offerings such as workshops, courses, and conferences can further enhance your understanding and mastery of management. The resources listed at the end of this chapter and others (see "For Further Reading") may be helpful in facilitating development of your management expertise.

Following in the Footsteps of Multiple and Short-Term Managers

When you inherit staff members who have been through a lot of change, problems abound. Initially, it may be best to observe before making changes of your own. In addition, the staff may feel you will be another short-term manager and may be skeptical. Considering the numerous changes, the setting may need some structure. One way to provide structure is to improve the organization of the unit. Look at your office and talk to peer nurse managers to determine which files are truly needed. Use aids such as accordion binders or a scheduling board to help you feel more organized. The simple acts of organizing the mess may help you and your staff feel less overwhelmed. Get vertical files, bookcases, and whatever else is needed to gain some control over your new environment. Remember and practice organizational skills. Integrating these skills into your daily work life will result in the following:

1. A sense of accomplishment.
2. A feeling of control over your space.
3. More time to do the task at hand; namely managing the unit.
4. Demonstrating organization for your staff.

It may take your staff time to believe that you will be the manager for an extended period. Sometimes such frequent changes create strong and effective staff members because they have functioned as the leaders for their unit throughout the gaps and turnover of managers. This staff may also have had to adjust to very different management styles and expectations over time and may know what works best for the unit. Because of these factors, the staff members can be knowledgeable resources about their unit. They may have good ideas about the stability and direction needed on the unit and contribute positively to these goals. Encourage staff members to share their ideas. For a more in-depth discussion on organizational skills, see Chapter 6, "Effective Time Management."

Your Supervisor's Negative Evaluation of You

Performance evaluations can be difficult for both the evaluator and the employee being evaluated. If your supervisor gives you a poor or average evaluation, you must, with her/his help, determine the cause or causes. Try to be objective and put yourself in the evaluator's position. Does your supervisor feel uninformed? Are you generally late with work projects? Are you loyal? Do you follow through when your supervisor delegates work to you? Does your supervisor feel respected by you?

Sometimes it is hard to remember that your supervisor is your supervisor and, as such, must be considered correct. If you are surprised by your supervisor's negative evaluation, you can ask for additional feedback on an ongoing basis to gauge your progress. Ask what specific behaviors are problems and how you can demonstrate improvement to your supervisor. If you are in a new position, it is important to remember that you probably will not perform exceptionally from the start. Stress your interest in learning and improving and ask for your supervisor's help.

A disappointing performance evaluation can be particularly frustrating in those instances where the supervisor promoted you into the position or recruited you for the job. You may feel misled or even betrayed. If you feel that you did not receive an adequate management orientation, you may wish to request additional training. Look objectively at your job description and objectively demonstrate, in writing if need be, the ways you feel you meet the position standards. Whatever you do, especially in the current economic climate, do not tell your supervisor that she/he is wrong. Other mistakes to avoid are blaming others and constantly complaining (especially about issues over which your supervisor has no control).

Also, consider how your supervisor deals with other nurse managers she/he supervises. If she/he frequently praises a peer nurse manager, observe what your peer does differently from or better than you. Perhaps you have not gained recognition for your accomplishments. We all would like to believe that good work gets recognized and reinforced, but, in reality, sometimes the squeaky wheel gets the attention. In this case, the squeaky wheel also gets the positive strokes and evaluations. Some people have a knack for pointing out to their supervisors just what they are doing that is wonderful, helps the organization look good, and most importantly, makes the supervisor look great. No one likes to be self-congratulatory, but sometimes you may need to bring your achievements to your supervisor's attention.

When You Do Not Get the Recognition You Deserve

The questions in Box 10-1 may help you identify whether you are getting the recognition you deserve. Your supervisor may not know what you are doing, and it may appear that the work you are accomplishing is minimal. This situation particularly can be seen in some settings where there are bonuses. Workers who toot their own horns and come out ahead are not necessarily better workers; they may simply be better at public relations and at communicating to their managers what the managers want and need to hear.

WHEN YOU IDENTIFY THE NEED FOR A CHANGE IN YOUR JOB

Occasionally, your work situation may be so uncomfortable that you want to leave your position. When you are unhappy at work, you must try to determine specifically why you feel that way. Such information will help you identify the actions you need to take to improve the situation. All jobs have inherent pros and cons. The important issue is that the position meets your unique needs. The decision to leave is usually reached when all actions taken fail. Many skills are available to try to affect a negative work situation.

Problem-solving, conflict resolution, and other avenues towards finding solutions should be attempted when possible. However, note that sometimes, even when your

---

box 10-1

DOING YOUR PART TO RECEIVE RECOGNITION

The following questions can help you determine if you are doing your part to receive the recognition you deserve.

- Do people at different levels of the organization know who you are?
- Do you volunteer for assignments or opportunities to increase your visibility?
- Do you routinely tell your supervisor about your accomplishments?
- Sometimes we may be hassled or nervous when we meet with our supervisors, and we may neglect to refer to our accomplishments. Try to make it a point to always have three accomplishments to tell your supervisor about at the onset of your meetings. The supervisor wants to see objective results too, so in turn your boss's boss may hear those same items. This positive action reflects on your boss and can only help you.
- Do you share your unit's accomplishments with your staff and encourage them to share their individual accomplishments with you?
- Have your staff enumerate three accomplishments every week that you can then present to your supervisor. It will help your staff feel a part of the team. In addition, the knowledge that you share this information with your boss will increase their feeling that you are all working together.

job is fulfilling, it simply may be time for a change. At some point, people consider changing careers entirely. Knowing when to leave can sometimes result from intuition and honest discussions with trusted friends or colleagues.

Many businesses will welcome an RN on their staff's roster. Nurses have many job opportunities that tie together health interests and other activities. Some of these include health care–related sales such as computers, medical equipment, or supplies; programs for the aging; nursing staffing companies; medicolegal consulting; research; health or hospital administration; liaison between facilities; teaching; insurance utilization review; case management services; private practice; lobbying; and occupational health and wellness programs. For an in-depth discussion about other opportunities and marketing yourself and your skills, refer to Chapter 12, which specifies steps that may help you find the right position or identify the next professional stage in your career.

THE BOTTOM LINE

"It was much pleasanter at home, thought poor Alice, when one wasn't always growing larger and smaller, and being ordered around by mice and rabbits. I almost wish I hadn't gone down that rabbit hole...!"

The thoughts and experiences of Lewis Carroll's Alice are an eloquent parallel to those of nurses in middle management roles. Many wish to go 'home' to bedside nursing, where one is not accountable to, and responsible for, everyone above and below (all those mice and rabbits!), besides being responsible for quality patient care. The step into management, be it prompted by curiosity, ambition, or a desire to contribute, can mimic Alice's dreamlike fall down the rabbit hole, complete with changes in size and form, and encounters with all kinds of mysterious characters.[4]

Determine if your current position has the critical elements needed to make you happy and effectively use your special skills and abilities. It is important that you spend some time considering those aspects of the position that are satisfying as well as those that are not. Weighing these criteria will assist you in deciding whether to move on. This is also the time to reflect on your perception of problems. Those who frame problems as challenges and find solutions seem to enjoy their work more. In addition, although every setting has different problems, some types of problems are inherent in management and may follow you regardless of the setting in which you work.

SUMMARY

Problems appear in many facets of our worklives. It is important to realize and sometimes remind ourselves that we are not alone. The good point about addressing problems is that once we problem-solve or identify the action needed for resolution, we have one less problem to address. In addition, some problems, after initially being addressed, serve as precedents for our way of effectively handling similar problems. With these facts in mind, problem-solving becomes easier. For example, human relation problems are varied and can be addressed in many ways. However, your facility policy manuals and your supervisor are resources for guidance or responses needed during the period of transition to experienced nurse manager. Your peer nurse managers can be a source of support and of information about "how do you handle" issues. A peer manager meeting on problem-solving and conflict resolution may be a particularly effective method of increasing your comfort level, obtaining support, and increasing your job knowledge.

We learn from our experiences, and the problems become easier to solve with time and experience. Addressing the problems is what is important. We cannot have all the right answers all the time. There are resources in your chain of command to help you during this time, and it is important that you use them when needed. You must realize that being a manager is a continual growth process. This process can be facilitated through the reading of professional books or journals and participating in workshops or attending courses.

In your capacity as manager, you are the role model for your staff. This cyclical process of training members of your staff through delegation, empowerment, and their assumption of accountability develops their skills to professionally grow and perhaps become managers themselves.

References

1. Casey JL; Counseling nurse managers, *Nurs Manage* 20(9):53, 1989.
2. Pritchett P, Pound R: *Business as unUsual,* Dallas, 1988, Pritchett Publishing.
3. Lopez JA: The boss from hell, *Working Woman* page 69, December, 1991.
4. Boll ML: Middle management in nursing, *Nurs Manage* 21(2):54, 1990.

For Further Reading

Betancourt EK: Job sharing in nursing management: it can work, *Nurs Manage* 21(1): 47, 1990.

Bramson RM: *Coping with difficult people,* New York, 1981, Ballantine Books.

Clinical managers help agency staff cope with growth, stress. *Hospital Home Health* 9(8): 108, 1992.

Collyer ME: Resolving conflicts: leadership style sets the strategy, *Nurs Manage* 20(9): 77, 1989.

King P: *Never work for a jerk,* New York, 1987, Dell.

O'Neil KK: The head nurse's managerial role, *Nurs Manage* 20(6):39, 1989.

Perlman D, Takacs G: The 10 stages of change, *Nurs Manage* 21(4);33, 1990.

CHAPTER 11

THE NURSE MANAGER IN HOME CARE AND HOSPICE

T.M. MARRELLI

HOW HOME CARE IS UNIQUE

Home care itself is different for many reasons. The reasons center primarily around the fact that health care providers are guests in their client's homes. Unlike the inpatient setting, visiting hours are not set, and patients have control over their environment as well as numerous other choices within their homes, including their clothing, food, visitors, and lifestyle. The care provider must be the one to adjust whenever accommodation is necessary. This customer-oriented or service-driven philosophy is what makes the home setting so different from other clinical environments. To support this structure, we need to see how the nurses who make visits or provide care at home bring special skills to the home care position. This is not to say that nurses in inpatient areas do not have some or even all of these traits. Rather, this chapter concerns the attributes that must be developed by effective home care managers for professional nurses to remain in home care and addresses the specifics of home care management that are not integrated into the other chapters.

HOME CARE AND HOSPICE CONSIDERATIONS

The multifaceted administrative and clinical operations that must be maintained to provide patient care are the core of the home care manager's responsibilities. Be aware that all the chapters, for example, Chapter 7, "Resource Management and Budgeting Basics," and Chapter 9, "Taking Care of Yourself and Your Staff," are relevant to home care managers. Stress management skills are needed by all managers, and the budgeting discussions are particularly relevant in home care. In fact, one example of productivity in the budgeting chapter is a home health agency (HHA) example.

The management skills needed in home health and hospice are many and varied. They range from effective recruiting and hiring of skilled and interpersonally effective clinicians to the ongoing duties needed to achieve timely and correct billing submissions. Although the term *home care* is used throughout this discussion, this discussion is germane to all care provided in the patient's place of residence. There-fore this information is also relevant for hospice care or other special programs that emphasize providing care at home. Because many hospices are affiliated or otherwise associated with a home care agency, the term *home care* is used generically for ease of discussion. *Home care* is also used in this chapter for all home care programs, in-cluding HHAs. Regardless of the type of care program provided at home, the man-ager's duties and responsibilities are directed towards the maintenance of effective daily operations to provide high-quality patient care.

This chapter is organized with an overview of the hallmarks that make up the pro-fessional practice of home care, the regulatory aspects and requirements, and pa-tient care considerations. The overview includes important issues such as how pa-tient/nurse assignments are made, the practice models used, automated systems, the documentation requirements, and the unique billing/administrative functions that the manager must direct on a daily basis. A home care and hospice resource guide is located at the end of this book for your information and for continued professional growth.

How Home Care Management is Unique

You were probably promoted from being a staff home care nurse to being a manager because of your clinical competence, expertise, and other valued skills. However, in addition, the new home care manager must be willing to achieve or possess the fol-lowing skills and knowledge:

- An in-depth knowledge of the current regulatory environment, including the Medicare Conditions of Participation (COPs) and state surveyor interpretations for compliance, the state Certificate of Need (CON), and licensure laws, where applicable. Also, the manager must know the status (and source) of accredi-tation and the complex multifaceted "rules" that are synonymous with home care, including the HHA Health Insurance Manual (HIM-11), the specific pro-visions for coverage, and the documentation requirements in the HIM-11.
- Knowledge of the billing procedures and rules that dictate the administrative structures and processes necessary to support timely and effective billing. The administrative skills needed to orchestrate the many steps that must occur require flexibility. A structure that moves the process forward regardless of staffing problems or other operational problems is demanded. This is part of the manager's responsibility for being accountable for the fiscal health of the HHA. Please refer to Chapter 6, "Effective Management," for an in-depth dis-cussion about effective time management.
- A repertoire of service-driven and patient-oriented interpersonal skills. Unlike many inpatient facilities, where the structure defines the services, in home care, because the patient is at home, the patient's needs are the criteria that drive the program. These skills are also highly valued in the manager's role in

public relations or community liaison activities, which are a daily part of effective home care operations.

- The experience base and knowledge to successfully and credibly deal with complex situations that may be addressed exclusively over the phone and through documentation. In the inpatient setting, nurses are down the hall or closer for consultation or supervision. In home care, delegation, communication, or follow-up interventions are with staff members who may be four counties away or even across the state line. This is why there is such an emphasis on continuous quality improvement in home care, including the ongoing and systematic process of comparing patient episodes of care by like diagnoses or other similar factors affecting patient outcomes.

- Possession of an incredible attention to detail. This is especially true in the daily operations of (1) billing and (2) documentation. Because these two factors go hand in hand, they are equally important. An HHA manager who does not send bills or bills incorrectly is jeopardizing the credibility and viability of the organization. In addition, the HHA that does not have necessary documentation to support the bills not only faces problems from a risk-management standpoint, but also from the payer's viewpoint. The payer may view this situation as overutilization, a gray zone that may indicate abuse or even fraud. The documentation in billing and the clinical records must be correct for any audit trail.

Home Care Reimbursement Changes

As with all of health care, home health services have risen dramatically in the past 10 years. According to the Health Care Financing Administration (HCFA), the payer of Medicare benefits, the number of licensed home health agencies increased by 50% between 1990 and 1995, with freestanding, proprietary (for-profit) agencies accounting for 65% of that growth, with a resultant 50% of all agencies being for-profit. In addition, home health visits per beneficiary have increased from 28 visits per person to over 65 visits per person during the same time period; episodes of illness (length of certification and recertification periods) have increased 14% between 1990 and 1993. Patients are being seen for longer periods of time, with a greater number of home health aide visits being made. Finally, the HCFA reports that Medicare spending for home health services has grown 20% per year since the late 1980s, with a crest of 53% being reached in 1990.[1]

Beneficiaries who qualify for Medicare coverage are eligible for home health services if they have a need for either skilled nursing or physical, occupational or speech therapy; require intermittent or part-time services; are under the care of a physician; and are homebound. There is no need for prior hospitalization and there is no co-payment. Medicare pays Medicare-certified agencies the lower of aggregate costs or charges, up to an established cost limit. There is no incentive to control costs under this type of reimbursement.

With the budget deficit continuing to loom over the American economy and fierce debates occurring in a Republican-controlled Congress with a Democratic President, the Medicare program has come under pressure to reduce its allocations. Home care specifically has been targeted because of its tremendous growth over the past decade and the forecast of a 12% increase over at least the next 4 years if nothing is done to reform the reimbursement system. Congress has proposed a system that would set prospective rates for each type of home health visit but that would limit total payments per episode as of fiscal year 1997; payment would be based on national average costs in cost-reporting periods ending on or before June 30, 1994. Case mix categories would be developed with regional limits calculated for each, based on the average cost of up to 120 days of care. Episode limits would be applied to the first 165 days of care in an episode. The Democratic response would establish episode-based payments effective in 2000 with stop-gap measures to limit spending instituted each fiscal year under the turn of the century. Cost limits would be reduced from 112% of the mean to 105% of the mean by 1999. The per beneficiary amount would be calculated by blending 1994 agency-specific costs with the national average.[2]

The home health industry with national representation developed a counterproposal to both the Congressional and Administration plans that would gradually phase in a per-episode payment plan; this would act as an incentive for home care organizations to contain costs by receiving a percentage of the difference between the total per-visit payment and the agency's aggregate limit. During this time, the HCFA would be mandated to begin collecting home care statistical data, which is more reliable and therefore more valid, for establishing payment criteria to be used in determining future per-episode costs.

This shift in reimbursement will be a major challenge to home care managers who have become complacent. There will be a need to quantify outcomes of care and associated care interventions to resource usage (cost) in order to determine the best course for each patient, both clinically and financially, as per-episode payment is implemented. Administrative systems will need to be in place to track, control, and manage the care of patients and the resource usage associated with that episode of care.

HOW HOME CARE NURSES ARE UNIQUE

Box 11-1 lists some of the unique characteristics of nurses and the home care setting. Obviously, the management skills needed for success in home care are many and varied. They range from the effective hiring of skilled and interpersonally strong clinicians to the ongoing orchestration of duties to achieve timely billing submissions.

The nurses who choose home care must be able to function somewhat autonomously. Consider the inpatient critical care nurse who goes into home care thinking it will be "less stressful" and finds the culture so different that she/he cannot successfully make the transition to independent and successful home care nursing. With

---

box 11-1

UNIQUE CHARACTERISTICS OF NURSES AND THE HOME CARE SETTING

1. The staff must be flexible. It is home care staff members who must bend or renegotiate, not the patient, as members are guests in the patient's home. This usually includes visit times but can include aspects of the plan of care as well.
2. The staff member must not mind driving, even in inclement weather; have a good sense of direction; and be willing to take risks (e.g., get lost).
3. The staff members assume responsibility for the patient and the patient's plan of care. True primary nursing or case management occurs in home care. From the initial assessment visit to identifying and using appropriate nursing diagnoses, the nurse in home care assumes the planning and follow-through of care. Possibly only one or maybe a limited number of team members are involved in the care, depending on the patient's needs. These team members directly affect the care and see the results of care provided. Because of this, the outcomes may be more directly attributable to care rendered. This total patient management function, with its associated prioritizing and complex decision-making, renders this field unique. Note that in practice, the simple, positive patient and family outcomes and feedback are where many home care nurses receive a great deal of personal and job satisfaction. Because of this factor, this feedback also needs to be highly valued by all members of the management team.
4. Staff members must be generalists and specialists. This means that, although clinically the RNs may be able to competently and proficiently handle a wide range of patients and clinical problems, they usually have an area of expertise that can be called on for specialized clinical problems, for orientation of new staff, or as a resource for information.
5. The staff must be autonomous and able to function in a nonstructured atmosphere.
6. The staff must have effective time management skills regarding both visits scheduled and documentation/administrative duties required. The amount of detail management that must be mastered is key to long-term success for many nurses in home care. For example, the tracking of recertifications, 486 generation and visit schedules demand nurses who are detail-oriented and even value that detail. In addition, plans made between the nurse and patient must be followed up in actuality and on paper.
7. The staff must be open and accepting of people's unique and chosen lifestyles and the associated effects on their health. Judgments about lifestyle, the presence or absence of family support, and the choices patients make with which nurses do not agree must be diplomatically and carefully voiced when appropriate.
8. The staff must like to interact with patients and their families and caregivers. This teaching or consulting role also brings job satisfaction to nurses in home health.
9. The staff must be aware that a constant balance exists between the clinical and administrative demands and that they are equally important, but in different ways and for different reasons.
10. The staff must be aware that successful mastery of time management and delegation skills is essential to effective daily operations.

this in mind, plan orientation periods with the goal of the participant's having long-term success in the role. We know change is difficult, and the home care nurse culture and setting are different from the structure and on-site camaraderie, supervision, and peer consultation available from the structure of a facility. Similarly, your orientation as a new manager must be effective for you to efficiently carry out your new management responsibilities.

THE NEW MANAGER'S ORIENTATION TO HOME CARE

There are too many stories of home care managers who get no orientation and not surprisingly get burnt out or disillusioned and leave their position, home care, or even nursing. Do not let this "revolving door" phenomenon happen to you. All managers are entitled to an appropriate orientation period. No matter how understaffed the administrator says the agency is, protect yourself from being put in that position from the start. Try to define or address your orientation, including time span and content, before accepting the position. The following discussion addresses what details your orientation should include.

WHAT YOUR ORIENTATION SHOULD ENTAIL

The items in Box 11-2 are the *minimal* topics that can be considered to provide an effective orientation to home care. Obviously, if you have been in home care for some time, some of these may not be appropriate or needed, but all managers should have these "hallmarks" of home care as a base of information. In addition, these items will give you information about the HHA's internal operations.

Orienting a new manager should take at least as long as it does for a new clinical nurse in home care. Much of the above information is also appropriate for the new nurse in home care. Remember, the more managers communicate the program's goals or visions, the more staff members feel a part of the team and are thereby more effective.

It goes without saying that your staff members cannot be held accountable for what they do not or could not know if they did not get an effective orientation. With this in mind, and from your perspective as the risk manager and person responsible for implementing CQI, adequately train your home care clinical staff. Like you, their manager, they need to know the cornerstones of information about home care. These should **always** include such basic topics as home visits and what they entail, including buddying with an experienced, positive role model nurse; visit utilization; orientation to the forms used; infection control; and coverage and associated documentation requirements of home care services and CQI processes. The manager cannot be effective if she/he does not know the program, the key players, and the expected performance goals. Similarly, it is difficult and usually unfair to hold staff members accountable for information of which they were unaware. Be a prudent manager: orient your team effectively.

·· box 11-2 ··

HALLMARKS OF ORIENTATION

1. The HHA orientation manual.
2. The conditions of participation and state licensing regulations, as appropriate.
3. The HHA's continuous quality improvement program. The HHA should share its last quarterly or last few quarterly reports. This will help you to follow-up on areas that needed improvement before your tenure began. If no report exists or "one was not done last quarter, this could indicate why the agency needs your skills. Obviously, this can be a good or a bad sign!
4. The Home Health Manual-11,[3] especially Transmittal 222 and 227, the HHA Coverage Requirements section.
5. The clinical policy and procedure manuals.
6. The human resource policy manual, including position descriptions.
7. Organizational chart and current staffing needs. This includes who you report to and who has true (not just on paper) responsibilities for specific areas.
8. The staff education and in-service training log.
9. An overview of the medical records and documentation system.
10. An overview of the clinical/billing/administrative automated system information, where applicable.
11. A schematic diagram of the paper flow process from patient intake/admission to billing and discharge.
12. The HHA's fiscal statements and accounts pending, and the most recent cost reports, where appropriate.
13. The caseload of the previous months/year.
14. The HHA's annual report.
15. Their interest in, or their actual accreditation status.
16. The HHA's strategic plan.
17. Community linkage and involvement.
18. The HHA's denial rate.
19. The HHA's participation in state and national industry organizations.
20. Other information as needed.

IF YOU HAVE TO NEGOTIATE FOR AN ORIENTATION

If you are in the unfortunate position of bargaining for an adequate orientation, there is a problem. Most professional nurses want to be affiliated with high-quality programs. However, believing that all home care programs are functioning at the same (high-quality) level would be naive. There may be instances when your supervisor uses the word "quality," but that same supervisor's actions concern you. Trust your nursing knowledge and experience. Look to the professional standards of care for guidance and more information.

If you are always needing information to do your job, if you cannot do your job effectively because of no orientation or support, or if you are a manager in "title" but are continually in the field seeing patients because of incredible turnover, you are experiencing problems that may not be resolved by your management. Note that you cannot be expected to be continually in the community making visits and also be in the office supervising agency operations. This could be a prescription for failure in a busy HHA setting. Clinical and administrative demands are so different that to attempt both is ineffective.

Another uncomfortable position that a manager can be involved in entails the admission of patients clearly needing home care services and not having the personnel resources available to provide them. For example, the admitting nurse appropriately identifies a patient's need for skilled intermittent services and, because of extensive personal care needs, frequent home health aide visits. Your agency does not have the aides (or the speech/language pathologists or the physical or occupational therapists) to adequately meet the patient's care needs. Admit only those patients whose care needs can safely and adequately be met. It is most unfortunate, and certainly not fair to the patients or their families, if patients do not receive the services they need because of the HHA's administrative problems. The necessity of demonstrating quality outcomes in patient care delivery must not be underestimated. As competition continues, as more programs receive accreditation, and as HHA licensure increases throughout the country, HHA operations will appear to be more uniform. However, as both inpatient and HHA days of care continue to be shortened, only those HHAs that are truly responsive to patients and payers and that provide high quality cost-effective care will survive.

MEASURING OPERATIONAL QUALITY

Discussion is underway about accreditation in home care, and both the NLN and the JCAHO accredit home care programs of all auspices. The design and implementation of a continuous quality-improvement program in your organization must meet your agency's unique clinical focuses. Many organizations incorporate CQI operational aspects into their daily operations. Often it encompasses tracking patients and patient information regarding episodes of hospital readmissions within 31 days, complaint trends, ongoing clinical record reviews, infection surveillance and rates, and focused studies. It may also include patient, physician, and referral source satisfaction surveys. The manager in home care must be very involved in the organization's CQI program. In addition, home care staff need to have a voice in operations.

The educational preparation and clinical knowledge and experience of home care staff can be another measure of quality. A new certification in home care is being offered by the American Nurses' Credentialing Center for home care nurses. This new specialty certification is a way to help ensure that nurses in home care know and practice within standard quality parameters.

The nursing care delivery system model used in the HHA can also affect the quality of the care provided by affecting patient outcomes.

MODELS OF NURSING CARE DELIVERY SYSTEMS IN HOME CARE

Various models in home care describe how care is delivered to HHA patients. Primary nursing through assignment of client/patient care managers (or case managers in some settings) is a model frequently seen in home care. We all recognize that continuity through primary nursing care models promotes professional accountability and increased effectiveness in communications and outcomes. The manager's knowledge of each staff member's preparation, experience, and capabilities promotes the fullest use of skills and provides a basis for continued growth.

Regardless of the model used, assigning a nurse who has the overall responsibility for assessing, planning, implementing, and evaluating the ordered plan of care is a key to positive patient outcomes. The purpose of assigning one nurse to this responsibility is to help ensure the quality of the care by providing a mechanism for consistent rapport and communications between patient and caregivers. Clearly, this is not to say that additional nursing staff such as "associate or revisit nurses" are not also involved in the care of the patient. In fact, involving another nurse can be helpful. For example, a nurse specialist, such as an enterostomal therapist, could consult on appropriate cases, thus assuring quality while providing patient care in a consultative role. Assigning home care nurses to patients, in keeping with your organizational philosophy, also supports patient care assignments that are directed towards meeting the specific physical, psychologic, cultural, social, and other defined needs of each patient.

This assignment is most effectively accomplished by the nurse case manager evaluating the projected assessed needs of patients as soon as possible after the referral process has occurred. The effective case manager accomplishes this by gathering all the available and pertinent information about the patient and her/his care needs. The manager then assesses the availability of RN resources. This includes the number of staff members and their clinical expertise, educational preparation, experience, and demonstrated capabilities. Matching of patients and nurses is sometimes referred to as "skill matching" or "care matching." In addition, the manager should also consider the individual preferences of staff members while evaluating the complexity or extent of patient needs. Consideration for the preferences of patient care staff members needs to be kept in mind and valued, since this positively influences the morale of the group.

Information concerning preferences needs to be acquired in a systematic way, such as regular individual staff meetings with the manager, to ensure all staff members are given equal consideration. The assignment process is also made with the primary nurse's current patient caseload in mind. Geographic location and equitable work distribution are two additional factors to consider. In addition, matching assignments to the abilities and growth potential of the professional staff member enhances the quality of care, is cost-effective, increases productivity, and promotes staff member satisfaction. Effective managers work with their staff to assist them, when possible, in understanding the rationale of assignments.

Depending on your chosen nursing or patient care model, the delegation of responsibility for planning, supervising, and evaluating the total nursing care of the patient occurs when the patient is assigned to the primary nurse or case manager.

Communication with staff on an ongoing basis is the key to a successful operation where all efforts are directed towards common goals. Although the bulk of daily communications with clinical staff will be over the phone, it is important that you interact with staff on a regular basis. Box 11-3 addresses the important role of staff meetings in home care and hospice.

STAFF MEETING EVALUATIONS

Regularly evaluate the staff meetings. On a written evaluation form, ask open-ended questions to elicit if staff needs are being met by the current forum. Some HHAs have only the nurses and home health aides at the meetings, others involve the MSWs as well. These choices and decisions are all based on your program's unique history and needs. Some HHAs do an annual (or more frequently if needed) evaluation of the staff meeting structure, agenda contents, physical space, and so on, to ensure, as part of the CQI process, that meetings are meaningful to all involved.

INTRADISCIPLINARY TEAM CONFERENCES

Some HHAs schedule their intradisciplinary team conferences immediately following the staff meetings. For example, if the staff meeting is held every other Wednesday at 11:30 A.M. and the meeting is conducted during lunch, the clinical case conferences begin promptly at 12:30 P.M., when the other service representatives appear for these meetings. Again, the staff meeting must end promptly, particularly if you are paying to have the professional associates, such as the physical therapist, speech/language pathologist, and the occupational therapist, who are waiting for the nurse and the home health aide who are in the meeting room next door. The rationale for scheduling such conferences in this way is (1) there may be new referrals for these colleagues, and the nurses can expect that they will be able to discuss these new patients with the appropriate colleague after the staff meeting, and (2) the staff members are already out of the field, and to bring them in another day means the nurse is not making needed visits in the community. Always try to get "the most mileage" out of an idea or process. In the above example, the nurses are already at the office. To bring them in another day and disrupt their schedule may not be cost-effective because it pulls the nurse out of the community again.

HOSPICE STAFF SUPPORT

Similarly, some hospices have the ongoing staff support sessions scheduled immediately following their hospice staff meeting. The meeting with the facilitator is

box 11-3

THE IMPORTANCE OF STAFF MEETINGS IN HOME CARE AND HOSPICE

The importance of regularly scheduled staff meetings in the home care or hospice office cannot be understated. Because the very nature and definition of the care provision is external, the staff members need to be, and feel, a part of the group. Staff meetings assist in meeting both the staff and manager's goals. Although you may define the agenda, ask your staff members for issues or concerns they want addressed and incorporate the items whenever possible. Make the staff meetings and their agenda items and ensuing discussions meaningful and valuable. Sometimes there is not enough time to address all the staff items. As the manager, you may need to prioritize requests, but you should communicate your shared concern about the item and ensure staff members it will be on the next agenda.

Staff meetings are an appropriate forum for staff members to share clinical information or "better ways of doing things," or to evaluate any process that affects their patient care or work life. For example, a typical staff meeting may consist of administrative agenda items: addressing the fact that the medical social worker (MSW) is on vacation on such dates and naming the MSW who will be covering the clients and available for new referrals, the new home health aide assignment form (the nurses and aides should see drafts first), and any problems that need resolution or clarification. Standing agenda items should also include safety, continuous quality improvement activities, and educational opportunities.

These meetings can also foster camaraderie and trust among members. Any manager in home care or hospice knows that the nurses must feel that other staff members are clinical peer professionals, or problems can arise with long-term coverage or assignments. In addition, some nurses, if they are sick or on vacation, have other nurses they usually want to cover their patients. As long as the patients are cared for appropriately and cliques do not develop, nothing is inherently wrong with this practice.

These meetings can also influence positive morale as the nurses in the community realize they are not alone and that the other home care nurses share the same concerns. Some HHAs hold their meetings at lunchtime and have food there for their staff or the staff brings their own lunch. Others hold meetings in the morning. The common complaint about early morning meetings in home care is that patients with IVs or receiving insulin must be seen in the morning. Schedule meetings at whatever time seems best for the consensus of the staff. It is difficult, if not impossible, to listen and **hear** what is being said in a staff meeting if the nurse is worried about her/his next three patients. Always include evening and weekend staff. This allows them a forum for issues even if they are unable to attend.

The manager must value the meetings and thus make them mandatory. Again, it is difficult to hold staff members accountable for what they were not told in the interviewing, hiring, and orientation processes. If a requirement for your program is that staff meetings are mandatory, this needs to be communicated clearly to all. However, the manager must be realistic about such a decision. Obviously, with an extensive traffic back-up or a patient problem in the community needed resolution, the actions of the home care nurse are clear. However, the nurse should call the manager as soon as possible and explain her/his absence. Minutes from these meetings should be typed and distributed to staff. This process reinforces items presented and resolves the "I wasn't at the staff meeting" comments and resulting problems.

Again, allow the home care staff input into the time and, if appropriate, place of the meetings. Try to make these meetings informative and valued. The meetings should start promptly and end at the designated time. If you note many absences, this may be a sign that the staff does not value the time and content of the meetings.

scheduled in this way for a few reasons. First, the staff is already on-site, having just attended the staff meeting. Second, the clinical and administrative issues that needed to be addressed were usually taken care of in the staff meeting. The resolution of the problems and the end of the staff meeting helped the staff members let go of those immediate concerns as they were completed. Third, the staff members may be in a more relaxed frame of mind than if they had just driven to the office, ran up the stairs, and sat down for staff support or were late or feel harassed. This also helps ensure that the group is all present at the onset of the meeting, which decreases or minimizes the interruptions or disruptions.

It is important in staff support meetings that the facilitator, the format and process, and the associated environment also be regularly evaluated by the manager and the hospice team participating in hospice support. In home care and hospice, it is of utmost importance that we care for the caregivers. The stress of the care provided must be identified and dealt with effectively and appropriately. The managers in home care and hospice must be aware and attuned to the stress levels and any overextension of involvement by the nurse with the patients and their families. For an in-depth review of stress of both manager and staff members, please refer to Chapter 9, "Taking Care of Yourself and Your Staff."

STAFF MEETINGS WITH ADMINISTRATIVE STAFF MEMBERS

In home care or hospice you may also have accountability for administration and operations subordinates who report to you. This can include clerical and secretarial staff, scheduling and intake staff, and billing and accounting personnel. Others may include patient coordinators, private pay schedulers, and miscellaneous staff members. It is important to hold meetings with this staff. Initially, meetings should be held weekly, until you understand the paper flow and work process across the organization. It is important that the staff who represent the agency or program on the phone (as well as in person) be articulate, helpful, and professional. Administrative functions should be included in the organization's CQI program. An example would be a policy of all phones being answered by the third ring. Referral sources want to call these types of service-driven organizations. Remember, how you sound on the phone forms an outsider's first impression of you. Clearly, a case manager who wants effective care, usually at the "best" price, will call a service-oriented organization. The perception here is that how things "look" is how they are.

All parts of your team must work together. Do not make references to outside (field, visiting) staff and inside (administrative) staff. The team works together. All team members should be equally busy. In addition, the office administrative staff reporting to you should be cross-trained whenever possible. Always keep this in mind when bringing in new administrative staff members. For example, the clerical staff should be able to enter data on patients as a backup to the billing staff. Remember, many vacations and holidays must be covered. Do not put yourself in the position of having only one person who can do a given function (e.g., data entry, intake, statistical report collation, phones, reception, aide scheduling, record review).

Have your administrative staff function as small teams broken down into similar functions. Cross-train them all to know at least one other position. Do not wait until a crisis to discover the effectiveness of a staff member's cross-training. Plan for practice days and stagger the days so there is backup. These efforts will pay off significantly. It is also a way to develop your staff and see and value them for their range of skills.

Remember, part of your job as manager (and in home care this is a large part) is to help make the clinical staff members' jobs easier by the successful resolution of administrative problems. For example, if your home care field staff are being hassled by an archaic or duplicative documentation or operational system, address this concern. Have the administrative and clinical staffs work together with you to determine a more successful way to handle the process.

Fiscal Responsibilities in Home Care

In no other setting in health care are the billing functions as closely integrated with the clinical information as in the HHA. Because the HHA must have the physician's plan of care (POC) on the clinical record before billing for the care provided, this discussion begins with documentation.

Although not all patients are Medicare patients, Medicare sets the standard for documentation, and sometimes coverage, offered by other payers. Because documentation in home care can comprise an entire book, the following discussion is an overview of the topic to assist the home care manager develop the staff's documentation skills.

An Overview of Health Care Financing Administration

The HCFA has responsibility for the Medicare and Medicaid programs. Remember that Medicare is a medical insurance program and, like all medical insurers, there are exclusions to coverage of services. HCFA is administratively under the Secretary of Health and Human Services. HCFA contracts with insurance companies to process and adjudicate (make a payment determination or decision) Medicare claims. There are nine Regional Home Health Intermediaries (RHHIs); these process all the HHA and hospice claims nationally. These RHHIs are generally given the HHAs in certain geographic areas as their service area. (However, chain HHAs usually have one RHHI because these HHAs may have centralized billing.)

The HCFA created, with input from HHAs, the current 485/6/7 forms. In addition, the COPs are also part of Medicare requirements for HHAs. With this information in mind, be aware that HCFA, by law, can pay only for necessary and covered care. When admitting patients to your program, ensure that they meet all the criteria. For example, they must *meet* the homebound criteria, the skilled care criteria, and the intermittent/part-time criteria to be covered under the Medicare program. These criteria must be reflected in the clinical documentation.

DOCUMENTATION

All efficient HHAs must have their nurses and other care providers generate documentation that simultaneously does the following:

1. Demonstrates in the documentation the patient care provided and the patient's response to that care.
2. Shows that current standards of care are maintained.
3. Meets documentation requirements for Medicare and other payers.

The nurse's entries in the patient's clinical record are recognized as a significant contribution that documents the standards of care provided to a patient. As the practice of nursing has become more complex, so, too, have the factors that influence the roles of documentation. Some of these factors include requirements of regulatory agencies (e.g., the State Health Department), health insurance payers (e.g., Medicare), accreditation organizations (e.g., JCAHO, NLN), and consumers of health care and legal entities.

In home care, the nurse must try to satisfy these various requirements all at once, often with precious few moments in which to accomplish this important task. The book *Handbook of Home Health Standards and Documentation Guidelines for Reimbursement*[4] was written expressly to show how to ensure meeting the various requirements simultaneously. The manager should have these standards and guidelines available to the home care and discharge planning staff members. This will help ensure an understanding of the level and clarify of specific documentation required by any payer.

As manager, review a percentage of your staff's documentation on an ongoing basis to monitor the quality of care as demonstrated in the documentation and to ensure that other, particularly reimbursement, requirements are being met. This review can also be incorporated into your CQI program, and clinical factors may be identified through the review process that can become the subject of focused studies. In addition, areas for further education may be identified through this process.

In your sample review, ask the questions in Manager's Tip 11-1 to assess the quality of the home care medical record. Manager's Tip 11-2 on p. 276 presents some suggestions to help you help your staff improve their documentation.

THE IMPORTANCE OF REPORTS

Reports present information that is useful and objective for any manager. They track what is happening with the HHA or program. Many types of report tools are available. Following is a discussion of the report tools the new manager should find helpful. A

MANAGER'S TIP 11-1

NURSE MANAGER'S CHECKLIST
FOR DOCUMENTATION

✔ Try to look at the documentation objectively: does it tell the story of the patient's progress (or lack of progress) and the interventions implemented based on the initial assessment and plan of care?

✔ Are telephone calls and other communications with physicians and other team members documented? Do they explain what occurred with the patient; what actions were ordered, modified, and implemented; and the patient's response to these interventions?

✔ Is the nursing process demonstrated in the record? Look for the nursing diagnoses, the assessment, evidence of care planning, implementation or ordered interventions and actions, assessment of the patient's response, and continued evaluation.

✔ Is there documentation of goal achievement or progress towards predetermined, mutually set goals and outcomes? Are the goals realistic, quantifiable, and patient-centered?

✔ If progress has not occurred as planned, are the reasons explained in the documentation?

✔ Is the patient's/caregiver's response to care interventions or actions documented?

✔ Are the interventions modified, based on the patient's response, where appropriate?

✔ Is there evidence of intradisciplinary team conferences and discussions?

✔ Does the chart show continuity of care planning goals and consistent movement towards goal achievement?

✔ Generally, does the record tell the story of the patient's care and progress while receiving home care services?

✔ Do the entries and overall information reflect care of the level expected by today's health care consumers and their families?

✔ Finally, does the clinical documentation demonstrate compliance with regulatory, licensure, and quality standards?

prudent manager is up-to-date on the status or health of the HHA. Keeping current helps ensure the early and easy identification of problems or trends that should be watched closely before they become risk management problems or financial disasters. Reports ensure objective findings of different components of the operations in an HHA. This helps the manager by showing information in an organized format that assists and improves managerial effectiveness. Reports can quantify information you may need. For example, if you believe that the nursing visits are up significantly over the last 2 weeks (e.g., by viewing the nurse visit logs or the number of referrals), the actual report that integrates the information by nurse, by week, and by total visits by day or week would validate that finding. This report and the rationale would then help justify an increase in FTEs to your supervisor. The ability to show the increase in care and visits to meet the patient's needs is a key to successful HHA operations.

SUGGESTIONS TO HELP YOU HELP YOUR STAFF IMPROVE DOCUMENTATION

✔ As a manager, show by your actions that you value effective documentation. This attitude will be conveyed to staff and become the standard of the performance expected.

✔ Remember that writing effective documentation is a learned skill and, as with any skill, improvement comes only with practice.

✔ Recognize that in home care, at the first visit the nurse usually begins the process of claims payment (or denial) with the initial 485 and then 486/7 forms.

✔ Have your nurses read their own documentation objectively. They should ask themselves, "Does this 485/6/7 or visit record say why the patient is homebound (if Medicare or another insurer that has that criteria)?" and "How or why are the skills of a nurse or therapist needed?" Involve your staff in peer review of clinical charts. This will significantly help develop their documentation skills, and they will be able to objectively read their own documentation.

✔ As a manager, look at who is admitted to the home care program. Do the patients meet your admission criteria? (This is also a quality assurance function.) If the nurse cannot clearly identify the skilled, covered service needed but does know the requirements, the patient may not be appropriate for insurance coverage. This patient may still have care needs that another program may provide.

✔ Have your staff focus on the patient's problems in their documentation. That is why home care is being provided, and it is what the payers must see to justify reimbursement.

✔ Have your nurses demonstrate through their documentation that the care provided is patient-centered. Make the patient goals quantifiable and outcomes patient-centered and specific to the patient's unique problems and needs. Whenever possible, the patient should help set these goals.

✔ Emphasize to the nurses that anyone else who picks up their patient's chart does not have the information they have from actually being there and seeing the patient in her/his own home setting. Encourage your staff to write information that is objective and clearly paints a picture of the patient, the problems, the needs, and where the care is directed for goal achievement and discharge.

✔ Have the clinical records reviewed overall by the nurse when the initial admitting information has been completed. Use a checklist form to make it easier. This is the best time to check that all identifying information is completed and consistent across the various admission forms. For example, if allergies are noted on the referral information, this same information, after being validated by the patient on the admission visit, should be noted on the medication list and the 485 form (POC). This way, you as the manager know that if the state or HCFA should make an unannounced onsite visit, your charts have met minimal requirements.

✔ Remember to tell your staff that effective documentation does not have to be lengthy or wordy. However, it should convey to any reader the status of your patient, the plan for care, and the consistent movement towards predetermined patient-centered goals.

✔ Have the nurses check that the information on the record flows well and that you can tell by objective evidence what is happening with the patient. This includes the prob-

Continued.

lems, projected plans, and the skilled services that are needed, based on the clear picture presented in the documentation.

✓ Emphasize that paperwork needs to be legible, neat, and organized consistently.

✓ Remind your staff that the payers generally only know as much as is communicated on the 485/6/7 forms. They are painting a picture for the payer/reviewer of why the patient needs nursing or other skilled services. Emphasize that the forms must document why the care was initiated, what the professional nurse is doing (i.e., what are the skilled nursing interventions), where the patient's plan is going (patient-centered goals), and the plans for discharge (rehabilitation potential) and why the case should continue for recertification.

✓ Encourage and appoint a staff nurse representative to your HHA's regularly scheduled CQI committee meetings. This nurse can communicate to peers the important role of documentation.

✓ Instruct your home care nurses to complete admissions and most of the documentation in the patient's home whenever possible. This is particularly true for new admissions to home care or hospice care. Patients clearly know that third-party payers (except in private pay service home care) generally pay for the care the HHA is providing. Complete the 485 and begin the 486 through to item 12 (which is identifying types of information). Complete the visit record and all the initial admitting forms. The nurse should not rely on memory to complete needed documentation. In addition, tell your nurses to explain on the initial visit that requirements must be met for the payers and that the last few minutes of the visit are for the nurse to complete these requirements. Some agencies have implemented this standard very successfully, and it is reflected in the quality of the detailed documentation.

✓ Emphasize that the POC is the most important part of the home care clinical record. All other information flows from the identified skilled needs ordered on the plan. Hold training sessions on the correct completion of the 485 (and the 486/7). If you identify gaps on the data elements on the POC or if the content is not appropriate or detailed enough for effective patient care, such training will be timely.

Management Report Tools for New Managers

1. Use your referral logs as an important source of information at least weekly. The weekly information may be tabulated by your staff for monthly or cumulative reports. Look at:

   • Who and where your referrals are coming from. Are there trends in the diagnoses, types of patients, payer sources, or other information (i.e., visits per referral may indicate level of acuity)?

   • Who are the specific hospitals, physicians, discharge planners, and inpatient nurses? Compare this current information to that of the previous period. If a change exists, try to determine its cause. Have your own HHA coordinator involved in the causes.

   • The referral log's information should not be underestimated. Use this as a working management tool to track your referrals or nurse care manager caseloads or to project future work assignments. In addition, it is the one place, at a glance, to see your payer mix or geographic spread or to identify trends.

2. Readmission (if within 31 days) to hospital reports.
3. Patient or family complaint logs.
4. Accident/incident logs.
5. HCFA form 488 requests or additional data requests (ADRs). These forms generated by the RHHI request more clinical information. It should include the date received and the date the information is requested. In addition, look at the entire process: locating, copying, and collating the information. Analyze these findings on a quarterly basis, since these requests for information cost time and money. In addition, share the request with the primary nurse, not in a negative or punitive way, but as an educational opportunity and as a way to perhaps avoid such information requests in the future.

   Clearly, an increase in ADRs or 488s may signify the need for in-service training on documentation and the correct completion of the HCFA 485/6/7 forms.
6. Reports generated from automated systems. Many HHAs now have specialized software systems to assist them in their daily operations in such important and time-consuming areas as intake/referrals or billing data entry. Many of these systems are capable of generating useful information for managers. An example is categorizing patients by diagnosis, geographic area, or primary nurse. In addition, nurse productivity reports or financial reports (e.g., status and aging of accounts) assist the manager in planning daily and future operations. Still others include status of budgeted versus actual expenditures and numerous fiscal information. Such reports can be generated for your weekly or monthly review to assist in making decisions.
7. Monthly or quarterly quality report/update/activities. This report should include all continuing education sessions held since the last report and all ongoing research or special-focus studies. These findings, or a synopsis of the findings, may be appropriate for inclusion in the utilization review committee meeting report or in the HHA annual report.
8. Referral source, patient and family satisfaction surveys.

The information to be found in reports is important. An effective automated system that meets your HHA's needs can prove invaluable once you and the staff have learned to use it. The following is a brief discussion about these programs and their applicability in home care.

Computerization

The list below is of factors that need to be addressed before purchasing HHA computer software or choosing software vendors. The more defined your needs, requirements, and knowledge on this issue, the better your decision will meet your agency's requirements.

- Volume.

- Current paper processes and workflow.
- Budget for this endeavor.
- Specifically defined primary need(s) for computerization (usually began as a needs/wish list).
- The staff component of using the product (e.g., current and new staff computer comfort levels).

Before making any such capital purchase decisions, consider the following. Believing that automation will streamline all operational functions is naive. Undoubtedly, a software system that simultaneously generates the 485/6/7 forms and the Medicare Part A billing form (UB-82/92) is a great idea and clearly cuts down on duplicative paper and errors. But effective automated paper processes must be in place before smooth transition to any new system is possible. There is a wide variance in the products, price, and features of computer systems. The recommendation that you network with other HHA managers is especially true in this area.

Automation in scheduling and particularly in billing is emphasized as HCFA and other payers move towards an electronic, paperless claims process in the effort to cut costs. This has become an especially heightened issue as the U.S. Congress passes legislation to pay electronic media claims (EMC) faster than claims on paper. EMC can include tape-to-tape, on-line, modem, or other electronic routes. The RHHIs are also working towards the goal of increasing EMC claims from HHA and hospice providers.

In addition, as nursing informatics addresses more issues that affect the provision of care in the community and how such automated nursing needs are different, we may see the proliferation of more options to assist professional nurses in their care of patients at home.

SPECIAL PROGRAMS
Hospice

Hospice care is a very special type of care and is now receiving deserved recognition. The nurses, social workers, chaplain, volunteers, and other hospice team members all bring skills to assist patients and their families in meeting their unique needs. This discussion focuses on the special needs unique to hospice management.

Managers in hospice are unique for several reasons:

1. They provide direction and support to a staff whose patient population, by definition, has an illness of a terminal nature.
2. They interface daily with the processes of dying and death. Therefore the feedback about feelings of anger, denial, and sadness are incorporated into their management role.
3. They must have specialized skills to work successfully with volunteers.
4. They must have training skills to train and successfully maintain volunteers.
5. They must have specialized knowledge of hospice reimbursement systems (e.g., the Medicare Hospice program and all its specific nuances).

6.   All these functions demand effective interpersonal communication skills and the ability to talk and teach about hospice factually and sensitively.

In addition, because of the nature of hospice care, funding has historically been problematic. Many hospices are involved in fund-raising to support their continued services in communities. The manager in hospice must have or develop the skills to work with fund-raising committee representatives or other associated entities that do this important work for the hospice. There is an ongoing need to be able to articulate clearly the special needs and costs of hospice care.

Hospices must have systems capable of tracking needed information for such important components of hospice care as bereavement counseling and the associated anniversary or remembrance information. In addition, many hospices keep detailed statistics about their programs and the patients and families served in the community. These functions also generate the need for effective tracking through automated systems.

Personal Emergency Response System Programs

Some HHAs also have another special program that is a part of their organization and that the HHA manager may also have responsibility for—the personal emergency response system program (PERS).

Such PERS systems are a unique application of technology that allow some patients the ability to remain in their home alone or give them a heightened sense of security. Most nurses in home care are familiar with this technology, since most have the subscriber (patient) wear the PERS button around the neck or on a belt clip. This technology is tied into the phone system and, once activated, contacts one or more preselected family members or friends of the subscriber to come over immediately. The responders then go to the home, since they have access, and address the problem. Sometimes the responders are municipal services—the fire department or ambulance service. Falls engender the most calls for help in this patient population.

Many of these programs have volunteers who do some of the actual installation and explanation of this important service and technology. Reports should be available to you, as the manager, about the number of subscriber calls, equipment inventory, current or projected purchase needs, public relations associated with the service, and other factors that ensure a safe and responsive program for subscribers and their families and friends.

In addition, most PERS programs have (at least) quarterly meetings that are advisory in nature. They may include the manager, the operators who receive the calls (the response center), a representative of the company that sells and services your PERS equipment, a representative consumer of the service (if possible), the volunteers who assist with the program, and others in the program who are key factors in the effective functioning of this 24-hour service. Some programs have hundreds of these PERS units in the community because the programs allow some frail or elderly people to remain at home. Otherwise, they could not be at home and alone.

The HHA manager may have responsibility for numerous other programs (e.g., Meals on Wheels, private duty services, or durable medical equipment and supply services) in day-to-day operations. With the increasing population of the older elderly (over 85 years), and as community service becomes more the pattern of care, these types of programs can be expected to grow.

A Word About Human Resource Records

HHAs maintain files on their personnel. Such files must be maintained in an orderly and consistent method. There should be a standard format for keeping performance evaluations, PPD or x-ray results, status on hepatitis B information, physical, completed safety in-service programs, orientation checklist, and competency evaluations on all employees. This not only reflects internal organization and the value placed on needed detail, but should surveyors or other external visitors appear, you know that all information is complete and in order. A tickler file system can be used to generate a monthly list of information due, including performance evaluations, CPR recertifications, license renewals, PPDs, and so on.

In addition, as part of the CQI program, pull the personnel records of the caregivers noted in the patient clinical records you are reviewing. This is how the surveyor will do it, so practice these methods to identify your internal problems so they are not a bigger problem for the HHA.

Review Chapter 3, "Human Resource Management," because it is germane to this discussion about home care and the special needs of the managers.

Summary

The home care manager of the future must be flexible, have vision, and be committed to a service-oriented management style. This manager will use newer technologies with the staff to ensure increased communications and safety for the staff. Even 5 years ago, who would have imagined the number of car phones, voice mail, and beepers in use as there are today for home care staff?

All of those involved with home care are aware of the incredible growth in dollars, patients, and provided services over the past few years. Home care and hospice will continue to grow as patients become more proactive consumers—they will continue to demand care in their own home setting. However, as managed care continues to grow and sometimes appears to rachet down the number of patient visits, the home care manager must be able to articulate the clinical needs of the patient for that patient to receive quality care while remaining at home. Who would have thought that Dobutamine drips, PICC lines, or ventilators would be daily occurrences in home care? These and other types of complex patient problems will increase as the health care technology explosion continues.

The proactive manager who can quantify and communicate staff needs and explain to superiors the needs based on objective information will be successful in home care. This chapter is a brief overview of what you need to know to manage a quality program. Many good resources are available to the new manager in home care. The hope is that you will locate or create them.

References

1. *Health Care Financing Administration,* Office of Survey and Certification and Office of the Actuary.
2. Reports and Recommendations to the Congress, printed in *Insider.* American Federation of Home Health Agencies, Silver Spring, Md, 3/22/1996.
3. *Health Insurance Manual—11:* Washington, DC, 1989, Government Printing Office.
4. Marrelli TM: *Handbook of home health standards and documentation guidelines for reimbursement,* St Louis, 1994, Mosby.

CHAPTER 12

WHERE TO FROM HERE?

T.M. MARRELLI

During the course of your career, there may be times when you question your level of job satisfaction. Your questioning might begin in the form of occasional nagging doubts such as, "Why did I ever accept this position?" or "Management is nothing like the recruiter told me it would be." Maybe you find yourself not laughing as much, dwelling on work problems when at home, or answering the phone at home with the name of your unit. All of these are clues that it may be time to reevaluate your job satisfaction. If, like many workers today, you are seeking personal fulfillment, this introspective evaluation may be a difficult process. However, you should start the process when you want to, not when you are stressed out and are forced to address the issue. So where do you start?

Nurses, by nature and education, have a strong tendency to take care of others. However, this chapter's focus is on you and your needs and goals. You must realize that the perfect job does not exist. All positions have their own unique strengths and drawbacks. This review includes what your aspirations were when you accepted your current position, your dreams of being a nurse when you were a student, and your perspectives on the realities of nursing now. Put simply, are your professional and self-fulfillment needs being met in your current position and environment? Are your expectations realistic?

ASSESSING JOB SATISFACTION

The types of questions to ask to assess your satisfaction with your job may be broken down into two areas: (1) the work and the associated environment or culture of the setting in which you manage, and (2) your professional and personal needs and where these fit in your life in relation to other responsibilities. These questions are best answered initially with a quick "yes" or "no" without much thought (this is your "gut" feeling). You can then go back and reconsider your answers after the overall evaluation is complete.

Asking yourself the questions in Manager's Tip 12-1 may help you assess your position and determine if management and this particular position are suitable for you.

It is important to note that some of us have a tendency to give and take care of everyone and everything except ourselves. This can lead to exhaustion and burnout. Our work life must be successfully integrated into other parts of our lives.

Part of the personal growth process is the identification of problem areas in our lives and the identification of actions for resolution. Maslow's needs identify the basic needs that must initially be attained before self-actualization can be achieved. The setting, evaluation, and reevaluation of personal and professional goals on a regular basis can be an effective tool in achieving what we want.

Focusing on the answers to the questions in Manager's Tip 12-2 can help you decide how well a management position fits with your personal needs. The direction your career takes is up to you. It is always okay to reconsider and ultimately readjust career goals to meet your unique needs. After a thorough review of your answers, your next step is to reaffirm or reevaluate your stated goals. In this way you can begin implementing changes to work towards achieving them. Only you know what will contribute to the feeling of self-fulfillment in your life. It has been said that, "Nurses leave the profession because they experience a lack of personal fulfillment, stemming from their inability to meet the unrealistic expectations imposed by this

MANAGER'S TIP 12-1

THE WORK AND ITS ENVIRONMENT

Ask yourself these questions to help you determine whether management and your present position are suitable for you:

✔ Do you enjoy the actual work tasks? In management this includes the human management activities of dealing with difficult personalities, conflict resolution, and having the position of power (whether or not you want it). This also includes the satisfaction of being part of a special team providing care to patients and being able to effect needed change or being appreciated by patients' families.

✔ Overall, do you like going to your job every day?

✔ Do you feel you have some control over outcomes and the tasks accomplished?

✔ Generally, are the obstacles to completion outweighed by the work accomplished?

✔ Generally, do you feel that you have the support you need to accomplish your work? If you decide that you enjoy the actual work responsibilities but still are not happy at work, consider whether your supervisor provides sufficient support for your team to get tasks accomplished. Continual frustration of goal achievement is very disheartening and leads to nurse manager and staff turnover. You may wonder, "Who else cares, so why should I?"

✔ Does your job leave you feeling energized or drained? Does your family see you enough? When they do, are you emotionally available, or are you redoing the staffing schedule in your head while having dinner?

ever-changing environment."[1] Nurse managers do not always have to leave their current work environment to feel more fulfilled in their professional roles. Skills that nurses use daily outside the work realm lend themselves to other potentially fulfilling professional or personal activities. The following are examples of such endeavors:

1. *Organizational skills*—Are you the family member who is, by nature, the organizer? You can use these skills in professional association activities in various administrative capacities.
2. *Writing skills*—Do you edit the community newsletter or contribute to the local newspaper? This can be developed into a resource for the nursing news at your facility or for publication in a professional nursing journal.
3. *Public speaking skills*—This needed communication skill can be used by speaker's bureaus, the local community college for health classes, support groups, or for speeches to elementary school students on subjects such as "Why I Like Being a Nurse."
4. *Persuasive skills*—Consider running for office or campaigning for the candidate of your choice.

Any of these special skills can be effective in assisting you in meeting your goals and helping you match them with your unique talents.

In the beginning of this chapter, you evaluated your satisfaction with your current work position and where it fits in your life. This chapter also discusses the importance of recognizing available employment choices. Specific ways to succeed and make yourself uniquely qualified for a position are addressed, and examples of choices and qualifications that may be helpful to you are included.

CHOICES

Choices are options that you give yourself. People tend not to give themselves the luxury of choices. In addition, even when we know that we may be unhappy in our

MANAGER'S TIP 12-2

YOUR PERSONAL NEEDS

To help you decide how well a management position fits with your personal goals, ask yourself these questions:
- ✔ Do you find the actual activities of the manager stimulating while being able to integrate the rest of your responsibilities into your life (such as your family and friends)?
- ✔ Are the rewards appropriate to the energy expended?
- ✔ Are you able to fulfill your own personal goals in this position (e.g., go back to school, have a family, complete certification, teach Sunday school class, or be a volunteer firefighter or paramedic in your community)?

work environment, we may procrastinate about taking the steps needed to change and grow. You are not alone. (The Procrastinator's Club has approximately 10,000 members!)

Once you recognize that professional nurses have numerous choices for employment, you can begin to explore your many options. Even if you have a satisfying job, considering your options can provide growth opportunities important to your professional career in the future. This is also a way to help market yourself and your skills. Being open to and considering your choices enables you to (1) keep some perspective on your current job (this is particularly important when you are unhappy in your position), (2) receive objective feedback about yourself and the external professional environment, and (3) receive information on possibilities for the future. This feedback can be received through the interview process, through networking with professional associates, and through other methods of communication.

MARKETING YOURSELF

Marketing is broadly defined as the theory and practice of selling. In reality, we market ourselves in any interpersonal or written encounter. However, when we consciously market ourselves, we focus on the unique skills that we bring to a work environment and offer to a prospective employer, enhancing our desirability to that employer. Examples of assets that make a nurse uniquely qualified include advanced degrees or certification in a specialty area. Still other examples include awards, experience, and other types of recognition in a chosen field. We sometimes tend to underestimate our own unique skills. The credit and acknowledgment of others can be of important benefit in achieving your long-term professional goals.

A large part of successfully marketing yourself is your projection of your belief in yourself. This is your self-confidence. We know that feelings follow thoughts. Therefore even if on a bad day you are not feeling self-assured, your acting that way may contribute to your feeling more confident. Use available resources to develop or improve such self-promoting skills. Look at role models who seem self-assured; watch how they act, dress, and behave. It is important that you recognize your strengths and areas for improvement. This level of self-knowledge leads to an increased self-assurance that is communicated as belief in yourself.

IDENTIFYING YOUR UNIQUE OR SPECIAL SKILLS

Although professional RNs must pass nursing boards for licensure, and thus meet specific standards, the following section addresses additional ways to help you grow professionally.

Certification

In the 1940s, nurse anesthetists were the first nurses required to meet specific standards to enter professional practice. Since then, certification has grown to encompass those nurses who meet high standards through experience and expertise in nursing practice. Certification is a validation of clinical or administrative skill. The process of certification generally requires an RN license, a set amount of years or hours in practice in a specific specialty, and documented continuing education credit hours. A major benefit of professional certification is the recognition that sets certified nurses apart. Several nursing organizations have boards for certifying nurses. These boards set the criteria, determine scoring, validate credentials, and confer certification in over 50 nursing specialties. Examples of organizations that certify nurses include the American Nurses Association (ANA), the American Association of Critical Care Nurses, and the National Certification Corporation. These and other unique credentials you have as a nurse contribute to your power base as a nurse and nurse manager.

Writing for Professional Publication

Because of their clinical expertise and communication skills, all nurses, particularly those in management, have something important to share with other nurses and nurse managers. In addition, the initiative and perseverance necessary to research and develop an idea and then create and submit a completed manuscript reflect other desirable traits to a prospective employer. Publication in a nursing journal, for example, sets you apart from other candidates who may be similarly qualified. This has been particularly true for some time in the academic environment.

Workshops, Seminars, and Other Development Activities

Some people attend classes and expect to absorb all the information by listening quietly. Yet, it has been demonstrated that we forget most of what we learn within days, particularly when there is no active participation on our part. The 10 suggestions in Manager's Tip 12-3 on p. 288 can help you make the most of learning and networking opportunities at professional workshops or seminars.

NETWORKING

The contacts made and developed through professional organizations can be very advantageous. In time, these professional colleagues may become your peer support group, your friends, and sources of information on viable job alternatives when you want to move on professionally.

Working with Recruiters

As your management expertise and your networking contacts grow, your name will inevitably be given to a health care recruiter who is assisting an organization in locating potential candidates for middle to senior management positions. There are recruiters who specialize in physician, senior management, middle management, and hard-to-recruit staff positions. There are as many different types of recruiters as there are nurse managers, each with varying styles of accomplishing goals.

MANAGER'S TIP 12-3

10 TIPS FOR LEARNING

✔ Set three learning goals. Develop a list of three to six overall goals in attending the educational session. This will help you focus your thinking. Your goals generally will be oriented towards getting specific questions answered or utilization or practical application of skills or theory.

✔ Think about specific questions you want answered. Develop a list of 10 to 15 specific questions. (Consider giving this list to the seminar leaders in advance.)

✔ Meet other participants at the program. Network with them. Each attendee has a specific area of expertise. Make a note of it. Start your own network. Exchange cards (bring along plenty). Go to breakfast, lunch, and dinner with those with whom you can share information and learn.

✔ Develop a plan of action. Make a list of anything you want to consider doing differently when you get back on the job. This will help you apply what you learned and help you achieve objective benefits.

✔ Participate. Ask questions and make contributions. Comment. Be visible. You will benefit in two ways. First, your mind will almost automatically start working on information, problems, and solutions. Second, the speaker and other attendees will also contribute by finding answers for you.

✔ Make contact with the seminar leader personally (and early) when possible. She/he will think more of and about you. It will also be easier to follow up with questions and problems after the program.

✔ Take clear, detailed notes. Not only will this be helpful for future reference, but the very act of taking good notes and organizing your thoughts will keep you more involved. Take notes legibly and coherently the first time to eliminate any need for rewriting them later.

✔ Write a brief report—one to three pages—based on your plan of action and notes. Consider sharing your report with your supervisor.

✔ Hold a staff meeting when you get back and share the useful information you have gained. Implement a plan of action using your new ideas.

✔ Enjoy yourself—we all learn more when we are having a good time.

Recruiters are inherently interested in whether you would like your resume presented to a search committee or manager and, if not, if you are aware of any similarly qualified professionals who may be in the market for a change or new position. Recruiters should be treated with the same respect as any vendor or other professional that you deal with. Even though you may not be job-hunting at this time, you may need assistance in the near future. Recruiters are a potential resource in your job hunt. Manager's Tip 12-4 offers some pointers for dealing with recruiters.

MANAGER'S TIP 12-4

POINTERS FOR DEALING WITH RECRUITERS

- ✔ Be open and honest about whether you are interested in pursuing a position.
- ✔ If no position is available now, ask them to hold your resume and assist them if you know of other possible candidates.
- ✔ Do your homework and research the reputation of the recruiter or parent firm.
- ✔ Treat the recruiter with respect and professionalism.
- ✔ Recruiters usually are paid on a commission or retainer basis, dependent on the amount of business done with a client; they need to be assertive but not aggressive.
- ✔ The recruiter is "working for the employer." The goals will be aligned as such and you are under no obligation to take a job that does not interest or will not compensate you as you desire.
- ✔ Outline your salary and benefit requirements early in initial negotiations, based on skills, job requirements, market demand, and personal desires.
- ✔ Get a clear description of job responsibilities before the interview.
- ✔ Do not try to negotiate with a potential employer without the consent or knowledge of the recruiter.

RESUMES AND CURRICULUM VITAE

Resumes, curriculum vitae, and associated cover letters all represent you. Remember, they are sometimes the only communication about you that a prospective employer receives. These first impressions do count. Resumes are used in most business settings, whereas curriculum vitae are used primarily in the educational and teaching realms. Always type your resume or curriculum vitae, and print the document on the best quality paper available. It is a good idea to have someone proofread your resume or curriculum vitae and cover letter for content, implications, format, clarity, and typographic errors. If no one is available to provide objective comments, put your materials aside for a day or two and then reread them. You may be amazed at the findings. Most print or copy shops will print your resume or curriculum vitae on quality paper fairly inexpensively. The outcome may be worth the cost if it results in additional interviews scheduled. About now, you might be saying, "I do not have the time to do all this and pay attention to such details." Remember the resumes and cover letters that have come across your desk? You have probably been drawn to those that are short and neat, and that communicate clearly. Use your time management skills to ensure that the documents you provide any prospective employer are clear, complete, accurate, and professional.

Resume Preparation

A resume is a synopsis of an individual's educational and career experiences. Its purpose is to give enough information to the potential employer to initiate a first interview; therefore it must be concise, factual, and targeted to the position being sought. With the availability of word processing, resumes should be reviewed and revised based on the focus of the position in question. This is not to imply that one should document untrue statements on a resume, but rather target specific career and educational achievements to what is potentially needed in a desired position.

Resumes should be no longer than three pages, unless there are extensive professional experiences and accomplishments. They can be organized in a number of different manners; however, it is best to organize positions, experiences, and accomplishments chronologically. For the individual who is contemplating a career change, or who has been out of the job market for an extended period of time, the resume should focus on functionality, listing the skills possessed that can transcend different industries.

Do not list any salary information or reasons for leaving any positions. It is not a good idea to list family, gender, or other personal information. And NEVER, NEVER stretch the truth, lie, or fabricate information on your resume—at some point, it will come back to haunt you. Manager's Tip 12-5 lists the basic elements to include in a resume.

Your resume, particularly for management positions, should indicate the number and types of staffs you have been responsible for in your current and previous positions. Be clear about your level of responsibility (e.g., "24-hour responsibility for over 50 nurses and for over 25 professional associates [speech-language pathologists, occupational therapists, medical social workers, physical therapists, etc.] who cared for over 400 patients in the home setting"). When writing your resume, always use verbs that express management in action. Appropriate verbs include *created, developed, implemented, evaluated, supervised, problem-solved,* and *analyzed.* Examples of a resume and cover letter, the introductory letter about you and your skills that accompanies your resume or curriculum vitae, are given in Boxes 12-1 and 12-2.

MANAGER'S TIP 12-5

BASIC ELEMENTS TO INCLUDE IN A RESUME

When preparing a resume, be sure to include the following basic information:
- ✔ Identifying information: name, address, home and work phone numbers.
- ✔ Career objectives (aligned with position requested).
- ✔ Academic degrees and honors; applicable credentials.
- ✔ Pertinent education (do not list high school if college degree is noted) and skills.
- ✔ Progressive career experience, with both accomplishments and job functions listed.
- ✔ Publications, awards, and presentations as applicable.
- ✔ Professional affiliations.

box 12-1

EXAMPLE OF A RESUME

Name, Credentials
Address
Phone Number

Career Objectives:

Professional Experience:
Dates: Most Current Position, Employer Name, City, State
(Continue for all positions—up through 10 years)

Major Accomplishments:
List major accomplishments of career (e.g., expense control, revenue growth, development of service line or program, etc.)

Education:

Professional Affiliations:

Awards, Presentations, Publications, etc.

References (upon request)

box 12-2

EXAMPLE OF A COVER LETTER

June 14, 199•
Alice Campbell, RN, MSN
Recruitment Office
St. Elsewhere General Hospital
Anytown, Maryland 11111-2222

1212 Mockingbird Lane
Anytown, Maryland 11111-2222

Dear Ms. Campbell,

I am writing in response to your ad for a nurse manager in the Sunday Anywhere Paper of June 12, 199•. I believe my 4 years of experience in the St. Elsewhere General Hospital telemetry unit as evening shift coordinator, as well as other accomplishments, make me uniquely qualified for this position.

I have attached my resume, which highlights my experience, for your confidential review. I look forward to hearing from you. I can be reached at (410) 222-1234.

Sincerely,

Jennifer Brown, RN

Curriculum Vitae

A curriculum vitae (CV) differs from a resume in that it is a written progression of your career that is used primarily for academic purposes or in such settings. A CV outlines in more detail than a resume and includes all educational opportunities that have affected your career positively, as well as a listing and description of all positions you have held.

BEFORE THE INTERVIEW

Consider *any* communication that occurs with a prospective employer as an opportunity to shine and market yourself. Even if you suspect that the employer may not be considering you or have a position available for someone with your unique qualifications, remember that this person might consider you in the future. What you do and say today can position you for a future job. Your interactions can influence early deliberations about such future opportunities.

At the beginning of this chapter you considered and identified what is important in order for you to meet your unique needs in a nursing position. The following sections will discuss the active process of the job search and offer tips for finding and getting the job you want. Manager's Tip 12-6 offers suggestions to help you prepare for the interview.

Your responses should reflect your professionalism, job knowledge, management skills, and goals. Being well prepared will also help decrease any interview jitters or nervousness.

THE INTERVIEW

The interview process is appropriately valued as the most important factor in getting a job. In addition, the interview is an important step in the information-gathering process about the prospective employer. Through active listening to someone who knows the system and manages there, you can learn needed information about the actual nursing and management philosophy. Manager's Tips 12-7, 12-8, and 12-9 on pp. 294-295 provide general suggestions for interviewing, taking advantage of opportunities that the interview offers, and concluding the interview.

THE INTERVIEW WITH YOUR PROSPECTIVE NEW STAFF

Many employers now schedule the nurse manager candidate finalists to meet with and be interviewed by representatives of the staff they may be managing on accepting the position. Usually the staff chooses representatives. The number may vary based on the facility's philosophy. This can be a very useful opportunity for the prospective nurse manager to determine more about the actual day-to-day operations and culture of the clinical area. Usually the nurses chosen are leaders in the

MANAGER'S TIP 12-6

PREPARING FOR THE INTERVIEW

✔ Find out all you can about your prospective employer.

✔ Talk to employees, including nurses you know who no longer work there.

✔ Recognize that the advertisements in the newspaper communicate important information about the position and the facility. For example, does the ad describe where you would live and work geographically (urban, rural, etc.)? Does the employer sound progressive? Does the ad mention clinical ladders, collaborative practice models, or other progressive nurse-oriented activities that are important to you? Ads sometimes communicate the management philosophy. Ads may provide information that can help you determine whether or not you would fit in as a team member in a particular setting.

✔ Obtain written materials. Most health care facilities produce flyers or brochures, available to the community, about their services. Read the factual information listed. This may include the size of the facility or program, the number of beds (if an inpatient setting), the mission statement or goals, the specific services or programs provided (e.g., maternity care, ambulatory care, hospice, home health), and the geographic area they serve.

✔ Write and send a cover letter with your resume to the person identified in the newspaper ad. This may be the nurse recruiter, the nursing office supervisor, or an administrator for the clinical area. In the letter clearly request consideration and an interview at this person's earliest convenience. Set the tone to sound professional and enthusiastic.

✔ Think about and prepare a written list of questions for the interview. Your questions might relate to the nursing philosophy, the mission statement of the program, the average staffing ratios on the unit you would be managing, the kind of documentation system used, computerization status, the average length of stay for the hospital or for the specific unit, or information about the nursing newsletter.

✔ Make a list of questions you think you might be asked and practice answering them. Think of those questions that you ask prospective applicants. Practice before the interview so that you will not need to have your notes with you. Questions commonly asked in interviews include:

   ✔ Where do you want to be professionally in 5 to 10 years?

   ✔ What are your strengths and weaknesses?

   ✔ Give an example of a particularly difficult management situation and how you addressed the problem.

   ✔ Why are you looking for another position?

   ✔ Tell me about your nursing management style.

   ✔ Why do you want to work here?

   ✔ What is your background?

   ✔ Why do you believe you are the best person for this job?

MANAGER'S TIP 12-7

GENERAL TIPS FOR INTERVIEWING

✔ The more prepared you are, the more self-assured you will be, and this will be projected to any prospective employer.

✔ It is a good idea to bring along an extra resume should the interviewer not be able to locate her/his copy. (If this happens, it may give you important insight into the work environment, such as disorganization, tight resources, or poor communication between human resources and nursing [or it may be that this is just a bad day].)

✔ It is okay to ask for a copy of the specific position description should one not be offered. Since usually more functions are required than those listed on the position description, consider asking the interviewer to describe the daily routine of the area.

✔ As part of your preparation, bring a typed list of professional and personal references. List the names, professional degrees, addresses, and telephone numbers of your references. The three professional references should be people you have worked with and/or who have supervised your work. Be sure to notify your references that you will be actively interviewing and that they may receive a call. Of course, you should ask if they are willing to serve as references before you list them.

✔ It is important that you appear as calm and composed as you can for an interview. This gets harder the more you want a specific job. Therefore plan to arrive at the setting at least 20 minutes ahead of time, assume you will not find a parking place anywhere near the facility, and plan to complete some paperwork, such as an application, before the actual interview begins.

✔ Be punctual, dress professionally in a suit that you feel good in, get a good night's sleep the night before, and tell yourself that you will have a successful interview.

✔ Use your interpersonal skills and good judgment throughout the process. Allot plenty of time; some interviews can be lengthy depending on who else the interviewer wants you to meet with or on whether the interviewer gives you a tour of the clinical setting.

✔ Many interviews with potential employers include a variety of interview panels (e.g., peer managers, subordinates, managers, or select group of senior managers). Be prepared to speak before a small group of people with different information needs and interview focus.

staff hierarchy. The interview with representatives of your prospective staff will also give you needed information about the staff and should be looked on as a positive and information-finding meeting. This is your time to be professional, positive, and persuasive. You might practice with a trusted friend the speech about why you are the best candidate for the job and about your style of management.

FOLLOWING UP THE INTERVIEW

If the interviewer or the nurse recruiter does not call by the discussed date, call her/him to determine whether a decision has been made and, if not, when you

MANAGER'S TIP 12-8

MAKING THE MOST OF THE INTERVIEW

✔ Use your active listening skills.

✔ If you determine that the interviewer is having a bad day and seems very hassled (e.g., there may be numerous interruptions), know that this could be indicative of the interviewer's personality or of the setting. Try to use your intuitive skills during the encounter to know the difference between a bad day and what is "normal" for the functioning of the setting (e.g., crisis management).

✔ Do not smoke (even if the option is offered).

✔ Try to bring the conversation to the style of management practiced (e.g., "Are the staff nurses involved in shared governance or other aspects of departmental decision-making?").

✔ Do not share negative feelings or experiences about your current or past work settings. Although these occur to all of us, discussing them, particularly during a first meeting, may be perceived as indicating failure to appropriately address and handle identified problems.

✔ Act enthusiastic and you will feel that way. This will be communicated.

✔ Smile, use eye contact appropriately, take some deep breaths, try to relax, and listen.

✔ Communicate to the interviewer that you want this job (if indeed you want it) and that you are right for it.

MANAGER'S TIP 12-9

CONCLUDING THE INTERVIEW

✔ Allow the interviewer to wrap up the interview.

✔ Make sure that your correct phone number is on your resume and application.

✔ Have your questions ready when the interviewer asks, "Do you have any questions for me that I have not covered?"

✔ Thank the interviewer for the time and information.

✔ Ask how soon a decision will be made or what the next step will be (e.g., how soon the interviewer plans to fill the position and when you will be hearing about the decision or a second interview). In addition, ask who you will be hearing from (e.g., the interviewer or the nurse recruiter).

✔ Offer a verbal affirmation of wanting the job at the end of the interview (if you do, or think you do).

should call back. When you call, be brief and pleasant. Communicate that you are still interested in the position and want to know if a candidate has been selected. Offer to call back the following week. Remember that if you really want the job, be assertive and let the interviewer know that you are available for a second interview if she/he so desires. It is important to be patient. Getting the position you want may take time but will be well worth the wait if the position meets your identified needs.

THANK-YOU LETTERS

Send a thank-you letter to the interviewer within a week after the interview. Even when you call and speak to the interviewer, it is courteous to follow up with a letter. Two sample thank-you letters are provided in Box 12-3. The second letter gives you an idea of what to say if you are certain you are not interested in the position.

KEEPING A RECORD OF YOUR JOB SEARCH AND INTERVIEW INFORMATION

In your search, you will be in contact with and interviewed by various prospective employers. While you are trying to determine why you prefer one position or setting over another, it can be difficult to remember your thoughts and impressions without a written record. A notebook or log can be an easy way to help you remember details and your overall reactions to a specific facility.

Columns can be drawn vertically down a page with the following kinds of overhead information across the top horizontally. An example is:

NAME OF FACILITY   INTERVIEWER   BENEFITS   FOLLOW-UP   OUTCOME

Other variables that may be tracked in the log or notebook include dates (or copies) of letters, positions interviewed for, parking problems, commute time, the actual physical plant, other perceptions, and the interviewer's management or organizational style. Your record could also include your perceptions of such things as the level of cooperation when you called the facility, the human resources office, the security guards, the interviewer's receptionist, and how long you were kept waiting. Overall, did you feel like an intruder or that they were glad to have a promising candidate and communicated that to you? It is hard to go back and recreate details, so keeping the log in the car with you enables you to write your perceptions and objective facts immediately following the interview.

AFTER THE INTERVIEW

Identify whether this position has the critical job elements needed to make you happy and feel as if your best skills are being used. Brainstorm those factors you identified in your self-evaluation process that would help you achieve your professional goals. These may include the location (state, city, rural, urban, etc.), staff

·· box 12-3 ···

SAMPLE THANK-YOU LETTERS

LETTER 1:

June 21, 199•

Alice Campbell, RN, MSN   1212 Mockingbird Lane
Recruitment Office   Anytown, Maryland 11111-2222
St. Elsewhere General Hospital
Anytown, Maryland 11111-2222

Dear Ms. Campbell:

Thank you for interviewing me yesterday for the position of nurse manager on the B-4 telemetry unit. As you know, I am very interested in assuming this position. I believe I have the skills and experience to be a great asset to St. Elsewhere General Hospital and would welcome the opportunity to join the management team.

I look forward to hearing from you; I can be reached at (410) 222-1234.

Sincerely,

Jennifer Brown, RN

LETTER 2:

June 21, 199•

Alice Campbell, RN, MSN   1212 Mockingbird Lane
Recruitment Office   Anytown, Maryland 11111-2222
St. Elsewhere General Hospital
Anytown, Maryland 11111-2222

Dear Ms. Campbell:

As I said in today's phone conversation, and after further thoughtful consideration, I realize that the nurse manager position is not the job I am seeking at this time. It sounds as if you have a great team working on the B-4 telemetry unit. Thank you for your time. I wish you success in filling your open position and in your other professional endeavors.

Sincerely,

Jennifer Brown, RN

development program, professional growth opportunities, and any other factors, such as shared governance or nursing representation at the board level, that you value as criteria preferred in a prospective work setting.

NEGOTIATING

Salary is not the determinant of the best job, but in nursing, as in other fields, it sometimes can be a harbinger of the amount of work you will be responsible for. In addition, although starting nurses' salaries are usually fixed, experienced nurses, particularly managers, may consider negotiating for more based on their unique qualifications. Remember that you may never get what you do not request. Assessing a prospective employer's needs gives you information on which skills to emphasize. Remember:

1. You both want something. You want a fulfilling position that uses your talents effectively, and they want a competent manager who has the skills needed to accomplish the work at hand.

2. You are a competent manager who brings experience to this position. Be positive and enthusiastic about the position, and stress what you can do for them.

3. Know their specific needs. Often in an interview, the interviewer will share information about where the unit or organization is going. In fact, if this information is not shared, this is a good question to ask when the interviewer asks if you have any questions. The actual question could be phrased as, "What is St. Elsewhere General Hospital's vision for the future?" Many times you can use this information to promote your qualifications that make you the best candidate for the position. Examples are described in Manager's Tip 12-10.

Before you accept a position, know what you need to be happy and to meet your goals. You may need to negotiate for what you want. People do respect people who negotiate for what they believe they deserve. Many settings now offer "cafeteria style" benefit packages to more successfully meet an individual's needs. This contributes to position retention. Some of these items may be the salary, tuition reimbursement, professional workshops and development, or flexibility in your work hours. Remember that successful negotiations are "win/win" (i.e., you both get what you want).

WHEN YOU RECEIVE AN OFFER

Listen to what is said, and know that you do not have to make a decision immediately. In fact, it may be helpful to "try on" what it would feel like to work at the facility for a few days before giving them an answer. This could include driving 20 miles to the prospective setting for a few consecutive days to see if the commute would be a problem or other behaviors that might help you in your decision-making process.

MANAGER'S TIP 12-10

HOW ASKING ABOUT THE INSTITUTION CAN HELP YOU WIN THE JOB

✔ *Recognize and take advantage of unique opportunities.* The interviewer states that the facility is currently completing long-term plans for one of its medical-surgical units to become a designated hospice unit. She/he goes on to say that it looks as if the state planning process is almost completed and that conversion could occur as soon as 3 months from now. If you have the skills or experience and express the desire to be of assistance, this could place you at an advantage over other candidates. In addition, in this current era of working to increase effectiveness with fewer resources, you could offer this prospective employer flexibility and options they may need.

✔ *Offer any relevant special knowledge that you might have.* The interviewer shares the information that the facility is undergoing a transition to make all the units more decentralized and autonomous. If you have experienced a similar process at another setting, your special knowledge could be valuable to a new employer to help ensure a successful change.

✔ *Do not be afraid to share your accomplishments.* Remember that the resume is only the introduction that gets your foot in the door. There is much more that must be communicated. Identify your special skills and accomplishments, such as serving on the local health department board, being a member of a speaking organization or a speaker's bureau, attaining certification, and publishing. (These special skills and accomplishments should be listed on your resume.)

ACCEPTING THE OFFER

The job acceptance process can be as individual as the work setting. However, to protect yourself, as a general rule, ask to receive the offer in writing and wait until you receive a written validation of your job offer from your new employer before giving notice to your current employer. This should be done even in instances when the position has been offered verbally and you have verbally accepted. It has happened in some settings that because of disorganization or a miscommunication, it was said that the offer never was extended. If this occurs, it does not matter why it happened; you still do not have the job and will not be working there.

GIVING NOTICE

Read your facility's manual about the procedure for giving notice of resignation in your particular setting. This usually ranges from 2 to 4 weeks depending on the setting and culture. If you have signed a contract, consult your contract. In addition, some nursing agencies, particularly in the sales or community health setting, may have non-compete clauses as part of the nurse's contract or as a separate agreement that was signed on employment. You must address these and other unique situations for your own protection and for professional integrity.

Sample Resignation Letter

The actual resignation letter can be brief and to the point. Your letter should be directed to your immediate supervisor. The following is an example of the language that should be clearly stated:

> "It is with regret that I inform you that effective (specify date), I will be resigning from my position as (position, unit)."

Some people also state that they have enjoyed working in their position, when this is appropriate. It may not be appropriate if your supervisor knows that you have been stressed out and looking for a position for some time.

About "Not Burning Bridges"

All managers grow and change and sometimes need to move on, but we have all heard the saying "never burn bridges." This is true in all industries, but particularly in the nursing profession. The cohesiveness of the nursing profession, particularly in one specialty or state, ensures that in the future there will be interaction with past employers. For these reasons, and for your own professional growth, always try to leave the area for which you were responsible in better shape than when you first took the position. This will help you be successful in your future professional endeavors.

Guilt and Grooming Your Successor

Supervisors may try to make you feel guilty once you have made the decision to leave official. You have been in their shoes as a manager, so you already bring insight into this common phenomenon. One way to assuage any guilty feelings you may have is to have already begun the process of developing skills in a few nurses who will be ready to assume your role. When your manager says, "You know I can't fill your position for at least (hyperinflated) weeks and besides. . .," you can offer a suggestion for an appropriate successor. If you have used effective team-building and participatory management skills, your group is sure to have a few staff members qualified to act in your position should there be a delay in replacing you. Remember that you have a choice about whether or not to accept guilt about leaving a job.

SUMMARY

Changes and choices can be difficult but do present new opportunities for growth. Personal and professional development, active involvement in professional nursing associations, and networking with leaders in your specialty field can be occasions for growth. The process of learning, integrating new behaviors, and changing positions can be difficult. Once the choice has been made to accept a new opportunity, you have the challenge of creating a special environment for your team where your management style blends with your employer's organizational goals. Remember that effective nurse managers have been described as a "wonder in action." Being a nurse manager can be very fulfilling and exciting. You may have the good fortune of working with a highly competent and sensitive team.

There is no perfect job, only jobs that meet your needs and aspirations at particular times in your life. Only you can evaluate your unique needs, goals, and dreams and work towards achieving them.

References

1. Butler J, Parsons RJ: Hospital perceptions of job satisfaction, *Nurs Manage* 20(8):46, 1989.

For Further Reading

Bolles RN: *What color is your parachute?* Berkeley, Calif, 1992, Ten Speed Press.

Butler J, Parsons RJ: Hospital perceptions of job satisfaction, *Nurs Manage* 20(8):45, 1989.

Carroll MF: *Credentialing in nursing: contemporary developments and trends,* Kansas City, Mo, 1987, American Nurse's Association.

Cosgray RE et al: Getting started on your first manuscript, *Hosp Top* 67(5):28, 1989.

Fisher P, Vry W: *Getting to yes: negotiating agreement without giving in,* New York, 1981, Penguin Books.

Flores DW: Marketing yourself in an interview, *Nurs 92* 22(8):100, 1992.

Kaplan SM: The nurse as change agent, *Pediatr Nurs* 16(6):603, 1990.

Krouse HJ, Holleran SD: Nurse managers and clinical nursing research, *Nurs Manage* 23(7):62, 1992.

Levesque RF: Business planning in home health agencies: a guide for nurse executives, *Columbia University Teachers College,* 1991, Ed.D.

Newcomb BJ, Murphy PA: The curriculum vitae—what it is and what it is not, *Nurs Outlook* 27(9):580, 1979.

O'Connor P: Resumes: opening the door, *Nurs Econ* 2:428, 1984.

Pearlman D, Takacs GJ: The 10 stages of change, *Nurs Manage* 21(4):33, 1990.

Perry L: Nursing supervisors continue to lead climb up the ladder, *Mod Healthcare* 21(21):27, 1991.

Sher B: *Wishcraft,* New York, 1983, Random House.

Taylor T: Healthcare marketing and the nurse manager, *Nurs Manage* 2(15):84, 1990.

INDEX